AIDS-Related Cancers and Their Treatment

BASIC AND CLINICAL ONCOLOGY

Editor

Bruce D. Cheson, M.D.

National Cancer Institute
National Institutes of Health
Bethesda, Maryland

1. Chronic Lymphocytic Leukemia: Scientific Advances and Clinical Developments, *edited by Bruce D. Cheson*
2. Therapeutic Applications of Interleukin-2, *edited by Michael B. Atkins and James W. Mier*
3. Cancer of the Prostate, *edited by Sakti Das and E. David Crawford*
4. Retinoids in Oncology, *edited by Waun Ki Hong and Reuben Lotan*
5. Filgrastim (r-metHuG-CSF) in Clinical Practice, *edited by George Morstyn and T. Michael Dexter*
6. Cancer Prevention and Control, *edited by Peter Greenwald, Barnett S. Kramer, and Douglas L. Weed*
7. Handbook of Supportive Care in Cancer, *edited by Jean Klastersky, Stephen C. Schimpff, and Hans-Jörg Senn*
8. Paclitaxel in Cancer Treatment, *edited by William P. McGuire and Eric K. Rowinsky*
9. Principles of Antineoplastic Drug Development and Pharmacology, *edited by Richard L. Schilsky, Gérard A. Milano, and Mark J. Ratain*
10. Gene Therapy in Cancer, *edited by Malcolm K. Brenner and Robert C. Moen*
11. Expert Consultations in Gynecological Cancers, *edited by Maurie Markman and Jerome L. Belinson*
12. Nucleoside Analogs in Cancer Therapy, *edited by Bruce D. Cheson, Michael J. Keating, and William Plunkett*
13. Drug Resistance in Oncology, *edited by Samuel D. Bernal*
14. Medical Management of Hematological Malignant Diseases, *edited by Emil J Freireich and Hagop M. Kantarjian*
15. Monoclonal Antibody-Based Therapy of Cancer, *edited by Michael L. Grossbard*
16. Medical Management of Chronic Myelogenous Leukemia, *edited by Moshe Talpaz and Hagop M. Kantarjian*
17. Expert Consultations in Breast Cancer: Critical Pathways and Clinical Decision Making, *edited by William N. Hait, David A. August, and Bruce G. Haffty*
18. Cancer Screening: Theory and Practice, *edited by Barnett S. Kramer, John K. Gohagan, and Philip C. Prorok*

ADDITIONAL VOLUMES IN PREPARATION

ADDITIONAL VOLUMES IN PREPARATION

AIDS-Related Cancers and Their Treatment

edited by

Ellen G. Feigal

National Cancer Institute
National Institutes of Health
Bethesda, Maryland

Alexandra M. Levine

University of Southern California School of Medicine
and USC/Norris Cancer Center
Los Angeles, California

Robert J. Biggar

National Cancer Institute
National Institutes of Health
Bethesda, Maryland

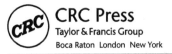

CRC Press
Taylor & Francis Group
Boca Raton London New York

CRC Press is an imprint of the
Taylor & Francis Group, an **informa** business

CRC Press
Taylor & Francis Group
6000 Broken Sound Parkway NW, Suite 300
Boca Raton, FL 33487-2742

First issued in paperback 2019

© 2000 by Taylor & Francis Group, LLC
CRC Press is an imprint of Taylor & Francis Group, an Informa business

No claim to original U.S. Government works

ISBN-13: 978-0-8247-7669-5 (hbk)
ISBN-13: 978-0-367-39901-6 (pbk)

**Visit the Taylor & Francis Web site at
http://www.taylorandfrancis.com**

**and the CRC Press Web site at
http://www.crcpress.com**

Series Introduction

The current volume, *AIDS-Related Cancers and Their Treatment,* is Volume 21 in the Basic and Clinical Oncology series. Many of the advances in oncology have resulted from close interaction between the basic scientist and the clinical researcher. The current volume follows, expands on, and illustrates the success of this relationship as demonstrated by new therapies and promising areas for scientific research.

As editor of the series, my goal has been to recruit volume editors who not only have established reputations based on their outstanding contributions to oncology, but also have an appreciation for the dynamic interface between the laboratory and the clinic. To date, the series has consisted of monographs on topics such as chronic lymphocytic leukemia, nucleoside analogs in cancer therapy, therapeutic applications of interleukin-2, retinoids in oncology, gene therapy of cancer, and principles of antineoplastic drug development and pharmacology. *AIDS-Related Cancers and Their Treatment* is certainly a most important addition to the series.

Volumes in progress include works on secondary malignancies, chronic lymphoid leukemias, and controversies in gynecologic oncology. I anticipate that these volumes will provide a valuable contribution to the oncology literature.

Bruce D. Cheson, M.D.

Preface

Malignancies are a significant cause of illness and death in the population infected with the human immunodeficiency virus (HIV), the causative agent of acquired immunodeficiency syndrome (AIDS). As the management of retroviral disease and opportunistic infections improves, allowing patients to survive longer with severe immunocompromise, these individuals will increasingly come to the attention of the practicing oncologist. A multidisciplinary approach is essential for developing the appropriate therapeutic management options. This approach must utilize the expertise of oncologists, internists, infectious disease specialists, and other subspecialists. Furthermore, this approach will be enhanced by an understanding of the epidemiology, biology, immunology, virology, and pathogenesis of malignancy and the underlying HIV infection.

People with HIV/AIDS are at risk for three AIDS-defining malignancies: Kaposi's sarcoma, intermediate or high-grade B cell/non–Hodgkin's lymphoma, and cervical cancer. In addition, anogenital neoplasias and Hodgkin's disease are increasingly noted. With nearly 1 million adults with HIV infection in the United States the co-incidence of HIV and common cancers will rise. Diagnosis and treatment of AIDS-specific malignancies, as well as the common cancers, pose unique and special challenges in a setting where the underlying illness, HIV infection, has significantly destroyed the patient's immunity.

The book begins with a general introduction of the epidemiology of AIDS and AIDS malignancies, and then delves into the diagnosis and management of malignancies by signs and symptoms, based on the regional anatomy. A specific chapter describes cancer in children with HIV/AIDS. The many therapeutic challenges encountered in the AIDS population are addressed. Non–AIDS-defining cancers present unique problems in differential diagnosis and in clinical management of the patient who also has HIV/AIDS. Separate chapters outline future directions for prevention and therapy, summarizing approaches and agents currently being evaluated or envisioned.

Critical patient management and treatment decisions must address the underlying HIV-related immunosuppression and its related complications. For this reason the book includes comprehensive chapters on agents and approaches to attenuate side effects of therapy. The need for combining primary anti-HIV therapy with antitumor therapy is presented, along with ways to measure the effects of such therapy. Infections are a complication of HIV, and can increase with the use of antitumor agents that further exacerbate an already compromised immune system. A chapter focused on the management of infection in the AIDS patient with cancer is discussed. Separate chapters provide guidance in dealing with the psychological and social aspects of HIV infection, both for the individual patient and for the communities of urban poor, homosexuals, and drug users. The last chapter summarizes the National Cancer Institute's programs in AIDS and cancer research and provides patient and health care workers with website addresses for clinical trials information and research resources.

The book is designed to be comprehensive in scope, but focuses on clinical management issues that are of practical use to the health care provider involved with the care of patients with AIDS malignancies. This information is concisely but clearly presented, with ample tables, illustrations, and photographs. It should be of immediate use to practicing oncologists, general internists, infectious disease specialists, surgeons, radiologists, and other health care providers.

Ellen G. Feigal, M.D.
Alexandra M. Levine, M.D.
Robert J. Biggar, M.D.

Contents

Contributors

Robert J. Biggar, M.D.   Viral Epidemiology Branch, Division of Cancer Epidemiology and Genetics, National Cancer Institute, National Institutes of Health, Bethesda, Maryland

Cathy W. Critchlow, Ph.D.   Associate Professor, Department of Epidemiology, School of Public Health and Community Medicine, University of Washington, Seattle, Washington

Ellen G. Feigal, M.D.   Deputy Director, Division of Cancer Treatment and Diagnosis, National Cancer Institute, National Institutes of Health, Bethesda, Maryland

Mindy Thompson Fullilove, M.D.   Associate Professor of Clinical Psychiatry and Public Health, Department of Psychiatry, New York State Psychiatric Institute and Columbia University, New York, New York

Nancy B. Kiviat, M.D.   Professor of Pathology and Medicine, School of Medicine, University of Washington, Seattle, Washington

Susan E. Krown, M.D.   Member and Attending Physician, Clinical Immunology Service, Division of Hematologic Oncology, Department of Medicine, Memorial Sloan-Kettering Cancer Center, and Professor of Medicine, Cornell University Medical College, New York, New York

Fa-Chyi Lee, M.D.   Division of Hematology–Oncology and UCLA Center for Clinical AIDS Research and Education, Department of Medicine, University of California, Los Angeles, Los Angeles, California

Alexandra M. Levine, M.D.   Professor of Medicine and Chief, Division of Hematology, University of Southern California School of Medicine, and Medical Director, USC/Norris Cancer Center, Los Angeles, California

Richard F. Little, M.D.   Senior Clinical Investigator, HIV and AIDS Malignancy Branch, National Cancer Institute, National Institutes of Health, Bethesda, Maryland

Mitchell Maiman, M.D.   Director of Obstetrics and Gynecology and Director of Gynecologic Oncology, Department of Obstetrics and Gynecology, Staten Island University Hospital, Staten Island, New York

Michael Marco   Director, Clinical Science, Treatment Action Group, New York, New York

Henry Masur, M.D.   Clinical Professor of Medicine, George Washington University School of Medicine, Washington, D.C., and Chief, Critical Care Medicine Department, Warren Grant Magnuson Clinical Center, National Institutes of Health, Bethesda, Maryland

Steven A. Miles, M.D.   Associate Professor of Medicine and Director, UCLA CARE Clinic, UCLA Center for Clinical AIDS Research and Education, Department of Medicine, University of California, Los Angeles, Los Angeles, California

Kirk D. Miller, M.D.   Associate Clinical Professor of Medicine, Georgetown University School of Medicine, Washington, D.C., and Staff Physician, Critical Care Medicine Department, Warren Grant Magnuson Clinical Center, National Institutes of Health, Bethesda, Maryland

Ronald T. Mitsuyasu, M.D., F.A.C.P.   Associate Professor of Medicine and Director, UCLA CARE Clinic, UCLA Center for Clinical AIDS Research and Education, Department of Medicine, University of California, Los Angeles, Los Angeles, California

Brigitta U. Mueller, M.D.   Associate in Medicine, Children's Hospital, and Assistant Professor of Pediatrics, Harvard Medical School, Boston, Massachusetts

Joel Palefsky, M.D., C.M.   Professor, Departments of Laboratory Medicine and Stomatology, University of California, San Francisco, San Francisco, California

Philip A. Pizzo, M.D.   Physician-in-Chief and Chair, Department of Medicine, Children's Hospital, and Thomas Morgan Rotch Professor of Pediatrics, Harvard Medical School, Boston, Massachusetts

Alice Reier, M.D.   Division of Hematology–Oncology and UCLA Center for Clinical AIDS Research and Education, Department of Medicine, University of California, Los Angeles, Los Angeles, California

David T. Scadden, M.D.   Director, Center for AIDS Oncology, Dana-Farber/Partners Cancer Care, Massachusetts General Hospital and Harvard Medical School, Boston, Massachusetts

Umberto Tirelli, M.D.   Director and Professor, Division of Medical Oncology and AIDS, Aviano Cancer Center, Aviano, Italy

Emanuela Vaccher, M.D.   Division of Medical Oncology and AIDS, Aviano Cancer Center, Aviano, Italy

Robert Yarchoan, M.D.   Chief, HIV and AIDS Malignancy Branch, Division of Clinical Sciences, National Cancer Institute, National Institutes of Health, Bethesda, Maryland

AIDS-Related Cancers and Their Treatment

1

The HIV/AIDS Epidemic

Robert J. Biggar
*National Cancer Institute, National Institutes of Health,
Bethesda, Maryland*

I. INTRODUCTION

The acquired immunodeficiency syndrome (AIDS) epidemic was first reported in
June 1981 in a brief summary of six cases of a normally rare pulmonary infection,
Pneumocystis carinii, in Los Angeles (1). Besides the temporal link, all these
cases occurred among young, apparently healthy homosexual men. About the
same time, physicians in New York notified the then Centers for Disease Control
(CDC) of a similar outbreak. In their experience, the conditions included *Pneumocystis* pneumonia (PCP) but also the rare cutaneous malignancy, Kaposi's sarcoma (KS). As in Los Angeles, the patients were preponderantly homosexual
men, but they noted that nonhomosexual intravenous drug users were also affected (2).

    These two almost simultaneous reports provided the basic description of
the emerging epidemic of what soon became known as AIDS. The physicians
caring for these patients recognized immediately that the common thread linking
these diseases was immunosuppression, predominantly involving severe deficits
of cellular immunity. However, known causes for such immunodeficiency included only rare genetic disorders and iatrogenic immunosuppression from
therapies specifically formulated to suppress transplant rejections or to treat
cancer. There were no known causes for this type of epidemic immunodeficiency.

    The next 3 years were spent both in further defining the disease and its
underlying immune dysfunction, but most urgently, in trying to discover the etiology. In addition to homosexual men and intravenous drug users, persons receiv-

ing blood or blood products were soon recognized to be at risk. This led to a growing certainty that an infectious agent caused this epidemic. Despite intensive efforts, it was not until 1983 that a plausible candidate, a novel human retrovirus, was discovered (3) and 1984 before it was shown in cross-sectional (4–7) and prospective cohort (8,9) studies to be the cause of AIDS.

II. HUMAN IMMUNODEFICIENCY VIRUS

This virus was given a variety of names during the 1980s. The initial name given was the "lymphadenopathy virus (LAV)" which judiciously identified the virus as isolated from a subject with enlarged glands, not AIDS (3). Others reisolated this and other strains of the same virus from persons with AIDS and, in recognition of its structural similarity, related it to two other known human retroviruses by using the name "human T-lymphotropic virus type III (HTLV-III"; 10). The early confusion in nomenclature was resolved by the adoption of the name "human immunodeficiency virus (HIV)."

Although not always stated, HIV is generally understood to mean the type 1 variant, a distinction that needed to be clarified when it was reported in 1986 that at least one other closely related virus, HIV-2, existed in West Africa (11). Despite being about 60% homologous with HIV-1, HIV-2 has a somewhat different pathophysiology, leading to much slower disease progression and lower rates of transmission (12). This virus remains confined almost exclusively to West Africa and has little potential for becoming epidemic elsewhere. Studies describing HIV in this book can be accepted as meaning HIV-1, unless it is specifically identified as HIV-2.

In contrast with the HTLV viruses, which apparently have been endemic in humans for many millennia, the HIV outbreaks were probably occasional zoonoses arising from primates until the current epidemic (13,14). This is well established for HIV-2, a virus that resembles almost indistinguishably a simian immunodeficiency virus found in sooty mangabey monkeys of West Africa (15,16). This virus appears to have had multiple independent introductions into humans. Because HIV-2 is relatively poorly transmitted, secondary spread is limited. Establishing this link to primate retroviruses was undoubtedly simplified by the limited spread of HIV-2 in humans. In contrast, HIV-1 is readily transmitted between humans, and its origins are obscure. The primate virus most closely related to HIV-1 was found in a chimpanzee from Gabon (17,18), but further work needs to be done to establish the source. It is possible that simian-to-human transmission of HIV-1 happened many times over thousands of years, but only the rise of the major urban areas in Africa during the current century permitted the occurrence of a sustained epidemic.

III. DEMOGRAPHICS OF THE HIV–AIDS EPIDEMIC

Identification of HIV as the cause of AIDS resulted in major advances in quantifying the epidemic and in tracking its transmission and natural history. The results
of these studies led to a grim understanding of the reality of this epidemic. In
the United States, initial estimates suggested 1.5 million persons were already
infected by 1985. Recently, more reliable studies have lowered these estimates
to about 1 million persons ever infected as of 1993 (about half by 1985; 19,20),
which, nevertheless, represents a staggering number of persons. Without great
improvements in therapy, the vast majority of these persons will, over time, succumb to the immunodeficiency resulting from HIV infection.

   For purposes of public health reporting, AIDS was initially defined by a
list of clinical conditions related to immunodeficiency. This list of conditions
was expanded in 1985 and 1987, and in 1993, the definition was further modified
to include persons with HIV positivity who have laboratory evidence of profound
immunodeficiency (CD4+ count < 200, or < 14%). The 1993 changes recognized that prophylactic therapies were delaying the onset of clinical AIDS and
enabled persons needing health care to obtain insurance coverage. However, in
spite of the expanding definition, the number of newly identified AIDS cases has
declined markedly (Fig. 1). This decrease has occurred primarily because the

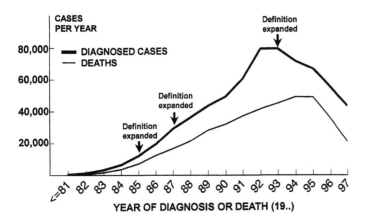

Figure 1   The annual numbers of AIDS cases and deaths from AIDS in the United States
through December 1997: For 1997, numbers are incomplete; therefore, midyear numbers
were doubled to estimate the full-year numbers. Cumulatively, through 1997, there have
been 652,721 cases and 396,668 deaths. At the indicated points, the definition of AIDS
was expanded to accommodate the changing understanding of the clinical profile. (From
Ref. 31.)

incidence of HIV infection decreased considerably during the 1980s, but additionally, because new and more effective antiretroviral agents are now slowing the progression to AIDS among those already infected.

IV. RECENT HIV INCIDENCE

New infections are still occurring, although their recent incidence is difficult to determine. As of the early 1990s, there were probably about 30,000–60,000 new infections annually in the United States alone (19,21). This transmission has occurred despite intensive efforts to modify behaviors in ways that would reduce transmission. In part, the sustained epidemic results from the high prevalence of HIV in some groups practicing high-risk behaviors for transmission, such as receptive anal intercourse among homosexual men and sharing of needles and syringes among injection drug users. However, heterosexual transmission, especially among minorities, is becoming an increasing problem among young persons (22).

Thus, although at-risk groups have modified behaviors in ways that lower risk, there remains considerable infection risk for persons continuing to engage in risk-taking behaviors. Notably, the groups now becoming infected are young, in contrast with the wide age range infected in the initial wave of the infection. In the United States, the median age for AIDS in the late 1980s was about 25 years old (Fig. 2) and about a quarter of newly infected persons were younger than 23 years old (23). More recent estimates suggest the peak period of transmission is now even younger (22).

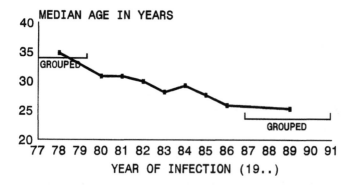

Figure 2   Median age of HIV infection in the United States by year, estimated by backcalculation techniques. Backcalculation models the HIV infection curve from reported AIDS cases and the incubation period between HIV infection and AIDS (From Ref. 24.)

The routes of HIV transmission (Fig. 3) will determine which groups have already become infected and are likely to be infected in the future. Transmission by both homosexual and heterosexual intercourse is well established. In the early phase of the AIDS epidemic, HIV transmission associated with receptive anal intercourse among homosexual men overwhelmingly dominated the exposure statistics in the United States (Fig. 4; 24). In recent years, this route probably accounts for about half the new infections (19,22) in men. However, among young men, the incidence of HIV attributable to homosexual contact declined nearly 50% between 1988 and 1993, a major success of prevention and education programs (22).

Unfortunately, an increasing transmission risk among heterosexuals has offset this prevention success. Worldwide, spread among non–drug-using heterosexual partners is the predominant (> 90%) route of exposure among the 30 million thought to have been infected with HIV (25). In the United States, heterosexual transmission is now the leading mode among young women and is especially a problem in minorities (22). Unfortunately, these infections also expose unborn children to HIV infection. Mother-to-child transmission occurs in utero, at delivery, and during breast feeding. Without intervention, about a quarter of nonbreastfed infants born to infected women become infected (26,27). With breastfeeding, an additional 5–10% of infants become infected (28). Antiretroviral therapies and avoidance of breastfeeding can greatly reduce this risk.

In recent years, transmission within the community of injection drug users appears to have stabilized (22). Besides the risks of exposure from contaminated

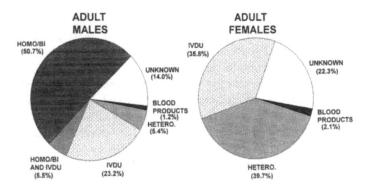

Figure 3 Distribution of HIV exposure categories for adult and adolescent AIDS cases in the United States occurring among 47,056 males and 13,105 females: Most (91%) of the 473 children (< 13 years old) with AIDS were infected from their mothers, 8% were infected by blood or blood products, and 2% had no source of exposure specified. Because of the long incubation period between infection and AIDS, exposure sources reflect events that happened many years earlier. (From Ref. 31.)

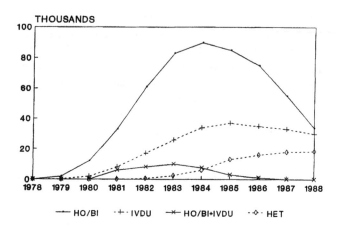

Figure 4 Distribution of HIV infections estimated by backcalculation for the 1980s
(24): More recent estimates become increasingly unreliable because few persons progress
to AIDS within the first few years after HIV infection. However, among young persons
(18–22 years old), who probably constitute the majority of new infections, 22,000 males
and 11,000 females became infected in 1993, the last year for which this can be estimated
(22). Among homosexual men, incidence declined nearly 50%, but among intravenous
drug users, incidence was fairly stable, and among heterosexuals, incidence increased.
Overall, between 1988 and 1993, transmission in this group declined 14%.

needles and syringes, sexual exposures to HIV-infected persons may also occur
in exchange for drugs, although the proportion of transmissions related to sexual
acts, rather than equipment sharing, is difficult to determine. Transmission by
exposure to contaminated blood products, although associated with a high risk
of infection, has almost ended with the introduction of HIV testing into blood
banks in the mid-1980s. It is estimated that 18–27 units of the 12-million units
of blood collected each year in the United States are infected, most occurring
because the blood was obtained from very recently infected persons who were
viremic but not yet making antibodies at a level that could be detected by screening assays (29).

This distribution of risk groups and the long incubation period between
HIV infection and AIDS led to the characteristic age profile of the AIDS epidemic, which shows a peak incidence in the 30–40-year-old age range. Even
though the overall male/female ratio of cases (Fig. 5) is 11.5:1 for all years of
the epidemic, it is 3.6:1 in 1997, largely because of the declining transmission
among homosexual men, but also because of rising heterosexual transmission,
particularly in minorities. By race group, 45% were white, 36% were black, 18%
were Hispanic, and 1.0% were Asian/Pacific Islanders and American Indians

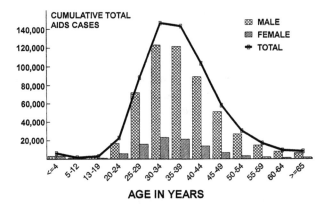

Figure 5 Age and sex distribution of 633,000 AIDS cases in the United States through 1997: Among infants infected from their mothers, the male/female ratio is equal, but in older children, males predominant because hemophilia is male dominated. Among adolescents infected heterosexually, women are infected earlier than men, but this is offset because homosexual contact also occurs in this age group. (From Ref. 13.)

(30). African-Americans and Hispanics are two- to threefold more likely to be AIDS cases than whites. Minority populations in inner-city urban areas have an especially high AIDS incidence (22,31).

V. THE EFFECT OF DEMOGRAPHIC CHANGES ON CANCERS IN AIDS

These demographic realities will influence the cancer profile in HIV–AIDS patients during the next decade. There are many reasons why this occurs. Younger persons have lower cancer risk than older persons. Furthermore, they develop severe immunodeficiency more slowly (32), and younger HIV-infected persons will also be at lower risk of developing cancer because they are not as immunosuppressed. Homo- or bisexual men have a much higher risk of KS than other transmission groups (33,34), and as homosexual AIDS cases decline as a proportion of HIV–AIDS population, the incidence of KS will decline. Similarly, because non–Hodgkin's lymphoma (NHL), the other major AIDS-related malignancy, is less common in minority populations (32), the incidence of NHL in AIDS patients may also decline. However, as the number of women with AIDS increases, cervical cancer will become more common. Finally, improvements in therapy may result in improved immune status, which may lead to lower cancer risks (see Chapter 2). Overall, the number of cancer cases in persons with

HIV/AIDS is likely to decline with these demographic changes. However, this decline could be offset because improvements in therapies will also permit more persons with AIDS to survive long enough to develop a malignancy. Finally, in the social dimension, the decreasing proportion of cases from more affluent, educated, and politically connected groups may result in fewer activists able to influence public policies that support HIV and AIDS research on cancer and outreach efforts to support the care of such patients.

REFERENCES

1. Centers for Disease Control. Kaposi's sarcoma and *Pneumocystis* pneumonia among homosexual men—New York City and California. MMWR 30:305–308, 1981.
2. Centers for Disease Control. *Pneumocystis* pneumonia—Los Angeles. MMWR 30: 250–252, 1981.
3. F Barré-Sinoussi, JC Chermann, F Rey, MT Nugeyre, S Chamaret, J Gruest, C Dauguet, C Axler-Blin, F Vezinet-Brun, C Rouzioux, W Rozenbaum, L Montagnier. Isolation of a T-lymphotropic retrovirus from a patient at risk for acquired immune deficiency syndrome (AIDS). Science 220:868–871, 1983.
4. RC Gallo, SZ Salahuddin, M Popovic, GM Shearer, M Kaplan, BF Haynes, TJ Palker, R Redfield, J Oleske, B Safai, G White, P Foster, PD Maricham. Frequent detection and isolation of cytopathic retroviruses (HTLV-III) from patients with AIDS and at risk for AIDS. Science. 224:500–503, 1984.
5. MG Sarngadharan, M Popovic, L Bruch, J Schubach, RC Gallo. Antibodies reactive with human T-lymphotropic retroviruses (HTLV-III) in the serum of patients with AIDS. Science 224:506–508, 1984.
6. F Brun-Vézinet, C Rouzioux, F Barré-Sinoussi, D Klatzmann, AG Saimot, W Rozenbaum, D Christol, JC Gluckmann, L Montagnier, JC Chermann. Detection of IgG antibodies to lymphadenopathy-associated virus in patients with AIDS or lymphadenopathy syndrome. Lancet 1:1253–1256, 1984.
7. J Laurence, F Brun-Vezinet, SE Schutzer, C Rouzioux, D Klatzmann, F Barré-Sinoussi, JC Chermann, L Montagnier. Lymphadenopathy-associated viral antibody in AIDS. Immune correlations and definition of a carrier state. N Engl J Med 311: 1269–1273, 1984.
8. M Melbye, RJ Biggar, P Ebbesen, MG Sarngadharan, SH Weiss, RC Gallo, WA Blattner. Seroepidemiology of HTLV-III antibody in Danish homosexual men: prevalence, transmission, and disease outcome. Br Med J 289:573–575, 1984.
9. JJ Goedert, MG Sarngadharan, RJ Biggar, SH Weiss, DM Winn, RJ Grossman, MH Greene, AJ Bodner, DL Mann, DM Strong, RC Gallo, WA Blattner. Determinants of retrovirus (HTLV-III) antibody and immunodeficiency conditions in homosexual men. Lancet 2:711–716, 1984.
10. M Popovic, MG Sarngadharan, E Read, RC Gallo. Detection, isolation, and continuous production of cytopathic retroviruses (HTLV-III) from patients with AIDS and pre-AIDS. Science 224:497–500, 1984.

11. F Clavel, D Guetard, F Brun-Vezinet, S Chamaret, MA Rey, MO Santos-Ferreira, AG Laurent, C Dauguet, C Katlama, C Rouzioux, D Klatzmann, JL Champalimaud, L Montagnier. Isolation of a new human retrovirus from West African patients with AIDS. Science 233:343–346, 1986.

12. F Clavel, M Guyader, D Guetard, M Salle, L Montagnier, M Alizon. Molecular cloning and polymorphism of the human immune deficiency virus type 2. Nature 234:691–695, 1986.

13. TF Schulz. Origin of AIDS. Lancet 339:867, 1992.

14. Barre-Sinoussi F. HIV as the cause of AIDS. Lancet 348:31–35, 1996.

15. F Gao, L Yue, AT White, PG Pappas, J Barchue, AP Hanson, BM Greene, PM Sharp, GM Shaw, BH Hahn. Human infection by genetically diverse SIV related HIV-2 in West Africa. Nature 358:495–499, 1992.

16. F Gao, L Yue, DL Robertson, SC Hill, H Hui, RJ Biggar, AE Neequaye, TM Whelan, DD Ho, GM Shaw. Genetic diversity of human immunodeficiency virus type 2: evidence for distinct sequence subtypes with differences in virus biology. J Virol 68:7433–7447, 1994.

17. M Peeters, C Honoré, T Huet, L Bedjabaga, S Ossari, P Bussi, RW Copper, E Delaporte. Isolation and partial characterization of an HIV-related virus occurring naturally in chimpanzees in Gabon. AIDS 3:625–630, 1989.

18. W Janssens, K Fransen, M Peeters, L Heyndrickx, J Motte, L Bedjabaga, E Delaporte, P Piot, G Van der Groen. Phylogenetic analysis of a new chimpanzee lentivirus SIVcpz-gab2 from a wild-captured chimpanzee from Gabon. AIDS Res Hum Retroviruses 10:1191–1192, 1994.

19. PS Rosenberg. Scope of the AIDS epidemic in the United States. Science 270:1372–1375, 1995.

20. JM Karon, PS Rosenberg, G McQuillan, M Khare, M Gwinn, LR Petersen. Prevalence of HIV infection in the United States, 1984 to 1992. JAMA 276:126–131, 1996.

21. SD Holmberg. The estimated prevalence and incidence of HIV in 96 large US metropolitan areas. Am J Public Health 86:642–654, 1996.

22. PS Rosenberg, RJ Biggar. Trends in HIV incidence among adolescents and young adults in the United States. JAMA 279:1894–99, 1998.

23. PS Rosenberg, RJ Biggar, JJ Goedert. Declining age at HIV infection in the United States. N Engl J Med 330:789–790, 1994.

24. R Brookmeyer. Reconstruction and future trends of the AIDS epidemic in the United States. Science 253:37–42, 1991.

25. World Health Organization. Report on the Global HIV/AIDS epidemic, June 1998. United Nations, 1998.

26. DT Dunn, ML Newell, MJ Mayaux, C Kind, C Hutto, JJ Goedert, W Andiman. Mode of delivery and vertical transmission of HIV-1: a review of prospective studies. Perinatal AIDS collaborative transmission studies. J Acquir Immune Defic Syndr 7:1064–1066, 1994.

27. LM Mofenson. Epidemiology and determinants of vertical HIV transmission. Semin Pediatr Infect Dis 5:252–265, 1994.

28. DT Dunn, ML Newell, AE Ades, CS Peckham. Risk of human immunodeficiency virus type 1 transmission through breastfeeding. Lancet 340:585–588, 1992.

29. EM Lackritz, GA Satten, J Aberle-Grasse, RY Dodd, VP Raimondi, RS Janssen, WF Lewis, EP Notari 4th, LR Peterson. Estimated risk of transmission of the human immunodeficiency virus by screened blood in the United States. N Engl J Med 333: 1721–1725, 1995.
30. PS Rosenberg, ME Levy, JF Brundage, LR Peterson, JM Karon, TR Fears, LI Gardner, MH Gail, JJ Goedert, WA Blattner, CC Ryan, SH Vermund, RJ Biggar. Population-based monitoring of an urban HIV/AIDS epidemic. Magnitude and trends in the District of Columbia. JAMA 268:495–503, 1992.
31. Centers for Disease Control. HIV/AIDS Surveillance Report. U.S. HIV and AIDS cases reported through December 1997. Atlanta: U.S. Department of Health and Human Services. Public Health Service, Center for Disease Control, 1997; vol 9.
32. PS Rosenberg, JJ Goedert, RJ Biggar. Effect of age at seroconversion on the natural AIDS incubation distribution. AIDS 8:803–810, 1994.
33. RJ Biggar, CS Rabkin. The epidemiology of AIDS-related neoplasms. Hematol Oncol Clin North Am 10:997–1010, 1996.

2
HIV Infection, Immunity, and Cancer

Robert J. Biggar
National Cancer Institute, National Institutes of Health, Bethesda, Maryland

I. INTRODUCTION

One of the earliest manifestations of the AIDS epidemic was the abrupt increase in the incidence of Kaposi's sarcoma (KS; 1). Later review of cancer statistics showed KS diagnoses in young, single men to be a sensitive indicator of when the HIV epidemic first entered homosexual communities. In New York City the incidence of KS started to increase in 1977, at least 3 years before acquired immunodeficiency syndrome (AIDS) was formally recognized (2). The significance of these few cases was missed at the time because they were seen by different caregivers and because cancer registry data takes several years to be compiled and analyzed.

The appearance of KS provided an important clue to the pathogenesis of AIDS. Studies done long before the AIDS epidemic had documented that the incidence of KS was high in immunosuppressed persons (3). Almost from the onset of the AIDS epidemic, studies of phenotypic and functional immunity in persons with AIDS documented profound deficits of cellular immunity. Furthermore, prospective studies of persons at risk of AIDS, usually homosexual men, noted that HIV-infected subjects had, over time, progressively impaired cellular immunity that led to fatal opportunistic infections and cancers (4). Even before the human immunodeficiency virus (HIV) was discovered, these data were able to establish that the cause was likely to be infectious, and that the probable routes of transmission were sexual and bloodborne. These hypotheses were confirmed after the causal agent, HIV-1, was finally determined in 1983–1984.

II. HIV-1

The virus HIV-1 is a member of the lentivirus family of retroviruses. Other members that infect humans include HIV-2 and the human T-lymphotropic virus (HTLV) types I and II. As a group, these viruses are characterized by being RNA viruses that carry the enzyme reverse transcriptase within the viral particle. This enzyme translates the RNA virus genome into a DNA form that is transported into the nucleus and randomly inserted into the host DNA. Once there, the DNA instructs the replication of viral components, which are assembled in the cytoplasm and emerge from the cell membrane as new virus particles.

Although the HIV and HTLV groups of viruses are quite distant from each other (less than 5% homology), they share structural similarity in the placement of gene sequences as well as operational similarity. The major antigens recognized by antibodies are the Gag (involved in binding the RNA core), the Env proteins (involved in the envelope surrounding the intact virus), the enzyme reverse transcriptase, and various regulatory proteins that control the production and assembly of the virus. Although beyond the scope of this book to discuss these in detail, they may appear in the context of reports of antibody results and are potential targets for virus-specific therapies.

A. Viral Entry and Tropism

The virus was initially thought to attach to CD4 receptors on the cell surface (5). However, recent investigators have shown that viral binding involves at least two chemokine receptor sites, CCR5 and CXCR4 (6–8) in addition to CD4. These coreceptor sites are essential for infection, as indicated by the fact that persons who have genetically determined losses of these receptors are rarely infected (9), although there are exceptions (10). Surface receptors may help determine the tropism of the virus to certain cells. Macrophages (11) and glial cells (12,13) have both CD4 and coreceptors, rendering them susceptible to infection. Although unproved, strain variation in the ability of the virus to enter cells of specific types could influence clinical manifestations.

B. Reverse Transcriptase and Error Production

A major growth characteristic of HIV-1 is the high rate of replication and mutation, with over a billion new virons produced each day. It has been estimated that only a small fraction of the viral particles produced are complete and capable of infecting another cell (14,15). With large numbers of viral particles coming from each cell before its death, this replication rate is sufficient to create a constant proliferation over the entire time course of infection (16,17). Soon after initial infection there is an initial high level outburst of viremia, but by 1 year after infection, viral levels become established at a somewhat lower level. These levels increase slowly over time, rising particularly at the end stages of AIDS illness (18,19). High viral load levels are established in the initial years after infection and are associated with a more rapid onset of immunosuppression and subsequent AIDS-defining illnesses, probably including cancers (20,21). Fortunately, chemotherapy given to HIV-infected patients with cancer does not affect viral levels (22).

This high rate of replication has several implications. Reverse transcriptase, the enzyme used to convert viral RNA to the DNA form, is error-prone in its copy fidelity (23), which no doubt contributes to the relative low number of complete, infectious viral copies. However, the error-prone nature of the enzyme also introduces variations in the virus, such that within the same host, many new variants emerge from the initially infecting strain over time. Whether a particular variant becomes the dominant strain is a consequence of enhanced replication by the more efficient subtypes and of immunological pressure, since the residual immune system recognizes and responds to the presence of the emerging variant. Furthermore, there is controversial evidence that the HLA type of the host could influence the immunological control of the virus (24,25).

Within individuals and transmission-linked groups, the variants ("quasi-species") are closely related genotypes (26). However, in distant populations, new subtypes emerge. By definition, subtypes, also called clades, are more than 10% different from other viral types. In North America and Europe, the B subtype is the dominant clade (27), but in other geographic areas, different clades predominate (28). In some areas, two or more subtypes are circulating in the same population (e.g., A and D in East Africa and B and E in Thailand), which implies at least two sources of the infection for these populations. At least one subtype, found in central Africa, termed type O, is sufficiently divergent that infected persons may escape detection by standard antibody tests (29). The clinical significance of these subtypes is unknown.

C. Antiretroviral Therapies

The variations of the viral quasispecies within an infected person can lead to the emergence of strains resistant to antiretroviral therapies. Zidovudine (AZT), the first drug shown to have a significant antiretroviral effect, is a thymidine analogue that competes for reverse transcriptase. Patients treated with AZT typically have an initial measurable decline of viral load by 1/2 to 1 log. Surprisingly, this minimal effect is associated with clinical improvement. However, because of emerging resistant subtypes, the clinical benefits wane within a few months, and viral load returns to the previous levels (30–32).

Because of this rapid emergence of resistence, the current clinical approach to therapy advocates the simultaneous use of multiple agents, each acting against a different viral target, such as reverse transcriptase and the viral proteases, with the objective of stopping all viral replication so that resistance cannot emerge. Since 1995, several new drugs have become available for clinical use (33–35). These fall into two groups, the nucleoside analogues and the protease inhibitors. Although each alone may be only marginally, if at all, better than AZT, their benefit lies in the combination usage. As they have different toxicities, they can safely be given together at tolerable doses, while at the same time effectively reducing viral replication to the point that HIV cannot be detected in peripheral blood samples. In such patients, CD4+ lymphocyte levels typically improve (37). Even though functional immunity is not fully restored, the patients usually show clinical benefit relative to opportunistic infections (38), leading to longer survival (39) and a decline in deaths caused by AIDS (40).

Despite their potential efficacy, wide-scale application of these new combination therapies will be difficult. Persons with limited mental or physical abilities, including those with advanced HIV-related conditions, have difficulty complying with the complex regimens, which require the use of several drugs, each given on different schedules. Furthermore, the subjects must be monitored for potential side effects of these therapies. Finally, the expense of such therapy, which currently can cost up to $30,000/year per patient, may be prohibitive. Certainly, such therapies will not be applicable to many developing countries where millions of people are HIV-infected but health care is limited by financial constraints.

For such countries, prevention strategies, including vaccines, will be the only practical approach. Prevention efforts have shown some success in many parts of the developed and developing world, but so far, vaccine progress has been disappointing. Many factors contribute. There is almost no evidence to demonstrate that infected persons might rid themselves of established infections through their own immunological response. "Therapeutic vaccines," which are given in the hope of slowing progression in persons already infected, are under evaluation but have not yet been shown to be effective. However, preventive vaccines, which are aimed at preventing primary infection, present a difficult immunological problem and safety concerns that will require separate approaches to design and testing.

III. IMMUNITY

Following initial infection, there is a period when the virus is below the threshold of detection. Thereafter, a burst of viremia emerges, sometimes associated with acute but nonspecific symptoms, called the acute retrovirus syndrome or HIV seroconversion syndrome (Fig. 1) (41,42). Over several weeks to months, viral loads usually decline, presumably because of host immunity. This early infection is reflected in changes in the immune system, with the loss of about a quarter to

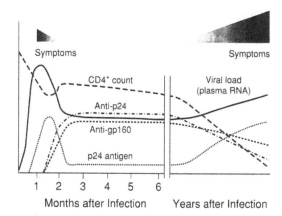

Months after Infection   Years after Infection

Figure 1 Schematic presentation of changes in virological and immunological parameters in relation to HIV infection and symptoms related to infection. The early symptoms are related to the initial viremia and described as "flu-like," often with a lingering lymphadenopathy. As immunity deteriorates in the years following infection, symptoms are related to opportunistic infections and malignancies. (From Ref. 68.)

a third of the CD4 cells in the peripheral circulation (43). Thus, the typical levels of CD4 cells are about 900/μL before infection, but within a year, cell levels are close to 600/μL, with persons who have a more dramatic decline having a faster course of subsequent immunosuppression. Thereafter, in the absence of antiretroviral therapies, the CD4 cell count will fall by 40–50/μL per year on average. After a median time of 8–9 years after infection, infected persons have about 100–200 cells per microliter, a level at which immunodeficiency-related illnesses start to occur (44,45).

The rate at which CD4 cell counts decline varies considerably among individuals. In addition, there is variation in the CD4 count at which immunodeficiency-related illnesses may occur. Having a high viral load 1–3 years after infection is a harbinger of faster CD4 cell count decline, but younger-aged persons develop AIDS at slower rate, even after adjusting for viral load (which does not appear to be age-related; 22). This may occur because CD4 stem cell replication capability is greater in the young, resulting in a slower rate of CD4 decline. Furthermore, young persons have fewer AIDS illnesses, even at the same level of immunodeficiency, probably because the young have had fewer exposures to environmental pathogens that might be reactivated with immunodeficiency. Interestingly, after adjusting for the CD4 cell count, increasing age was associated with an increased risk of AIDS-associated cancer, but not opportunistic infections in one study (46).

A. Implications for Cancer Epidemiology

The application of these observations to cancer epidemiology will be discussed in Chapter 3. Both KS and non–Hodgkin's lymphoma (NHL) require a setting of immunodeficiency to become manifest in HIV-infected patients. Thus, the HIV epidemic necessarily precedes the epidemics of associated cancers by several years. Because the number of persons with HIV-related immunodeficiency can be only estimated, the relative risks of these cancers have been compared with the expected rates in the general population. Therefore, relative-risk estimates become higher as the HIV epidemic matures and a higher proportion of HIV-infected persons are severely immunosuppressed. Among untreated persons, this trend will continue until the numbers of persons with HIV-related immunodeficiency reaches a steady state.

The advent of highly active antiretroviral therapies (HAART) will impinge on cancer risk both directly and indirectly. Two reports describe regression of already established KS in patients who responded well to antiretroviral therapy (47,48), presumably because of the improvements in immunity. Such remissions have previously been well documented in patients iatrogenically immunosuppressed, among whom reduction or cessation of immunosuppressive therapies have cured or caused regression in an established malignancy. The new therapies are also likely to reduce the incidence of cancer in HIV-infected persons. There is preliminary evidence that the incidence of KS in treated persons is already declining below that expected (38). In unpublished work described during a round table discussion at the second National AIDS Malignancy Conference, Washington, D.C., April 6–8, 1998, investigators suggested that the incidence of primary brain lymphoma has declined as well.

Presumably, if immunity were completely restored, the excess risk of cancer would entirely disappear. However, the cancer–incidence response pattern could be complex. If the deterioration in immunity is held at a level of only partial improvement, it is possible that, even though opportunistic infections are controlled and KS incidence is reduced, lymphomas might continue to be generated as the lymphoid system compensates for an ongoing, but smoldering, destructive process. The full effect of these therapies on cancer risk will require more follow-up time.

B. Cancer in Non–HIV-Related Immunodeficiency

When the AIDS epidemic first appeared in the United States, KS was a prominent manifestation in many of the earliest cases. This cancer, otherwise rare in the United States (49), had already been noted to occur in excess in organ transplant recipients who had been iatrogenically immunosuppressed to prevent rejection of transplanted tissue (50,51). Thus, its epidemic appearance in previously healthy young men was immediately recognized as a manifestation of an underlying epidemic of an acquired immunosuppression. However, KS was not the most common tumor associated with transplant-related immunosuppression, leading to concerns that other cancers would soon appear in AIDS patients.

Lymphomas were the most frequent tumor in the setting of iatrogenic immunosuppression (52–54), and they are also known to occur in rare genetic immunodeficiency syndromes (55). Lower, but still important, excess risks of many other tumor types (summarized in Ref. 56) have also been reported. Other frequently mentioned cancers in transplant recipients include lip and other skin (including squamous and basal cell carcinomas and melanoma) and renal and bladder cancers, but there are a variety of other cancer excesses reported. Overall, the 10-year risk of cancer in organ transplants is about 15–20%, providing a relative risk of about four to five fold compared with a general population of the same age (54,57).

Among patients in the United States, the median time to cancer onset after the onset of immunosuppressive therapy is about 22 months for KS, 32 months for NHL, and 67 months for other tumors (58). However, some cancers, especially KS, can appear within a few months of the onset of immunosuppression. As immunosuppressive regimens have become more powerful, the incidence of lymphomas in treated patients has risen, and the time to onset is generally more rapid (57,59–61).

Although the absolute risks of KS in transplant patients are much lower than for NHL, the relative risks are higher because KS is much rarer than NHL in the young persons typically undergoing transplantion. Unlike NHL risk, the KS risk varies geographically. Specifically, in a Scandinavian study, only 2 cases of KS were seen in 5692 renal transplant recipients (54), whereas in the United States, 307 of 7192 organ transplant patients developed KS (58). This variation indicated the existence of regionally distributed cofactors. The newly described human herpesvirus-8 may account for much of this variation (Chapter 3). Marrow transplant recipients are also at excess risk of malignancies, about half of which are NHLs, which tend to occur within the first few years (62). The relative risk of KS is increased, but the absolute risk is low; only 1 of nearly 20,000 marrow transplant recipients developed KS (63).

Even though transplantation-related cancers clearly occur in the setting of immunodeficiency, it is unclear if the malignancy can be attributed to immunosuppression alone. Many other factors may contribute, such as events causing the underlying condition necessitating the transplant, treatment with potent carcinogenic drugs and radiation that are used therapeutically, chronic antigenic stimulation provoked by the presence of the foreign transplanted organs, and for marrow transplants, the occurrence of graft-versus-host disease (GVHD) from imperfect matches. Bone marrow transplant recipients offer a good example. These patients may receive transplants following marrow ablation of the underlying leukemia and, therefore, have exposure to multiple potentially carcinogenic agents, including chemotherapies and radiation, in addition to immunosuppressive regimens to prevent rejection of the transplanted marrow. In this setting, excess risks of thyroid and brain tumors appear to be related to radiation, whereas graft-versus-host reactions were associated with squamous cell tumors of the buccal cavity and skin (63). Melanoma risk is also excessive, but it is not specifically associated with any known factor (63) and may also occur in excess in organ transplant recipients (64). These forms of cancer do not appear to be excessive in AIDS patients. Of interest, NHL risk in patients with renal transplants is associated with cadaveric (rather than sibling) kidneys, and with having multiple transplants, raising the possibility that antigenic stimulation could be related to the etiology (65).

Possibly, immunosuppression adds an additional factor that increases tumor expression in these settings. Regression or even remission of both KS and NHL has been reported after discontinuing immunosuppressive therapy (66,67). These observations strongly suggest that immune function may affect tumor expression, even after the emergence of the tumor.

IV. SUMMARY

Although some of these findings have become evident only in recent years, the occurrence of NHL and KS in immunosuppressed persons was well established before the AIDS epidemic. Finding excesses of KS and NHL, therefore was, consistent with the other laboratory and clinical evidence of immunodeficiency in AIDS. However, NHL and KS are not the only tumors to occur in other settings of immunodeficiency. The possibility that these other tumors might also appear among AIDS patients raised the specter of a broad-based epidemic of multiple cancers of many different types in conjunction with the emerging AIDS epidemic.

Fortunately, only a limited number of cancers have so far been associated with HIV–AIDS (68,69). Although it is still possible that new cancer associations will be discovered as larger numbers of people survive long-term with HIV-related immunodeficiencies, it is unlikely these cancers will occur in large numbers. Nevertheless, any relations found may lead to important new understandings of the pathogenesis of these malignancies.

REFERENCES

1. KB Hymes, T Cheung, JB Greene, NS Prose, A Marcus, H Ballard, DC William, LJ Laubenstein. Kaposi's sarcoma in homosexual men—a report of eight cases. Lancet 2:598–600, 1981.

2. RJ Biggar, PC Nasca, WS Burnett. AIDS-related Kaposi's sarcoma in New York City in 1977. N Engl J Med 318:252 1988.
3. I Penn. Kaposi's sarcoma in immunosuppressed patients. J Lab Clin Immunol 12: 1–10, 1983.
4. RJ Biggar, P Ebbesen, M Melbye, DL Mann, JJ Goedert, R Weinstock, DM Strong, WA Blattner. Low T-lymphocyte ratios in homosexual men. Epidemiologic evidence for a transmissible agent. JAMA 251:1441–1446, 1984.
5. AG Dalgleish, PC Beverley, PR Clapham, DH Crawford, MF Greaves, RA Weiss. The CD4 (T4) antigen is an essential component of the receptor for the AIDS retrovirus. Nature 312:763–767, 1984.
6. H Deng, R Liu, W Ellmeier, S Choe, D Unutmaz, M Burkhart, P Di Marzio, S Marmon, RE Sutton, CM Hill, CB Davis, SC Peiper, TJ Schall, DR Littman, NR Landau. Identification of a major co-receptor for primary isolates of HIV-1. Nature 381:661–666, 1996.
7. M Samson, F Libert, BJ Doranz, J Rucker, C Liesnard, CM Farber, S Saragosti, C Lapouméroulie, J Cognaux, C Forceille, G Muyldermans, C Verhofstede, G Burtonboy, M Georges, T Imai, S Rana, Y Yi, RJ Smyth, RG Collman, RW Doms, G Vassart, M Parmentier. Resistance to HIV-1 infection in Caucasian individuals bearing mutant alleles of the CCR-5 chemokine receptor gene. Nature 382:722–725, 1996.
8. JP Moore. Coreceptors: implications for HIV pathogenesis and therapy. Science 276: 51–52, 1997.
9. R Liu, WA Paxton, S Choe, D Ceradini, SR Martin, R Horuk, ME MacDonald, H Stuhlmann, RA Koup, NR Landau. Homozygous defect in HIV-1 coreceptor accounts for resistance of some multiply-exposed individuals to HIV-1 infection. Cell 86:367–377, 1996.
10. R Biti, R French, J Young, B Bennetts, G Stewart. HIV-1 infection in an individual homozygous for the CCR5 deletion allele. Nature Med 3:252–253, 1997.
11. P Westervelt, DB Trowbridge, LG Epstein, BM Blumberg, Y Li, BH Hahn, GM Shaw, RW Price, L Ratner. Macrophage tropism determinants of human immunodeficiency virus type 1 in vivo. J Virol 66:2577–2582, 1992.
12. DD Ho, TR Rota, RT Schooley, JC Kaplan, JD Allan, JE Groopman, L Resnick, D Felsenstein, CA Andrews, MS Hirsch. Isolation of HTLV-III from cerebrospinal fluid and neural tissues of patients with neurologic syndromes related to the acquired immunodeficiency syndrome. N Engl J Med 313:1493–1497, 1985.
13. JA Levy, J Shimabukuro, H Hollander, J Mills, L Kaminsky. Isolation of AIDS-associated retroviruses from cerebrospinal fluid and brain of patients with neurological symptoms. Lancet 2:586–588, 1985.
14. DS Dimitrov, RL Willey, H Sato, L Chang, R Blumenthal, MA Martin. Quantification of HIV-1 infection kinetics. J Virol 67:2182–2190, 1993.
15. DS Dimitrov, RL Willey, M Martin, R Blumenthal. Kinetics of HIV-1 transmission with CD4 and CD8+ cells. Implications for inhibition of virus infection and intial steps of virus entry into cells. Virology 187:398–406, 1992.
16. DD Ho, AU Neumann, AS Perelson, W Chen, JM Leonard, M Markowitz. Rapid turnover of plasma virions and CD4 lymphocytes in HIV-1 infection. Nature 373: 123–126, 1995.

17. X Wei, SK Ghosh, ME Taylor, VA Johnson, EA Emini, P Deutsch, JD Lifson, S Bonhoeffer, MA Nowak, BH Hahn, MS Saag, GM Shaw. Viral dynamics in human immunodeficiency virus type 1 infection. Nature 373:117–122, 1995.
18. Y Cao, L Qin, L Zhang, J Safrit, DD Ho. Virologic and immunologic characterization of long-term survivors of human immunodeficiency virus type 1 infection. N Engl J Med 332:201–208, 1995.
19. DD Ho. Viral counts count in HIV infection. Science 272:1124–1125, 1996.
20. JW Mellors, CR Rinaldo Jr, P Gupta, RM White, JA Todd, LA Kingsley. Prognosis in HIV-1 infection predicted by the quantity of virus in plasma. Science 272:1167–1170, 1996.
21. TR O'Brien, WA Blattner, D Waters, E Eyster, MW Hilgartner, AR Cohen, N Luban, A Hatzakis, LM Aledort, PS Rosenberg, WJ Miley, BL Kroner, JJ Goedert. Serum HIV-1 RNA levels and time to development of AIDS in the Multicenter Hemophilia Cohort Study. JAMA 276:105–110, 1996.
22. OT Rutschmann, M Pechere, J Krischer, L Perrin, B Hirschel. Chemotherapy for AIDS-related malignancies does not increase HIV viraemia. AIDS 11:944–945, 1997.
23. JD Roberts, K Bebenek, TA Kunkel. The accuracy of reverse transcriptase from HIV-1. Science 242:1171–1173, 1988.
24. RA Kaslow, M Carrington, R Apple, L Park, A Muñoz, AJ Saah, JJ Goedert, C Winkler, SJ O'Brien, C Rinaldo, R Detels, W Blattner, J Phair, H Erlich, DL Mann. Influence of combinations of human major histocompatibility complex genes on the course of HIV-1 infection. Nat Med 2:405–411, 1996.
25. AV Hill, HIV and HLA: confusion or complexity? Nat Med 2:395–396, 1996.
26. FE McCutchan, E Sanders-Buell, CW Oster, RR Redfield, SK Hira, PL Perine, BLP Ungar, DS Burke. Genetic comparison of human immunodeficiency virus (HIV-1) isolates by polymerase chain reaction. J Acquir Immune Defic Syndr 4:1241–1250, 1991.
27. SK Brodine, JR Mascola, PJ Weiss, SI Ito, KR Porter, AW Artenstein, FC Garland, FE McCutchan, DS Burke. Detection of diverse HIV-1 genetic subtypes in the USA. Lancet 346:1198–1199, 1995.
28. G Myers. Assimilating HIV sequences. AIDS Res Hum Retroviruses 9:697–702, 1993.
29. LG Gürtler, PH Hauser, J Eberle, A Von Brunn, S Knapp, L Zekeng, JM Tsague, L Kaptue. A new subtype of human immunodeficiency virus type 1 (MVP-5180) from Cameroon. J Virol 68:1581–1585, 1994.
30. Concorde Coordinating Committee. MRCANRS randomized double-blind controlled trial of immediate and deferred zidovudine in symptom-free HIV infection. Lancet 343:871–881, 1994.
31. PS Volberding, NM Graham. Initiation of antiretroviral therapy in HIV infection: a review of interstudy consistencies. J Acquir Immune Defic Syndr 7(suppl 2):S12–22 [discussion S22–S23]. 1994.
32. MS Saag, M Holodniy, DR Kuritzkes, WA O'Brien, R Coombs, ME Poscher, DM Jacobsen, GM Shaw, DD Richman, PA Volberding. HIV viral load markers in clinical practice. Nat Med 2:625–629, 1996.
33. R Yarchoan, JA Lietzau, BY Nguyen, OW Brawley, JM Pluda, MW Saville, KM

Wyvill, SM Steinberg, R Agbaria, H Mitsuya, S Broder. A randomized pilot study of alternating or simultaneous zidovudine and didanosine therapy in patients with symptomatic human immunodeficiency virus syndrome. J Infect Dis 169:9–17, 1994.

34. AC Collier, RW Coombs, DA Schoenfeld, RL Bassett, J Timpone, A Baruch, M Jones, K Facey, C Whitacre, VJ McAuliffe, HM Friedman, TC Merigan, RC Reichman, C Hooper, L Corey. Treatment of human immunodeficiency virus infection with saquinavir, zidovudine, and zalcitabine. AIDS Clinical Trials Group. N Engl J Med 334:1011–1017, 1996.

35. PA Volberding, SW Lagakos, JM Grimes, DS Stein, J Rooney, TC Meng, MA Fischl, AC Collier, JP Phair, MS Hirsch, WD Hardy, HH Balfour Jr, RC Reichman. A comparison of immediate with deferred zidovudine therapy for asymptomatic HIV-infected adults with CD4 cell counts of 500 or more per cubic millimeter. N Engl J Med 333:401–407, 1995.

36. CC Carpenter, MA Fischl, SM Hammer, MS Hirsch, DM Jacobsen, DA Katzenstein, JS Montaner, DD Richman, MS Saag, RT Schooley, MA Thompson, S Vella, PG Yeni, PA Volberding. Antiretroviral therapy for HIV infection in 1998: updated recommendations of the International AIDS Society—USA Panel. JAMA 280:78–86, 1998.

37. CM Gray, JM Schapiro, MA Winters, TC Merigan. Changes in CD4+ and CD8+ T cell subsets in response to highly active antiretroviral therapy in HIV type 1-infected patients with prior protease inhibitor experience. AIDS Res Hum Retroviruses 14:561–569, 1998.

38. HR Brodt, BS Kamps, P Gute, B Knupp, S Staszewski, EB Helm. Changing incidence of AIDS-defining illnesses in the era of antiretroviral combination therapy. AIDS 11:1731–1738, 1997.

39. RS Hogg, KV Heath, B Yip, KJ Craib, MV O'Shaughnessy, MT Schechter, JS Montaner. Improved survival among HIV-infected individuals following initiation of antiretroviral therapy. JAMA 279:450–454, 1998.

40. RS Hogg, MV O'Shaughnessy, N Gataric, B Yip, K Craib, MT Schechter, JSG Montaner. Decline in deaths from AIDS due to new antiretrovirals. Lancet 349:1294, 1997.

41. B Tindall, S Barker, B Donovan, T Barnes, J Roberts, C Kronenberg, J Gold, R Penny, D Cooper. Characterization of the acute clinical illness associated with human immunodeficiency virus infection. Arch Intern Med 148:945–949, 1988.

42. B Tindall, DA Cooper. Primary HIV infection: host responses and intervention strategies. AIDS 5:1–14, 1991.

43. JB Margolick, AD Donnenberg, A Muñoz, LP Park, KD Bauer, JV Giorgi, J Ferbas, AJ Saah. Changes in T and non-T lymphocyte subsets following seroconversion to HIV-1: stable CD3+ and declining CD3-populations suggest regulatory responses linked to loss of CD4 lymphocytes. J Acquir Immune Defic Syndr 6:153–161, 1993.

44. PS Rosenberg, JJ Goedert, RJ Biggar. Effect of age at seroconversion on the natural AIDS incubation distribution. AIDS 8:803–810, 1994.

45. PJ Veugelers, KA Page, B Tindall, MT Schechter, AR Moss, WW Winkelstein Jr, DA Cooper, KJ Craib, E Charlebois, RA Coutinho. Determinants of HIV disease

progression among homosexual men registered in the Tricontinental Seroconverter Study. Am J Epidemiol 140:747–758, 1994.

46. PJ Veugelers, SA Strathdee, B Tindall, KA Page, AR Moss, MT Schechter, JS Montaner, GJ van Griensven. Increasing age is associated with faster progression to neoplasms but not opportunistic infections in HIV-infected homosexual men. AIDS 8: 1471–1475, 1994.

47. FW Wit, CJ Sol, N Renwick, MT Roos, ST Pals, R van Leeuwen, J Goudsmit, P Reiss. Regression of AIDS-related Kaposi's sarcoma associated with clearance of human herpesvirus-8 from peripheral blood mononuclear cells following initiation of antiretroviral therapy. AIDS 12:218–219, 1998.

48. J Krischer, O Rutschmann, B Hirschel, S. Vollenweider-Roten, JH Saurat, M Pechere. Regression of Kaposi's sarcoma during therapy with HIV-1 protease inhibitors: a prospective pilot study. J Am Acad Dermatol 38:594–598, 1998.

49. RJ Biggar, J Horm, JF Fraumeni Jr, MH Greene, JJ Goedert. Incidence of Kaposi's sarcoma and mycosis fungoides in the United States including Puerto Rico, 1973–1981. J Natl Cancer Inst 73:89–94, 1984.

50. AR Harwood, D Osoba, SL Hofstader, MB Goldstein, CJ Cardella, MJ Holecek, R Kunynetz, RA Giammarco. Kaposi's sarcoma in recipients of renal transplants. Am J Med 67:759–765, 1979.

51. I Penn. Malignant lymphomas in organ transplant recipients. Transplant Proc 736–738, 1981.

52. I Penn. Cancers complicating organ transplantation. N Engl J Med 323:1767–1769, 1990.

53. C Hiesse, F Kriaa, P Rieu, JR Larue, G Benoit, J Bellamy, P Blanchet, B Charpentier. Incidence and type of malignancies occurring after renal transplantation in conventionally and cyclosporine-treated recipients: analysis of a 20-year period in 1600 patients. Transplant Proc 27:972–974, 1995.

54. SA Birkeland, HH Storm, LU Lamm, L Barlow, I Blohmé, B Forsberg, B Eklund, O Fjeldborg, M Friedberg, L Frödin, E Glattre, S Halvorsen, N Holm, A Jakobsen, HE Jørgensen, J Ladefoged, T Lindholm, G Lundgren, E Pukkala. Cancer risk after renal transplantation in the Nordic countries, 1964–1986. Int J Cancer 60:183–189, 1995.

55. N Mueller, PA Pizzo. Cancer in children with primary and secondary immunodeficiencies. J Pediatr 126:1–10, 1995.

56. IARC. Monographs on the Evaluation of Carcinogenic Risks to Humans. Vol. 50: Pharmaceutical Drugs. Lyon: World Health Organization, 1990.

57. SBM Gaya, AJ Rees, RI Lechler, G Williams, PD Mason. Malignant disease in patients with long-term renal transplants. Transplantation 59:1705–1709, 1995.

58. I Penn. Neoplastic complications of transplantation. Semin Respir Infect 8:233–239, 1993.

59. LJ Kinlen, AGR Sheil, J Peto, R Doll. Collaborative United Kingdom–Australasian study of cancer in patients treated with immunosuppressive drugs. Br Med J 2:1461–1466, 1979.

60. I Penn. The changing pattern of posttransplant malignancies. Transplant Proc 23: 1101–1103, 1991.

61. E Brusamoino, G Pagnucco, C Bernasconi. Secondary lymphomas: a review on lym-

phoproliferative diseases arising in immunocompromised hosts: prevalence, clinical features and pathogenetic mechanisms. Haematologica 74:605–622, 1989.

62. HJ Kolb, W Guether, T Duell, G Socie, E Schaeffer, E Holler, M Schumm, MM Horowitz, RP Gale, TM Fliedner. Cancer after bone marrow transplantation. Bone Marrow Transplant 10(supp 1):135–138, 1992.

63. RE Curtis, PA Rowlings, HJ Deeg, DA Shriner, G Socié, LB Travis, MM Horowitz, RP Witherspoon, RN Hoover, KA Sobocinski, JF Fraumeni, JD Boice. Solid cancers after bone marrow transplantation. N Engl J Med 336:897–904, 1997.

64. I Penn. De novo malignancy in pediatric organ transplant recipients. J Pediatr Surg 29:221–228, 1994.

65. RN Hoover. Lymphoma risks in populations with altered immunity—a search for mechanism. Cancer Res 52:5477s–5478s, 1992.

66. TE Starzl, MA Nalesnik, KA Porter, MS Ho, S Iwatsuki, BP Griffith, JT Rosenthal, TR Hakala, BW Shaw Jr, RL Hardesty, RW Atchison, R Jaffe. Reversibility of lymphomas and lymphoproliferative lesions developing under cyclosporin–steroid therapy. Lancet 1:583–587, 1984.

67. PL Bencini, L Marchesi, T Cainelli, C Crosti. Kaposi's sarcoma in kidney transplant recipients treated with cyclosporin. Br J Dermatol 118:709–714, 1987.

68. IARC. Monographs on the Evaluation of Carcinogenic Risks to Humans. Vol. 67: Human Immunodeficiency Viruses and Human T-Cell Lymphotropic Viruses. Lyon: World Health Organization, 1996.

69. JJ Goedert, TR Cote, P Virgo, SM Scoppa, DW Kingma, MH Gail, ES Jaffe, RJ Biggar. Spectrum of AIDS-associated malignant disorders. Lancet 351:1833–1839, 1998.

3
Epidemiology of Malignancies in HIV/AIDS

Robert J. Biggar
*National Cancer Institute, National Institutes of Health,
Bethesda, Maryland*

I. INTRODUCTION

Two malignancies, Kaposi's sarcoma (KS) and certain types of non–Hodgkin's lymphomas (NHLs) dominate the cancer types seen in patients with human immunodeficiency virus (HIV) or acquired immunodeficiency syndrome (AIDS). According to the official definition of AIDS (1), the presence of either is considered an AIDS diagnosis in a person known to be HIV-infected, as is KS in a person younger than 70 years old, unless the patient is known not to be HIV-infected. The extraordinary frequencies of either cancer in HIV-infected persons amply justify considering these to be AIDS, but each has a rather different epidemiology and, presumably, etiology. Invasive cervical cancer is also accepted as an AIDS-defining cancer according to official guidelines, although the evidence for an association with AIDS is more tenuous. A variety of other cancers have been reported somewhat more commonly in AIDS patients, including epithelial anal cancers, conjunctival tumors, Hodgkin's disease, and leimyosarcomas (in children), and these have been suggested to be AIDS-associated. The incidence rates for selected cancers in men (Fig. 1; 2) and women (Fig. 2; 3) at high risk of HIV infection show the influence of the AIDS epidemic on cancer incidence in some populations.

The following description will focus on the cancers most stronglay associated with AIDS, providing a brief description of the background, clinical features, and incidence, against which the AIDS-associated cases will be compared.

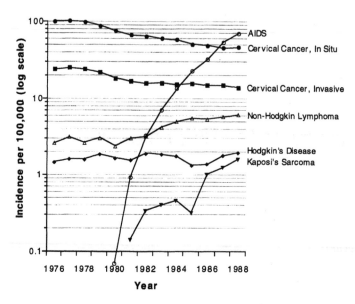

Figure 1   The incidence (log-scale) of selected cancers in never-married men (all races, but preponderantly white) aged 25–54 years old in San Francisco City, over time. Never-married men served as a surrogate for a likely homosexual lifestyle that was available in registry data. However, the authors estimate that only 24% of the observed population was HIV-infected in 1984. Thus, these rates understate the real risk in HIV-infected men. Incidences are presented on a log-scale because of the large increase in KS. Log-scale presentation makes variations in incidences for cancers with less dramatic changes appear minimal; however, a 1-log increase equates to a 10-fold increase and a half-log increase equates to a 3.2-fold increase in incidence. Increases in KS and NHL were most dramatic, but anal cancers and Hodgkin's disease also increased. (Data from Ref. 2.)

II. KAPOSI'S SARCOMA

A. Endemic (Non–HIV-Related) Kaposi's Sarcoma

1. Clinical Features

Classic KS was first described in 1872 by Moritz Kaposi, a Hungarian dermatologist. He reported that it was an idiopathic, multicentric, pigmented tumor more common in Jewish and eastern Mediterranean men. Over the next century, various "subtypes" of KS were described, first when this disease was found in Africa, then in younger, iatrogenically immunosuppressed transplant patients, and finally in persons with AIDS. KS is often still categorized according to these different subtypes, including "classic Mediterranean," "endemic Africa," "transplant-

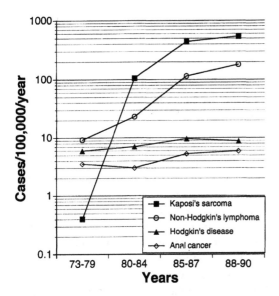

Figure 2 The incidence (log-scale) of selected cancer in black women (regardless of marital status) aged 20–49 years old in New York City, over time. The proportion estimated to be HIV-infected was not provided. However, the increase in AIDS cases in this group attests to their high risk of HIV infection. Although KS and NHL incidences increased, there was a decrease in both invasive and in situ cervical cancer and little change in the incidence of Hodgkin's disease. (Data from Ref. 3.)

related,'' and AIDS-related.'' These historical distinctions probably serve little purpose because there are only minor differences between these types. The classic form is typically seen in the elderly and usually has early "plaque" lesions on the limbs at presentation. In some parts of Africa, KS occurs at much higher incidence than in the United States; hence, patients present at younger ages and, because of poorer health care access, usually have the more advanced nodular disease. Neither the classic nor African types have documented immunological abnormalities; therefore, they are sometimes called "endemic KS" to distinguish them from immunosuppression-related KS. However, the emerging understanding of the common role of human herpes virus type 8 (HHV-8; KSHV) in all forms of KS suggests that they are the same condition in all settings.

The malignant cells are considered to be spindle cells, most likely of endothelial origins, although this is somewhat uncertain (4,5). Until recently, KS was often suggested to be a polyclonal response of vascular endothelial cells to an unknown stimulus. However, at least in nodular lesions (which could represent the more-advanced form of this disease), the cells have now been shown to be clonal in origin (6), with lesions at different sites all derived from the same clone, which suggests metastasis (7).

In nonimmunocompromised persons (endemic KS), KS generally first appears on the extremities, particularly the lower legs and feet (8,9). Initially, there may be flat, purplish lesions (plaques) that subsequently become more nodular and invasive of tissues around them. The purplish hue of the lesions is due to the rich vascularization of the KS tissue and extravasation of erythrocytes. Regional nodes may become involved. However, even in the absence of lymphadenopathy, lymphedema of the involved limbs may be pronounced. In patients with endemic disease, the disease is typically indolent or slowly progressive over years, although when it occurs in young persons, it may be more aggressive. It has been found in almost all organs except the brain, but internal tumors rarely cause serious clinical problems in nonimmunocompromised persons. Medical management is relatively easy when adequate facilities are available, and death of other causes is more likely than that of the tumor itself. In areas without adequate medical care, such as parts of Africa, secondary infections and disability are major contributors to mortality, even when the cancer is considered to be the primary cause of death.

2. Incidence

Before the AIDS epidemic, KS was already recognized to have peculiar epidemiological features. In the United States, it was a rare tumor, threefold more common in men (0.29:100,000, age standardized) than women (0.09:100,000) (10). Incidence rates in blacks are about half those of whites, but some of this difference may have been because of diagnostic bias. Figure 3 illustrates the geographic distribution of areas with higher incidences of endemic KS. In western Europe, rates were similar to American rates but were lower in England and Denmark and slightly higher in Sweden and Italy (11). In Mediterranean and eastern European areas, rates were threefold higher, about 1:100,000 persons, with persons of Jewish and perhaps also Arabic origin being at highest risk.

Even higher rates of KS occurred in parts of Africa (see Fig. 3), although quantifying the precise incidence is difficult because of lack of reliable data. Given the HIV epidemic in Africa and its effect on KS, it is now especially hard to determine the rates of non–AIDS-related KS in this region. The highest incidence for endemic KS has been reported for areas of East Africa, from Uganda to Zambia. In eastern Zaire, 8% of all tumors were reported to be KS in 1960 (12,13), long before the AIDS epidemic affected this area. In Africa, KS has been reported to occur up to tenfold more commonly in men than women, but some of the differences in gender found there may have been due to referral bias, because women may be less likely than men to obtain medical attention.

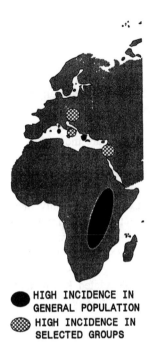

HIGH INCIDENCE IN
GENERAL POPULATION

HIGH INCIDENCE IN
SELECTED GROUPS

Figure 3 The distribution of high-incidence areas of endemic Kaposi's sarcoma. The highest incidence areas are in East Africa. Relatively high rates are found in older members of general populations of Greece, Sardinia, and perhaps parts of southern Italy. In Eastern Europe and Israel, rates are high in the Jewish populations. Rates in Asian populations are very low (even among persons with AIDS). Immigrants from these areas have rates similar to the original populations.

In all areas, endemic KS incidence increases markedly with age. In low-incidence areas, it is rarely diagnosed in immunocompetent persons younger than 70 years old. However, in Africa, where the incidence of endemic KS is high, cases regularly occur in adolescents and even in children (14,15). However, adults and children with non–AIDS-related KS in Africa appear to be immunocompetent, at least with available measurement of immunity (16). The clinical manifestations appear to be more aggressive in younger persons, and lymph nodes and internal organ involvement may be prominent (14,15). In the United States and Europe, endemic cases in childhood are very rare.

The high incidence of KS in younger persons with iatrogenic immunodeficiency related to transplantation is discussed in Chapter 2.

B. AIDS-Related Kaposi's Sarcoma

1. Clinical Features

Although KS in persons with and without AIDS has a similar appearance under the microscope, the clinical presentation of KS in AIDS patients is typically more abrupt and widespread than it is in non–AIDS-related KS. Lesions are usually purplish macules or only slightly raised papules. In contrast with endemic KS, multiple lesions often appear in AIDS-related KS and these are most often on the trunk or the head and neck. They may also appear in mucous membranes, sometimes as the only recognized site. These are most noticeable in the mouth, but internal lesions can be found throughout the gastrointestinal tract or in other organs (17,18). The KS lesions are rarely life-threatening, although involvement of internal organs, such as the lung, can be. The lesions on the skin are frequently cosmetically disturbing and may cause disability, requiring therapy for control. Median survival of patients with AIDS-related KS was 14–18 months in the early 1990s (19,20), which was relatively long for an AIDS-defining illness; it is likely to improve with advances in therapy. As with non–AIDS-related KS, patients usually die of another condition related to their immunosuppression.

2. Incidence

The incidence of KS in patients with AIDS varies considerably by HIV-exposure group (Fig. 4). Among homosexual and bisexual men, the risk is five- to tenfold higher than it is in other AIDS groups, even after adjusting for age, race, and calendar-time (21). Interestingly, incidence does not increase with age, as it usually does with cancers, even in the AIDS setting. Rather, in homosexual men,

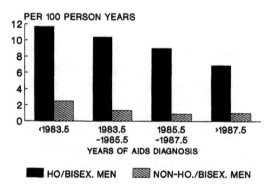

Figure 4 Declining risk of AIDS-related KS risk, over time: Data were adjusted for age and race differences in incidence. These declines were seen in both homosexual and nonhomosexual male AIDS cases. (From Ref. 21.)

KS peaks in 30–39 year olds, whereas in nonhomosexual men, younger adults have the highest incidence (Fig. 5). The relative incidence of KS has been well defined in cohorts of patients who present with another AIDS illness. During the period 6 months to 1 year after AIDS onset, the excess of KS is over 100,000-fold in homosexual men and 13,000-fold in nonhomosexual men, compared with age-, sex-, and race-matched rates in the general population during the pre-AIDS era (21). Never-married men in San Francisco, a surrogate for homosexual men, do not appear to have had an increased risk of KS before the AIDS era (22). Among nonhomosexual men or women with AIDS, only 2–3% of cases manifest KS as the first evidence of AIDS. Within HIV-exposure groups composed of both sexes (e.g., intravenous drug users and transfusion recipients), the relative risk of developing KS is lower in women than men (Fig. 6; 23).

The proportional and absolute risk of KS has also varied over time (24–26). Among the earliest cases of AIDS in homosexual men, 40% had KS as their first manifestation of AIDS, whereas, in the most recent years, it has been about 12%. This same variation by risk group is seen in KS incidence following another AIDS diagnosis, which is also falling in both homosexual and nonhomosexual men (see Fig. 5; 21). Intravenous drug-using men have a somewhat higher frequency of presenting with KS than other nonhomosexual men, but some of these could be men who have had sex with men in exchange for drugs, but who do not identify themselves as homosexual or bisexual. There may be several reasons for this decline. Minor lesions are now appreciated as non–life-threatening by both doctors and patients, and KS may be less completely reported to cancer registries. In addition, as the lifestyle of at-risk homosexual and nonhomosexual persons has changed to avoid HIV in the post-AIDS era, this may have also lowered exposure to other causal factors.

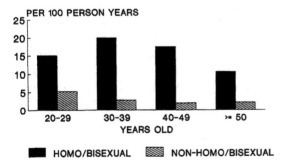

Figure 5 Percentage of AIDS cases who have ever had KS; by age: Data adjusted for differences in incidence by race. The peak incidence in homosexual men is 30–39 years old, whereas nonhomosexual men peak in their 20s and decline thereafter. (From Ref. 21.)

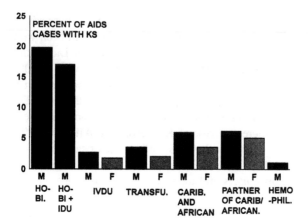

Figure 6 Percentage of men and women in different exposure categories who present with KS as the AIDS-defining illness: The higher risk in men with homosexual lifestyles is obvious. In addition, for exposure categories with both genders, males consistently have a higher risk than females. (From Ref. 23).

In patients with HIV infection, KS may appear at almost any stage of immunosuppression, but it is rare when immunity is near normal. Because KS can occur earlier than other AIDS-related illnesses in the course of HIV-related immune deterioration, the average CD4 counts are higher than are seen in many other AIDS illnesses. However, as immunity deteriorates, KS also becomes more frequent (20,27). Viewed as time from AIDS, the risk of KS nearly doubles in 12 months (21). During this period, immunity probably declined. As antiretroviral therapies become more effective, immunological improvements could lead to disappearance of KS lesions, given that spontaneous remissions of KS occur when immunosuppressive therapies are stopped in organ transplant recipients with KS. Thus far, this has been observed only occasionally in AIDS patients.

Cases of KS have been reported in homosexual men who are not HIV-infected and who are immunologically normal (28–30), but whether the number of cases exceeds those expected is unclear. Because of intensive medical surveillance of this population, there may be diagnostic bias in which early small KS lesions have been more commonly detected. However, these cases may also indicate the presence of causal factors, in addition to HIV, to which homosexual men may be exposed by their lifestyle.

3. Etiology

Over the past two decades, epidemiological studies have associated KS with various factors. These studies have been mostly conducted among homosexual men because of the high incidence of KS in this group. The findings have been difficult to interpret because they usually involve multiple associations that are, in turn, related to each other.

The common thread is that the most sexually active and "adventurous" subjects are at greater risk of KS, whether this is measured as a greater number of sexual partners (31), more oral–anal contact (32–34), more frequent infections with sexually transmitted infections (35,36), more drug use (especially of nitrite inhalants; 37,38), or sexual partners from communities of high HIV incidence (24,39). Despite attempts to disentangle the confounding by lifestyle, it has been difficult to discern which, if any, are the critically important factors or whether none of them really bears on the cause of KS. More impressive is evidence that women who were HIV-infected by bisexual partners were more likely to have KS as an AIDS illness than those infected by heterosexual partners (Fig. 7; 23,40,41).

The associations with sexual behavior were weak, and most findings were confounded by earlier exposure to HIV among persons with high-exposure–risk lifestyles. Thus, persons infected earlier will progress to immunosuppression sooner and manifest KS earlier. Furthermore, various sexually transmitted infections are spread by similar routes within these groups and thus could be considered as possible etiologic cofactors of KS by such studies. Many such candidate

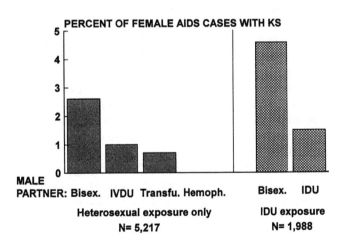

Figure 7 The difference in KS risk for women with AIDS, by exposure category of their sexual partners: Women were further separated into those without (heterosexual exposure only) and with exposure to intravenous drugs. For women in both categories, the KS risk was higher when they had bisexual partners, implying sexual transmission of a causal agent that is more common in bisexual men. (Data from Ref. 23.)

cofactors have been proposed: cytomegalovirus (42), *Rochalimaea henselae* (43), human papillomaviruses (HPV; 44), and *Mycoplasma fermentans* (45). However, only the recently described human herpesvirus-8 (HHV-8; see following section) meets the necessary criteria to be considered causal.

Although there may be an infectious etiology for KS, other noninfectious conditions could influence the development of the disease. Genetic susceptibility has been proposed. Initial studies suggested a higher risk in homosexual men with HLA-DR5 than in men with other HLA types (46,47). However, DR5 associations have not been confirmed in later studies of either non–AIDS-related or AIDS-related KS (48–50). Other HLA correlations have been reported, but none is consistently found in all studies (51).

Consistently higher rates of KS are found in men than in women, both with and without AIDS, when men and women of the same exposure groups are compared (see Fig. 4). This could indicate that hormonal factors are important. In vitro, hormones (human chorionic gonadotropin, or a closely related substance) appeared to accelerate apoptosis of KS cells (52). A recent study reported higher testosterone levels in homosexual men with KS than in those with other AIDS-defining illnesses, after adjusting for CD4 cell counts (53). In another study, however, lower testosterone levels were observed in KS cases, although the difference was not statistically significant (54).

Relation to HHV-8. In late 1994, investigators reported finding a new human herpesvirus (the eighth known human herpesvirus; hence, HHV-8) in KS tissues derived from AIDS patients (55). It was soon determined that this virus is also present in nearly all forms of KS, regardless of their geographic location, the age of the subject (56,57), or the degree of immunosuppression. Therefore, HHV-8 is often referred to as the "Kaposi's sarcoma herpesvirus (KSHV)." This strong association between KS and HHV-8 provides compelling evidence that KS in all areas and conditions are forms of the same disease process and that this virus is etiologically important to, and perhaps the cause of, both endemic and immunosuppression-related KS.

Human herpesvirus-8 is a member of the gamma herpesvirus group, along with Epstein–Barr virus (EBV) and the primate virus, herpesvirus saimirii. Both EBV and herpesvirus saimirii have been associated with NHL and, notably, HHV-8 is also strongly associated with a specific form of NHL called body–cavity-based lymphoma (BCBL) or primary effusion lymphoma (58).

The epidemiology of this new virus has yet to be well established. The primary difficulty relates to methods of detection, which have been molecular, largely based on polymerase chain reaction (PCR) tests performed on tissue. On average, BCBLs have 40–80 HHV-8 copies per cell, whereas KS cells have about a single copy per cell (58). HHV-8 can be detected in circulating peripheral B lymphocytes in only about 50% of persons with AIDS-related HHV-8–positive KS; in those with detectable virus, the number of copies per cell is on the order of 1:1000 cells.

A validated antibody test capable of detecting evidence of prior infection will be needed to determine the epidemiology and natural history of HHV-8 infection. First-generation assays, some using latent and others using lytic antigen, have provided diverse results. Overall, in high-risk subjects, such as homosexual men without KS, the prevalence varies from 20 to 40%, whereas in normal blood donors, the prevalence is between 2 and 20% (59,60). However, these assays often disagree about which individuals are seropositive in the normal population (personal data), limiting conclusions about the distribution of this virus in the general population.

Furthermore, the tests appear to be insensitive. Only about 70–80% of AIDS patients with KS cases have detectable antibodies (60,61). Almost all KS cases have HHV-8 detected by polymerase chain reaction and probably all are infected. Thus, antibody levels to this virus appear to be near the sensitivity of existing tests, perhaps because the level of the virus (and, hence, antibody levels) are low. Consequently, in population studies, it is still unclear whether some assays are giving nonspecific results, or others are specific, but insensitive, for detecting infection. Given the pace of development and the emerging ability to grow the HHV-8–infected cells in culture, there should be rapid improvements in these assays.

Despite the current inadequacy of serological tests, data about the routes of HHV-8 transmission are emerging. Analyses of subjects without disease consistently show that homosexual men have a higher prevalence of antibodies to HHV-8 than other groups (60,61), implying that some aspect of their lifestyle leads to an increased risk of exposure. Antibody prevalence is higher in men with more sexual partners, suggesting that sexual transmission is important. Both anal intercourse and oral–anal contact have been proposed as routes of transmission.

Finally, cohort studies appear to indicate that the risk of HHV-8 infection increased in the early 1980s and fell thereafter (62). This is consistent with the notion that HHV-8 became more widespread during the era when HIV and other sexually transmitted agents were also being spread epidemically, probably as a consequence of greater numbers of sexual partners among homosexual men in those years. The decline in recent years is also consistent with the decline in KS seen recently, presuming that the incubation period between infection and illness is short, as studies using polymerase chain reaction for detecting HHV-8 appear to indicate (59). However, all of these data must be viewed with caution for the sensitivity and specificity of the assays remain to be established.

III. NON–HODGKIN'S LYMPHOMA

Non–Hodgkin's lymphoma (NHL) is relatively common in young American adults in the age range for AIDS, having an incidence of 8 cases per 100,000 in males 20–54 in 1982 (statistics from Ref. 63 unless other specified). Thus, the increased incidence of NHL in AIDS patients was not as quickly appreciated as was the high incidence of KS. However, by 1982, it was appreciated that AIDS patients had a high risk of unusual, high-grade NHLs, including immunoblastic and Burkitt-like lymphomas (63a), an excess that was soon confirmed by registry surveillance studies (63b). Despite a high absolute risk of NHL in AIDS patients, the relative risk has been far lower than for KS because of the relatively high background rates of NHL.

The clinical and pathological profiles of NHL vary somewhat by the source of the data. Case series emphasize the more unusual manifestations of the tumors; therefore, reports may overstate their frequency because of investigator bias. However, registry-based data may contain only the initial or predominant NHL site or the site from which a biopsy was taken and thus be incomplete. For example, early in the AIDS epidemic, extranodal involvement was reported in 80% of patients with AIDS-related NHLs (63a). In contrast, registry data record 40% of AIDS-related NHLs as having extranodal involvement (63). This proportion is higher than is reported for non-AIDS NHLs (25%), which confirms the clinical impression that extranodal involvement is more frequent in AIDS patients, but it may understate the real frequency of this condition. Thus, sources of data should be noted when composing a clinical profile. The following discussion compares non–AIDS- and AIDS-related NHL using registry-based data.

A. Non–AIDS-Related NHL

1. Clinical Features

Non-Hodgkin's lymphomas account for about 4% of all cancers in the United States. About 85% are B cell in origin and the remainder are T cell or null cell. Almost all tumors are clonal, exhibiting uniform immunoglobulin heavy- and light-chain gene rearrangements, but biclonal or polyclonal tumors also have been reported (64,65). They include a large number of histological types that have different clinical courses. Different classifications have been used to categorize these tumors into related groups. However, these tumors may be pleomorphic and complex, making morphological classification difficult. For clinical convenience, NHL histologies that have progressively worse prognoses are grouped together by the Working Formulation by grade (66). This system is often used in studies of AIDS-related lymphomas. The grade categories include low (25%), intermediate (45%), or high (12%) grade, but some are not classified (18%) or grade is not specified (10%). The prognosis of NHL is relatively good. Nearly half (45%) of all patients surviving for 5 years. However, the median survival in patients with the high-grade (worst prognosis) NHL is about 18 months.

The most common presenting feature of NHL is lymph node enlargement, but extranodal lymphomas are frequent (20–30%) at presentation and may be found in a variety of sites (67). Nodal and extranodal tumors have a similar distribution by grade. About 2% of NHLs (10% of extranodal NHLs) in non–HIV-infected persons are primary lymphomas of the brain (68). The incidence of primary brain lymphoma is increasing in non–HIV-infected persons (69,70). Some but not all of this increase may be due to better ascertainment because diagnostic methods have improved in more recent years. When classified, most brain lymphomas have high (20%) or intermediate (50%) grade histologies in HIV-uninfected patients.

2. Incidence

In 1992, the overall age-standardized incidence of NHL in the United States was 15:100,000. In large part because of AIDS, incidence in young (20–54 years old) persons almost doubled (to 14:100,000) between 1982 and 1992. However, for several decades NHL incidence in the general population of non–HIV-infected persons has also increased, at a rate of about 4% per year (67,71). The reasons are unknown. This increase includes many subtypes of lymphoma, but high-grade NHLs are increasing most rapidly (72). NHL incidence increases exponentially with age, but the incidences of specific subtypes have different patterns and differ markedly by geographic areas. For example, Burkitt's lymphoma, a high-grade NHL, is the most common childhood tumor in tropical Africa and New Guinea, but rare elsewhere. Overall, the lymphomas as a group are about 1.5- to 2-fold more common in the persons of upper economic and educational status, in the white population and in men (26).

In both genetic and iatrogenic immunodeficiency conditions, about half of the cancers seen are NHL, with 22% of these involving the central nervous system (CNS; 73–75). Many of the lymphomas have high-grade histological classifications, usually of the immunoblastic type. In contrast with AIDS cases, they do not have a high risk of Burkitt's or Burkitt-like lymphomas (76). In organ transplant recipients, NHL incidence rises more slowly than the excess of KS, but faster than other transplantation-associated tumors (77). In bone marrow transplants, NHLs are also the most common cancer (78). Incidence is higher when HLA types were imperfectly matched (79), suggesting that chronic antigenic stimulation might be important.

3. Etiology

Whether all types of lymphoma are part of the same spectrum of disease (e.g., tumors arising at different points in the maturation of the cell type) or should be considered as tumors with different etiologies is unclear. In some settings, including AIDS, the incidence of several different types of NHL are increased, suggesting they are part of the same disease spectrum and could have a similar pathogenesis. However, other types have distinct epidemiological patterns; therefore, they presumably have different etiologies. Certainly, the specificity of some genetic and environmental associations, such as the 8:14 translocation in Burkitt's lymphoma and its association with EBV, argue that the molecular pathways promoting the growth of different NHL types are diverse.

Epidemiologically, non–AIDS-related NHLs have been associated with various environmental factors, such as farming occupations, herbicide exposure, and prolonged antigenic stimulation. In addition, infection with EBV, a B-cell tropic virus, appears to be important in some tumors, perhaps by enhancing the development of immortalized B cells that are susceptible to malignant transformation.

B. AIDS-Related NHL

1. Clinical Features

Clinicians caring for AIDS patients quickly appreciated that NHLs were occurring in excess. The lymphomas seen were most commonly high (40%) or intermediate grade (32%) or unclassified (27%), with only 2% being low grade. Among high-grade tumors, immunoblastic and Burkitt-like lymphoma predominate, whereas among the intermediate-grade tumors, most have diffuse, large-cell histologies. Extranodal distribution is more common (40%) in AIDS-related NHL, but the site distribution is generally similar to non–AIDS-related cases (80), with the exception of a marked excess of primary lymphomas of the brain, which represented 20% of all NHL cases in AIDS patients. Most primary brain lymphomas have high (40%) or intermediate (55%) grade histologies (68,70).

The grade classification of NHL was developed to clarify the relation between histology and prognosis. However, AIDS patients with lymphoma do poorly (median survival: 6 months) regardless of the grade of their NHLs (80). The median survival of primary lymphoma of the brain was even worse (median survival: 2 months; 68,70). The poor prognosis probably reflects the underlying immunosuppression of the patients with AIDS-related NHL. When NHLs occur in persons who are not severely immunocompromised, they may respond well to therapy; however, many tumors occur at a time when immunity is severely immunocompromised. These patients tolerate chemotherapy poorly and often die of other immunosuppression-related illnesses.

2. Incidence

Overall, about 3% of AIDS patients present with NHL (26). As with NHL in persons without AIDS, risk increases with age (Fig. 8). In AIDS patients who

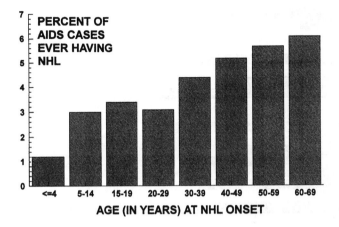

Figure 8 The risk of NHL in AIDS cases, by age (unpublished data from AIDS–cancer registry linkage studies): The rising risk is similar to that seen in persons without AIDS.

present with other conditions, the relative risk of developing NHL is 200- to 300-fold higher than in age-, sex-, and race-matched background population. NHL risk by exposure group varies modestly by group, being higher for men than women, and higher for whites than blacks (Fig. 9). These same demographic features are known to affect NHL risk in non-AIDS NHL. Although there is also some variation in NHL risk by HIV exposure category (see Fig. 9), these become minimal after adjusting for the demographic differences between the groups. Children have a lower risk of presenting with lymphoma, and among children and adolescents, Burkitt-like lymphomas are more frequent (26,76).

According to AIDS registry data, about two-thirds of all NHLs are diagnosed at the time of AIDS onset, and the remainder are diagnosed after another AIDS illness. However, about as many cases occur after AIDS as at the time of AIDS onset, but half of these later cases are never reported to AIDS registries (21,80). On death certificates, 5.7% of AIDS cases have NHL listed among their causes of death (81). The absolute risk of brain lymphomas is about 0.5–1%, which is 3600-fold higher than the risk in the general population (70). These tumors tend to have immunoblastic–plasmacytoid histological presentations (82).

By type, the highest relative risk is for high-grade NHL. Overall, the relative risk of NHL is about 200-fold above that of the general age-, sex-, and race-matched population: 377-fold for high-grade, 111-fold for intermediate-grade, and 17-fold for low-grade lymphomas. Even a small degree of misclassification could account for the small excess of low-grade tumors. By specific histological characteristics, the highest relative risks are for immunoblastic (650-fold), Burkitt-like lymphomas (250-fold), and large-cell, diffuse (145-fold) (80). AIDS-

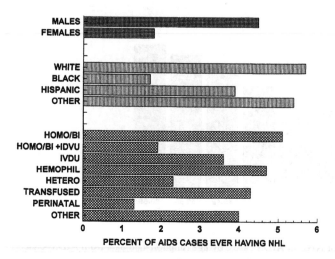

Figure 9 The risk of NHL in AIDS cases, by gender, by race, and by HIV exposure category (unpublished data from AIDS–cancer registry linkage studies): The higher risks in males and whites are similar to the pattern found for NHL risk in persons without AIDS. The majority of homosexual men and persons with hemophilia or transfusion exposure are white, whereas the majority of intravenous drug users are black, accounting for the differences seen between these groups.

related NHL tend to be more pleomorphic than non-AIDS NHLs (83) and may have plasmacytoid features (84). It is unclear if extranodal plasmacytomas are increased among the AIDS-related lymphomas (17). Miscellaneous (2%) or non-specific (25%) histological types are more commonly reported to registries, which could reflect difficulty in classification.

The added public health burden of AIDS-related NHL depends on the frequency of AIDS in the population. In 1990 in San Francisco, an epicenter of the AIDS epidemic, AIDS-related NHL accounted for about 60% of the NHL being diagnosed, whereas in Atlanta and New Jersey, about 24% of the NHL was AIDS-related (80). In areas where AIDS is less prevalent, the public health burden of the AIDS-related lymphomas is lower (80).

3. Etiology

The etiology of AIDS-related NHL is largely unknown. The NHL cells are almost all of B-cell lineage and not themselves HIV-infected. Chronic antigen stimulation may contribute, but cannot be causal alone, for excesses of NHL do not occur until immunity wanes, but HIV viral particles, which are highly immunogenic, are constantly produced throughout the course of infection (85,

86). Although associated with depressed immunity, it is unclear whether the etiology of NHL is related to immunosuppression itself, or to the immune dysregulation associated with the immunosuppression. In persons with AIDS, there is both immunosuppression of CD4+ T cells and intense immunostimulation of B cells (87).

Given that these tumors exhibit a range of chromosomal abnormalities and translocations similar to that in NHL among non–AIDS-related persons, these anomalies seem likely to be a common part of the pathway toward malignancy. Perhaps the rapid turnover of the cells increases the frequency of genetic errors. They may be driven by attempts to compensate for immunosuppression, by intense stimulation from antigenic exposure to circulating viruses, or by cytokines released from virally infected cells. However, in non-AIDS organ transplant recipients, NHLs may remit when iatrogenic immunotherapies are withdrawn, which argues that control of the malignant cells is possible, even if the malignancy is already a clonal outgrowth.

Epidemiological studies have not yielded dependable leads to the etiology of NHL. The demographic characteristics of the AIDS-related cases (older age, male, white, and higher socioeconomic status; 26) resemble those seen in non–AIDS-related cases. Geographically, there is little variation in incidence (88). NHL incidence in AIDS may be lower in Africa than elsewhere (89–92), but the data are weak. Unlike KS, the risk of NHL is generally similar in different risk groups. In the United States, the risk is somewhat higher in homosexual men, but this difference may be partly attributable to the demographic features of homosexual men, who tend to be affluent, urban, and white (26). In European AIDS cases, intravenous drug users have a slightly higher rate of NHL than homosexual men (93). No occupational exposures are known to influence NHL risk in AIDS. Hair dyes have been implicated as possibly etiologic factors, in other studies of NHL, but hair dressers who died of AIDS had no greater risk of NHL than other persons with AIDS (94). There is no indication that antiretroviral therapies increase the risk of NHL, a theoretical concern (95,96).

Of infectious agents, the virus most commonly associated with lymphomas is EBV. Almost all brain lymphomas have a clonal episomal EBV infection (97,98), as do many (50–70%) immunoblastic lymphomas and other NHLs (30–40%; 99,100). The association with EBV is thus stronger for the AIDS-related than non–AIDS-lymphomas, in which about 20% have clonal EBV infection. Furthermore, HIV-infected, immunocompromised persons have high numbers of circulating EBV-infected B cells (101) preceding the developing of lymphoma (102). Possibly the route to malignancy includes expansion of the EBV-infected B-cell clones that are then susceptible to another transforming genetic event (103).

One B-cell malignancy, primary effusion lymphoma (PEL), has special interest for its association with another herpesvirus, HHV-8. This is a rare malignancy even in the setting of AIDS. On the basis of some unusual clinical features and surface markers, it was first described as a specific type of tumor in 1989 (104). With the discovery of HHV-8 and its relations to KS, many NHL types were screened. Although this virus is not associated with other NHLs, it is strongly associated with PEL (58). Almost all PELs have this virus in high-copy number. Although there is no evidence that NHL incidence is higher in persons with KS, who are also HHV-8-infected, there are too few PEL cases to determine if this specific NHL is higher in KS patients. Most of the PELs are also EBV-positive (58).

A rare form of polyclonal tumors, called multicentric Castleman's disease, is closely associated with KS in AIDS patients and also harbors HHV-8 (105).

The T-cell malignancies in AIDS are rare (106). However, because T cells are susceptible to HIV infection, it has been possible to examine if HIV is clonally integrated. In a few instances, HIV integration has been reported to be adjacent to one of the proto-oncogenes (*c-fps/fes*) in the tumor cell genome (107,108). This could be a rare example of HIV acting through insertional mutagenesis.

IV. OTHER CANCERS

Many other tumors have been reported in persons with HIV–AIDS. Given the large number of persons with HIV and AIDS, now more than a million living and dead in the United States alone, it is no surprise that virtually any tumor can, by chance, appear in such a person. At issue is which tumors, other than the very obvious KS and NHL, are increased in frequency. Both cohort and registry-based approaches have been used to examine this question. However, few cohorts have enough HIV-infected persons to provide robust estimates of these rare events, whereas registry data do not generally include data about HIV-infection or risk factor data about groups possibly exposed to HIV. Study size concerns limit firm conclusions about which tumors occur in excess, but results in different studies have yielded generally similar findings.

Recently, it has been possible to link AIDS and cancer registry data directly, preserving confidentiality by erasing personal identifiers before data are taken for analysis. This provides a very large number of subjects known to be HIV-infected (because they had AIDS). Even these studies are not easily interpreted because of possible biases. Specific subgroups may have excess exposures to other potentially carcinogenic agents, such as greater levels of smoking and more exposure to hepatitis B and C in drug users and hemophilic persons. Because of health sensitivity and concern about sexually transmitted diseases, homosexual men may receive better than average medical care, for example, but drug-using persons and minorities may receive less than average care. Furthermore, doctors caring for HIV-infected persons or persons with AIDS may intensively screen patients at the time of AIDS, detecting cancers and other diseases at an unusual frequency. However, they may be less aggressive about pursuing possible signs of malignancy in late-stage HIV illness. Finally, many tumors are found only at the time of autopsy, but the autopsy rate in patients dying of AIDS may differ from those dying of other causes. Thus, both absolute and relative rates of difference between HIV-exposure groups and normal populations must be considered as estimates.

In one linkage study, the relative risk of all cancers other than NHL was marginally increased (1.5-fold, 95% confidence interval, 0.95–2.3) in a series of nearly 5000 persons followed after developing KS-related to AIDS (109). Specific types may occur in excess, as discussed later, but there has been no general increase in all cancers. However, tumors in profoundly immunosuppressed persons can be difficult to manage and will have a poor prognosis, reflecting the underlying conditions. This management dilemma does not indicate any difference in the fundamental tumor etiology or biology. In HIV-infected persons who are not severely immunocompromised, therapy may be very successful.

A. Cervical and Anal Cancers

During the late 1980s, women with AIDS were reported to have a high frequency of in situ cervical carcinoma, and unusually aggressive cases of invasive cervical cancer were noted (110,111). Among treated women, tumor recurrence was more common in the HIV-infected group (112). Several studies supported these findings by showing a higher frequency of cervical dysplasias, indicative of human papillomavirus (HPV) in HIV-infected women (113,114). In HIV-infected women, HPV infection was generally persistent, rather than self-limited, especially in immunosuppressed women (115,116), and carcinoma in situ was more common in women with immunosuppression (112,117). From this evidence, the Centers for Disease Control and Prevention (CDC) classified invasive cervical cancer in an HIV-infected woman as an AIDS-defining malignancy in 1993.

However, not all evidence supports considering cervical cancer to be AIDS related. Most studies have not adequately accounted for bias. Women with HIV infection are usually exposed by heterosexual activity or drug use. Often these women have many sexual partners or their sexual partners have many partners. Therefore, as a group, these women have a high frequency of sexually transmitted viruses, including HPV types associated with cervical dysplasia and cancer. When women with similar sexual exposures are compared, such as prostitutes in Africa, it is not clear if the HIV-infected group is more likely to be HPV-infected or to have abnormal cytological results (111,118). In registry-based studies, the incidence rates of invasive or in situ cervical cancers have not increased among women living in New York City (3), which is in contrast with the rates of AIDS and other AIDS-related malignancies in women (see Fig. 2). Similarly, in parts of Africa with rampant heterosexual HIV transmission and many women infected, cervical cancers have not increased (119,120). Furthermore, there is a quality of care bias. At one clinic, among women with abnormal cervical smears, those who were HIV-positive were significantly less likely to receive adequate follow-up because they returned for results less commonly (121). Thus, the advanced stages of cervical cancer seen in such women may reflect social problems, rather than biology.

In registry linkage studies, the incidence of cervical dysplasia in women with AIDS was elevated about fourfold, but in this group it was also elevated about fourfold for up to 5 years preceding AIDS (Fig. 10; 122), a time when they were probably relatively immunocompetent. Furthermore, although aggressive cases of invasive cervical cancer have been reported in women with AIDS, there does not appear to be a distribution of cases that is weighted toward unusual severity. These data suggest that cervical cancer is not epidemic, but it is possible that, at least in the United States, screening for early indications of HPV infection and aggressive early therapy of in situ disease might have blunted the appearance of invasive carcinoma. It is difficult to apply this explanation to African women,

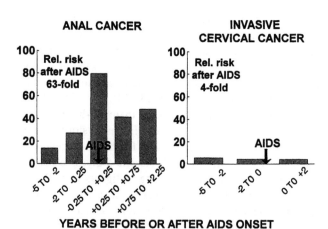

Figure 10 Changes in the relative risks of developing anal cancer in homosexual men (126) and cervical cancer in women in the pre-, at, and post-AIDS periods (149). For anal cancer, the high risk at AIDS is attributed to ascertainment bias. However, both the high relative risk and increasing relative risk as AIDS illness approached and past are consistent with anal cancer being related to HIV-infection or the related progressive deterioration of the immune system. However, there were no similar findings for cervical cancer in women. Prior screening and preventive care may have prevented a true association from being observed in women.

however. One might postulate that cervical cancer in Africa has a longer latent period than the expected survival from HIV-infection.

Contrary to the hypothesis that cervical cancer is unrelated to AIDS, the risk of epithelioid anal cancer, a condition also associated with HPV, is high in homosexual men with AIDS (123). Anal cancer was noted to be more frequent in homosexual men long before the AIDS epidemic appeared (22,124,125). However, the incidence rises as the HIV-infected population approaches and passes the time of AIDS (see Fig. 10), suggesting that it is related to the progression of immunosuppression (126). In contrast with cervical cancer, anal cancer risk does increase slightly among men approaching AIDS onset, even though it is a rare cancer (see Fig. 1; 2). Anal and cervical cancers appear to share major risk factors, including the associations with selected HPV types. These types are commonly found in sexually active homosexual men, with detection of HPV and findings of associated dysplastic lesions being more frequent in immunosuppressed men (127–129). Dysplastic lesions have not yet been reported to progress to invasive anal cancer, although the histological grade of the anal dysplastic lesions appears to increase over time in HIV-infected men (130), and disease progression may be only a matter of time. Despite these findings, anal cancer is not currently accepted as an AIDS-defining malignancy.

B. Hodgkin's Disease

Several reports indicate an increased frequency of Hodgkin's disease (HD) in patients with AIDS (2,131–133). Similarly, in a study linking 50,000 AIDS and cancer cases, there was an eight fold excess of HD, and the risk appeared to increase as AIDS onset was approached and passed (121). However, misclassification of NHL as HD occurred in up to 5% of NHL cases occurring in younger adults (134). Because the NHL excess is so high in AIDS, even a minor amount of erroneous classification either in the histology or the coding of NHL as HD would lead to a spurious association. In a very small series of followed-up reports, the histologies of 12 cases were reviewed at the National Institutes of Health, and 11 were confirmed to be HD (unpublished data). Therefore, it seems probable that HD is increased in AIDS.

Reported histological types are most commonly either mixed cellularity or, less commonly, lymphocyte-depleted (135). In non–HIV-infected persons nodular sclerosis is most common in young adults and only about 15% of HD will be of mixed cellularity or lymphocyte-depleted histological types (136). The presentation is at higher stages (80% have stage III or IV), and B symptoms (fever, weight loss, and night sweats) are more common in patients with AIDS (135,137). Mediastinal involvement appears to be infrequent (138). Given the advanced stages, HD in HIV-infected can be difficult to treat, and survival is less than in persons without AIDS who acquire HD (137).

No etiology is known for HD. EBV can be detected in the majority (60–80%) of HD cases in AIDS patients, which is about twice the frequency seen in non-AIDS HD cases (137,138).

C.　Leiomyosarcomas

Although very rare, the relative risk of leiomyosarcomas in children with AIDS is relatively high (139,140). This association has not been reported in adults with AIDS. This spindle cell sarcoma may involve the internal organs of the gastrointestinal tract and the lung, but it also occurs as a subcutaneous tumor. Malignant leiomyosarcoma and benign leiomyomas have both been associated with EBV in some (140,141), but not all (142), studies.

D.　Conjunctival Tumors

Several reports from Africa have found higher than expected numbers of invasive conjunctival carcinomas in persons with AIDS (92,139,143). This tumor is rare in the United States, but is slightly more frequent than expected in AIDS cases (144,145). Some conjunctival tumors are HPV-infected, but this has not yet been confirmed for conjunctival tumors in persons with AIDS.

E.　Testicular Cancer

Testicular tumor is relatively common in young men and, not surprisingly, it also occurs in men with HIV–AIDS. Seminomas are reported most commonly (50–70%; 146,147). However, registry-based studies have not supported the finding that there is an excess incidence of testicular cancers of any specific type (2,133). In one cohort study, a significant increase in testicular cancer was based on two gonad cases and one extra gonadal case (148). In a large registry-linkage study, seminoma was significantly increased (relative risk 2.9-fold; 149). However, the lower 95% confidence limit was 1.1, and the increase became significant only by including cases of mediastinal seminoma. In summary, the evidence for an association with AIDS is currently of borderline significance, but it may well be confirmed.

F.　Other Tumors

No other cancers have been firmly associated with HIV–AIDS, but a number are suspect. Because of its associations with hepatitis B and C, hepatoma incidence has been evaluated, but there is little to support an association in the United States or in Africa, where the tumor is more frequent. Similarly, because of their EBV association, nasopharyngeal carcinomas were examined, but no significant excess was found (150). Lung cancer incidence was increased slightly (2), but excess smoking by HIV-exposure groups could be contributing. Nonmelanoma tumors of the skin and lip have been reported to be more frequent in persons with non–HIV-related immunosuppression (73,74,151,152), but the incidence has not been well evaluated in HIV–AIDS patients. Data about nonmelanoma skin cancer is often not collected by registries because variations in diagnosis and reporting make it unreliable. However, one report suggests that there might be an increased incidence, especially of basal cells types (153).

G. Summary

The striking aspect of AIDS is that the range of cancers occurring in excess is highly limited. The relation between KS and HIV–AIDS is extraordinary (100,000-fold increase), in part because KS is otherwise very rare in healthy young men. The background rate of NHL in young adults is higher, but HIV–AIDS patients have an excess risk of 150- to 200-fold. Other than KS and NHL (including primary brain lymphomas), only Hodgkin's disease is firmly HIV–AIDS-related, having an excess risk of eightfold, and leiomyosarcomas in children. Anal and cervical cancers could be related, but the evidence is still inconclusive. Certainly, they occur in excess, but whether the excess occurs because of HIV–AIDS and immunosuppression or because HIV-infected populations have other HPV-related risk factors is unclear. Testicular cancer may also be HIV–AIDS-related (threefold excess of borderline statistical significance).

Numerically, more KS cases have occurred in AIDS patients than NHL cases, but KS is a disease seen tenfold more frequently in homosexual men compared with other risk groups with AIDS. As homosexual men become a smaller proportion of new AIDS cases, the frequency of this disease in all AIDS patients will decline. However, NHL occurs equally frequently in HIV-exposure groups and this disease will not decline as a consequence of the changing distribution of AIDS exposure groups.

The frequency of these diseases is expected to change with the advent of new, highly active antiretroviral therapies (HAART; 154). If therapies were able to restore immunity to normal, presumably there would be no excesses of cancer. However, thus far, the improvements have been partial, rather than complete. There is evidence that existing KS can be reversed and the incidence of new KS declines in persons responding well to HAART (see Chapter 2). Thus far, however, no changes in the frequency of NHL have been observed, although there is preliminary evidence that the incidence of primary brain lymphomas may be declining. Analyses are only now beginning to be possible as sufficient numbers of persons are being treated with HAART for periods long enough to observe changes in cancer incidence.

V. CANCERS ASSOCIATED WITH OTHER RETROVIRUSES OF HUMANS

Human Immunodeficiency Virus (HIV-2) is about 60% homologous with HIV-1. Infection causes a slowly progressive immunodeficiency condition. Laboratory studies have shown similar primate viruses can cause lymphomas in animals. In humans, NHL has been seen in HIV-2-infected persons, especially in autopsy material (155,156). However, the quantitative evidence is weaker because its distribution is confined to West Africa, where data about the distribution of HIV-2 and about cancer are both limited.

HTLV-I is also strongly associated with cancers, but of a very specific type: adult T-cell leukemia/lymphoma (ATLL). About 1–2% of HTLV-I-infected persons will develop ATLL during their lives (157). Some evidence suggested that infection early in life (mother-to-child transmission) is more likely to be associated with the later appearance of ATLL (158), implying that either the timing of infection is critical, or that the incubation period requires many years. HTLV-II has not been documented as causing cancers. HTLV-associated tumors have not been reported to occur excessively in persons coinfected with HIV and HTLV.

REFERENCES

1. Centers for Disease Control. 1993 revised classification system for HIV infection and expanded surveillance case definition for AIDS among adolescents and adults. MMWR Morb Mortal Wkly Rep 41:1–19, 1992.
2. CS Rabkin, FJ Yellin. Cancer incidence in a population with a high prevalence of infection with human immunodeficiency virus type 1. J Natl Cancer Inst 86:1711–1716, 1994.
3. CS Rabkin, RJ Biggar, MS Baptiste, T Abe, BA Kohler, PC Nasca. Cancer incidence trends in women at high risk of human immunodeficiency virus (HIV) infection. Int J Cancer 55:208–212, 1993.
4. K Rappersberger, E Tschachler, E Zonzits, R Gillitzer, A Hatzakis, A Kaloterakis, DL Mann, T Popow-Kraupp, RJ Biggar, R Berger, J Stratigos, K Wolff, G Stingl. Endemic Kaposi's sarcoma in human immunodeficiency virus type 1-seronegative persons: demonstration of retrovirus-like particles in cutaneous lesions. J Invest Dermatol 95:371–381, 1990.
5. EE Kaaya, C Parravicini, C Ordónez, R Gendelman, E Berti, RC Gallo, P Biberfeld.

Heterogeneity of spindle cells in Kaposi's sarcoma: comparison of cells in lesions and in culture. J Acquir Immune Defic Syndr Hum Retrovirol 10:295–305, 1995.

6. CS Rabkin, G Bedi, E Musaba, R Sunkutu, N Mwansa, D Sidransky, RJ Biggar. AIDS-related Kaposi's sarcoma is a clonal neoplasm. Clin Cancer Res 1:257–260, 1995.

7. CS Rabkin, S Janz, A Lash, AE Coleman, E Musaba, L Liotta, RJ Biggar, Z Zhuang. Monoclonal origin of multicentric Kaposi's sarcoma lesions. N Engl J Med 336:988–993, 1997.

8. JF Taylor, AC Templeton, CL Vogel, JL Ziegler, SK Kyalwazi. Kaposi's sarcoma in Uganda: a clinico-pathological study. Int J Cancer 8:122–135, 1971.

9. AC Templeton. Pathology. In: Kaposi's Sarcoma: Pathophysiology and Clinical Management. New York: Marcel Dekker, 1988.

10. RJ Biggar, J Horm, JF Fraumeni Jr, MH Greene, JJ Goedert. Incidence of Kaposi's sarcoma and mycosis fungoides in the United States including Puerto Rico, 1973–1981. J Natl Cancer Inst 73:89–94, 1984.

11. S Franceschi, M Geddes. Epidemiology of classic Kaposi's sarcoma, with special reference to Mediterranean population. Tumori 81:308–314, 1995.

12. AG Oettle. Geographical and racial differences in the frequency of Kaposi's sarcoma as evidence of environmental or genetic causes. Acta Unio Int Contra Cancerum 18:330–363, 1962.

13. MS Hutt. The epidemiology of Kaposi's sarcoma. Antibiot Chemother 29:3–8, 1981.

14. JL Ziegler, AC Templeton, CL Vogel. Kaposi's sarcoma: a comparison of classical, endemic, and epidemic forms. Semin Oncol 11:47–52, 1984.

15. JL Ziegler, E Katongole-Mbidde. Kaposi's sarcoma in childhood: an analysis of 100 cases from Uganda and relationship to HIV infection. Int J Cancer 65:200–203, 1996.

16. L Kestens, M Melbye, RJ Biggar, WJ Stevens,P Piot, AD Muynck, H Taelman, M De Feyter, L Paluku, PL Gigase. Endemic African Kaposi's sarcoma is not associated with immunodeficiency. Int J Cancer 36:49–54, 1985.

17. AM Levine. AIDS- related malignancies: the emerging epidemic. J Natl Cancer Inst 85:1382–1396, 1993.

18. JA Regezi, LA MacPhail, TE Daniels, YG DeSouza, JS Greenspan, D Greenspan. Human immunodeficiency virus-associated oral Kaposi's sarcoma. A heterogeneous cell population dominated by spindle-shaped endothelial cells. Am J Pathol 143:240–249, 1993.

19. J Casabona, T Salas, R Salinas. Trends and survival in AIDS-associated malignancies. Eur J Cancer 29A:877–881, 1993.

20. JD Lundgren, M Melbye, C Pedersen, PS Rosenberg, J Gerstoft. Changing patterns of Kaposi's sarcoma in Danish acquired immunodeficiency syndrome patients with complete follow-up. The Danish Study Group for HIV Infection (DASHI). Am J Epidemiol 141:652–658, 1995.

21. RJ Biggar, PS Rosenberg, TR Coté. Kaposi's sarcoma and non-Hodgkin's lymphoma following the diagnosis of AIDS. The Multistate AIDS/Cancer Match Study Group. Int J Cancer 68:754–758, 1996.

22. RJ Biggar, M Melbye. Marital status in relation to Kaposi's sarcoma, non-Hodg-

kin's lymphoma, and anal cancer in the pre-AIDS era. J Acquir Immune Defic Syndr Hum Retrovirol 11:178–182, 1996.

23. TA Peterman, HW Jaffe, V Beral. Epidemiologic clues to the etiology of Kaposi's sarcoma. AIDS 7:605–612, 1993.

24. V Beral, TA Peterman, RL Berkelman, HW Jaffe. Kaposi's sarcoma among persons with AIDS: a sexually transmitted infection. Lancet 335:123–128, 1990.

25. J Casabona, T Salas, C Lacasa, M Melbye, A Segura. Kaposi's sarcoma in people with AIDS from an area in Southern Europe. J Acquir Immune Defic Syndr 3:929–930, 1990.

26. RJ Biggar, CS Rabkin. The epidemiology of acquired immunodeficiency syndrome-related lymphomas. Curr Opin Oncol 4:883–893, 1992.

27. B Schwartländer, CR Horsburgh Jr, O Hamouda, H Skarabis, MA Koch. Changes in the spectrum of AIDS- defining conditions and decrease in CD4+ lymphocyte counts as AIDS manifestations in Germany from 1986 to 1991. AIDS 6:413–420, 1992.

28. AE Friedman-Kien, BR Saltzman, YZ Cao, MS Nestor, M Mirabile, JJ Li, TA Peterman. Kaposi's sarcoma in HIV-negative homosexual men. Lancet 335: 168–169, 1990.

29. YQ Huang, A Buchbinder, JJ Li, A Nicolaides, WG Zhang, AE Friedman-Kien. The absence of Tat sequences in tissues of HIV-negative patients with epidemic Kaposi's sarcoma. AIDS 6:1139–1142, 1992.

30. D Zucker-Franklin, YQ Huang, GE Grusky, AE Friedman-Kien. Kaposi's sarcoma in a human immunodeficiency virus-negative patient with asymptomatic human T lymphotropic virus type I infection. J Infect Dis 167:987–989, 1993.

31. JJ Goedert, RJ Biggar, M Melbye, DL Mann, S Wilson, MH Gail, RJ Grossman, RA DiGioia, WC Sanchez, SH Weiss, WA Blattner. Effect of T4 count and cofactors on the incidence of AIDS in homosexual men infected with human immunodeficiency virus. JAMA 257:331–334, 1987.

32. WW Darrow, TA Peterman, HW Jaffe, MF Rogers, JW Curran, V Beral. Kaposi's sarcoma and exposure to faeces. Lancet 339:685, 1992.

33. V Beral, D Bull, S Darby, I Weller, C Carne, M Beecham, H Jaffe. Risk of Kaposi's sarcoma and sexual practices associated with faecal contact in homosexual or bisexual men with AIDS. Lancet 339:632–635, 1992.

34. P Matondo. Kaposi's sarcoma and faecal–oral exposure. Lancet 339:1490, 1992.

35. C Urmacher, P Myskowski, MJR Ochoa, M Kris, B Safai. Outbreak of Kaposi's sarcoma with cytomegalovirus infection in young homosexual men. Am J Med 72: 569–575, 1982.

36. WL Drew. Is cytomegalovirus a cofactor in the pathogenesis of AIDS and Kaposi's sarcoma. Mt Sinai J Med 53:622–626, 1986.

37. M Marmor, AE Friedman-Kien, S Zolla-Pazner, RE Stahl, P Rubinstein, L Laubenstein, DC William, RJ Klein, I Spigland. Kaposi's sarcoma in homosexual men. A seroepidemiologic case–control study. Ann Intern Med 100:809–815, 1984.

38. HW Haverkos, PF Pinsky, DP Drotman, DJ Bregman. Disease manifestation among homosexual men with acquired immunodeficiency syndrome: a possible role of nitrites in Kaposi's sarcoma. Sex Transm Dis 12:203–208, 1985.

39. CP Archibald, MT Schechter, KJP Craib, TN Le, B Douglas, B Willoughby, M O'Shaughnessy. Risk factors for Kaposi's scarcoma in the Vancouver lymphade-nopathy–AIDS study. J Acquir Immune Defic Syndr 3(suppl 1):S18–S23, 1990.

40. V Beral. Epidemiology of Kaposi's sarcoma. In: Cancer, HIV and AIDS. New York: Cold Spring Harbor Laboratory, 1991:5–22.

41. D Serraino, S Franceschi, L Dal Maso, C La Vecchia. HIV transmission and Kaposi's sarcoma among European women. AIDS 9:971–973, 1995.

42. G Giraldo, E Beth, ES Huang. Kaposi's sarcoma and its relationship to cytomegalo-virus (CMW) III. CMV DNA and CMV early antigens in Kaposi's sarcoma. Int J Cancer 26:23–29, 1980.

43. J Bignall. Rochalimaeas from cat-scratch to Kaposi. Lancet 342:359 1993.

44. YQ Huang, JJ Li, MG Rush, BJ Poiesz, A Nicolaides, M Jacobson, WG Zhang, E Coutavas, MA Abbott, AE Friedman-Kien. HPV-16-related DNA sequences in Kaposi's sarcoma. Lancet 339:515–518, 1992.

45. RY Wang, JW Shih, SH Weiss, T Grandinetti, PF Pierce, M Lange, HJ Alter, DJ Wear, CL Davies, RK Mayur. *Mycoplasma penetrans* infection in male homosexu-als with AIDS: high seroprevalence and association with Kaposi's sarcoma. Clin Infect Dis 17:724–729, 1993.

46. MS Pollack, B Safai, PL Myskowski, JW Gold, J Pandey, B Dupont, Frequencies of HLA and GM immunogenetic markers in Kaposi's sarcoma. Tissue Antigens 21:1–8, 1983.

47. C Papasteriades, A Kaloterakis, A Fihotou, J Economidou, G Nicolis, D Tricho-poulos, J Stratigos. Histocompatibility antigens HLA-A, -B, -DR in Greek patients with Kaposi's sarcoma. Tissue Antigens 24:313–315, 1984.

48. M Melbye, L Kestens, RJ Biggar, GMT Schreuder, PL Gigase. HLA studies of endemic African Kaposi's sarcoma patients and matched controls: no association with HLA-DR5. Int J Cancer 39:182–184, 1987.

49. L Strichman-Almashanu, S Weltfriend, O Gideoni, R Friedman-Birnbaum, S Pol-lack. No significant association between HLA antigens and classic Kaposi sarcoma: molecular analysis of 49 Jewish patients. J Clin Immunol 15:205–209, 1995.

50. DL Mann, C Murray, M O'Donnell, WA Blattner, JJ Goedert. HLA antigen fre-quencies in HIV-1 related Kaposi's sarcoma. J Acquir Immune Defic Syndr 3 (suppl 1):S51–S55, 1989.

51. JP Ioannidis, PR Skolnik, TC Chalmers, J Lau. Human leukocyte antigen associa-tions of epidemic Kaposi's sarcoma. AIDS 9:649–651, 1995.

52. Y Lunardi-Iskandar, JL Bryant, RA Zeman, VH Lam, F Samaniego, JM Besnier, P Hermans, AR Thierry, P Gill, RC Gallo. Tumorigenesis and metastasis of neo-plastic Kaposi's sarcoma cell line in immunodeficient mice blocked by a human pregnancy hormone. Nature 375:64–68, 1995.

53. N Christoff, C Winter, S Gharakhanian, N Thobie, E Wirbel, D Costagliola, EA Nunez, W Rozenbaum. Differences in androgens of HIV positive patients with and without Kaposi's sarcoma. J Clin Pathol 48:513–518, 1995.

54. S Klauke, H Schoefer, PH Althoff, B Michels, EB Helm. Sex hormones as a cofactor in the pathogenesis of epidemic Kaposi's sarcoma. AIDS 9:1295–1296, 1995.

55. Y Chang, E Cesarman, MS Pessin, F Lee, J Culpepper, DM Knowles, PS Moore.

Identification of herpesvirus-like DNA sequences in AIDS-associated Kaposi's sarcoma. Science 266:1865–1869, 1994.

56. Y Chang, J Ziegler, H Wabinga, E Katangole-Mbidde, C Boshoff, T Schulz, D Whitby, D Maddalena, HW Jaffe, RA Weiss, PS Moore. Kaposi's sarcoma-associated herpesvirus and Kaposi's sarcoma in Africa. Uganda Kaposi's Sarcoma Study Group. Arch Intern Med 156:202–204, 1996.

57. FM Buonaguro, ML Tornesello, E Beth-Giraldo, A Hatzakis, N Mueller, R Downing, B Biryamwaho, SD Sempala, G Giraldo. Herpesvirus-like DNA sequences detected in endemic, classic, iatrogenic and epidemic Kaposi's sarcoma (KS) biopsies. Int J Cancer 65:25–28, 1996.

58. E Cesarman, Y Chang, PS Moore, JW Said, DM Knowles. Kaposi's sarcoma-associated herpesvirus-like DNA sequences in AIDS-related body-cavity-based lymphomas. N Engl J Med 332:1186–1191, 1995.

59. SJ Gao, L Kingsley, M Li, W Zheng, C Parravicini, J Ziegler, R Newton, CR Rinaldo, A Saah, J Phair, R Detels, Y Chang, PS Moore. KSHV antibodies among Americans, Italians and Ugandans with and without Kaposi's sarcoma. Nat Med 2:925–928, 1996.

60. ET Lennette, DJ Blackbourn, JA Levy. Antibodies to human herpesvirus type 8 in the general population and in Kaposi's sarcoma patients. Lancet 348:858–861, 1996.

61. SJ Gao, L Kingsley, DR Hoover, TJ Spira, CR Rinaldo, A Saah, J Phair, R Detels, P Parry, Y Chang, PS Moore. Seroconversion to antibodies against Kaposi's sarcoma-associated herpesvirus-related latent nuclear antigens before the development of Kaposi's sarcoma. N Engl J Med 335:233–241, 1996.

62. M Melbye, PM Cook, H Hjalgrim, K Begtrup, GR Simpson, RJ Biggar, P Ebbesen, TF Schulz. Risk factors for HHV-8 seropositivity and progression of Kaposi's sarcoma in a cohort of homosexual men, 1981–96. Int J Cancer 77:543–548, 1998.

63. CL Kosary, LAG Ries, BA Miller, BF Hankey, A Harras, BK Edwards. SEER Cancer Statistics Review, 1973–1992: Tables and Graphs. NIH Pub. No. 96-2789 ed. Bethesda, MD: National Cancer Institute, 1995.

63a. JL Ziegler, JA Beckstead, PA Volberding, D Abrams, AM Levine, RJ Lukes, PS Gill, RL Burkes, PR Meyer, CE Metroka, J Mouradian, A Moore, SA Riggs, JJ Butler, FC Cabanillas, E Hersh, GR Newell, LJ Laubenstein, D Knowles, C Odajnyk, B Raphael, B Koziner, C Urmacher, BD Clarkson. Non–Hodgkin's lymphoma in 90 homosexual men. Relation to generalized lymphadenopathy and the acquired immunodeficiency syndrome. N Engl J Med 311:565–570, 1984.

63b. RJ Biggar, J Horm, JH Lubin, JJ Goedert. MH Greene, JF Fraumeni Jr. Cancer trends in a population at risk of acquired immunodeficiency syndrome. J Natl Cancer Inst. 74:793–797, 1985.

64. DM Knowles, RD Dalla-Favera. AIDS-associated malignant lymphoma. In: S Broder, TC Merrigan, and D Bolognesi, eds. Textbook of AIDS Medicine. Baltimore: Williams & Wilkins, 1994:431–463.

65. B Shiramizu, B Herndier, L Meeker, L Kaplan, M McGrath. Molecular and immunophenotypic characterization of AIDS-associated, Epstein–Barr virus-negative, polyclonal lymphoma. J Clin Oncol 10:383–389, 1992.

66. C Percy, G O'Conor, LG Ries, ES Jaffe. Non–Hodgkin's lymphomas. Application

of the International Classification of Diseases for Oncology (ICD-O) to the Working Formulation. Cancer 54:1435–1438, 1984.

67. SS Devesa, T Fears. Non–Hodgkin's lymphoma time trends: United States and international data. Cancer Res 52(supp 19):5432S–5440S, 1992.

68. M Krogh-Jensen, F D'Amore, MK Jensen, BE Christensen, K Thorling, M Pedersen, P Johansen, AM Boesen, E Andersen. Incidence, clinicopathological features and outcome of primary central nervous system lymphomas. Population-based data from a Danish lymphoma registry. Ann Oncol 5:349–354, 1994.

69. NL Eby, S Grufferman, CM Flannelly, SC Schold, S Vogel, PC Burger. Increasing incidence of primary brain lymphoma in the US. Cancer 62:2461–2465, 1988.

70. TR Coté, A Manns, CR Hardy, FJ Yellin, P Hartge. Epidemiology of brain lymphoma among people with or without acquired immunodeficiency syndrome. AIDS/Cancer Study Group. J Natl Cancer Inst 88:675–679, 1996.

71. P Hartge, SS Devesa. Quantification of the impact of known risk factors on time trends in non-Hodgkin's lymphoma incidence. Cancer Res 52(supp):5566S–5569S, 1992.

72. CS Rabkin, SS Devesa, SH Zahm, MH Gail. Increasing incidence of non–Hodgkin's lymphoma. Semin Hematol 30:286–296, 1993.

73. SA Birkeland, HH Storm, LU Lamm, L Barlow, I Blohmé, B Forsberg, B Eklund, O Fjeldborg, M Friedberg, L Frödin, E Glattre, S Halvorsen, N Holm, A Jakobsen, HE Jørgensen, J Ladefoged, T Lindholm, G Lundgren, E Pukkala. Cancer risk after renal transplantation in the Nordic countries, 1964–1986. Int J Cancer 60:183–189, 1995.

74. LJ Kinlen, AGR Sheil, J Peto, R Doll. Collaborative United Kingdom–Australasian study of cancer in patients treated with immunosuppressive drugs. Br Med J 2:1461–1466, 1979.

75. I Penn. De novo malignancy in pediatric organ transplant recipients. J Pediatr Surg 29:221–228, 1994.

76. V Beral, T Peterman, R Berkelman, H Jaffe. AIDS-associated non-Hodgkin lymphoma. Lancet 337:805–809, 1991.

77. G Frizzera. Immunosuppression, autoimmunity and lymphoproliferative disorders. Hum Pathol 25:627–629, 1994.

78. G Socié, M Henry-Amar, A Bacigalupo, J Hows, A Tichelli, P Ljungman, SR McCann, N Frickhofen, E van't Veer-Korthof, E Gluckman. Malignant tumors occurring after treatment of aplastic anemia. N Engl J Med 329:1152–1157, 1993.

79. R Lowsky, J Lipton, G Fyles, M Minden, J Meharchand, I Tejpar, H Atkins, S Sutcliffe, H Messner. Secondary malignancies after bone marrow transplantation in adults. J Clin Oncol 12:2187–2192, 1994.

80. TR Coté, RJ Biggar, PS Rosenberg, SS Devesa, C Percy, FJ Yellin, G Lemp, C Hardy, JJ Goedert, WA Blattner. Non–Hodgkin's lymphoma among people with AIDS:incidence, presentation and public health burden. AIDS/Cancer Study Group. Int J Cancer 73:645–50, 1997.

81. RM Selik, SY Chu, JW Ward. Trends in infectious diseases and cancers among persons dying of HIV infection in the United States from 1987 to 1992. Ann Intern Med 123:933–936, 1995.

82. SC Remick, C Diamond, JA Migliozzi, O Solis, H Wagner, RF Haase, JC Ruck-

deschel. Primary central nervous system lymphoma in patients with and without the acquired immunodeficiency syndrome. A retrospective analysis and review of the literature. Medicine 69:345–360, 1990.

83. M Raphael, O Gentilhomme, M Tulliez, P Byron, J Diebold, for the French Study Group of Pathology for Human Immunodeficiency Virus-Associated Tumors. Histopathologic features of high-grade non–Hodgkin's lymphomas in acquired immunodeficiency syndrome. Arch Pathol Lab Med 115:15–20, 1991.

84. NL Harris, ES Jaffe, H Stein, PM Banks, JKC Chan, ML Cleary, G Deisol, C De Wolf-Peeters, B Falini, KC Gatter, TM Grogan, PG Isaacson, DM Knowles, DY Mason, HK Muller-Hermelink, SA Pileri, MA Piris, E Ralfkiaer, RA Warnke. A revised European–American classification of lymphoid neoplasms: a proposal from the International Lymphoma Study Group. Blood 84:1361–1392, 1994.

85. DD Ho, AU Neumann, AS Perelson, W Chen, JM Leonard, M Markowitz. Rapid turnover of plasma virions and CD4 lymphocytes in HIV-1 infection. Nature 373:123–126, 1995.

86. X Wei, SK Ghosh, ME Taylor, VA Johnson, EA Emini, P Deutsch, JD Lifson, S Bonhoeffer, MA Nowak, BH Hahn, MS Saag, GM Shaw. Viral dynamics in human immunodeficiency virus type 1 infection. Nature 373:117–122, 1995.

87. HC Lane, H Masur, LC Edgar, G Whalen, AH Rook, AS Fauci. Abnormalities of B-cell activation and immunoregulation in patients with the acquired immunodeficiency syndrome. N Engl J Med 309:453–458, 1983.

88. J Casabona, M Melbye, RJ Biggar. Kaposi's sarcoma and non–Hodgkin's lymphoma in European AIDS cases. No excess risk of Kaposi's sarcoma in Mediterranean countries. Int J Cancer 47:49–53, 1991.

89. F Sitas, CV Levin, D Spencer, RA Odes, W Bezwoda, I Windsor, R Sher, AA Wadee. HIV and cancer in South Africa. S Afr Med 83:880–881, 1993.

90. MT Bassett, E Chokunonga, B Mauchaza, L Levy, J Ferlay, DM Parkin. Cancer in the African population of Harare, Zimbabwe, 1990–1992. Int J Cancer 63:29–36, 1995.

91. HR Wabinga, DM Parkin, F Wabwire-Mangen, JW Mugerwa. Cancer in Kampala, Uganda, in 1989–1991: changes in incidence in the era of AIDS. Int J Cancer 54:26–36, 1993.

92. R Newton, P Ngliimana, A Grulich, V Beral, B Sindikubwabo, A Nganyira, DM Parkin. Cancer in Rwanda. Int J Cancer 66:75–81, 1996.

93. D Serraino, S Franceschi, U Tirelli, S Monfardini. The epidemiology of acquired immunodeficiency syndrome and associated tumors in Europe. Ann Oncol 3:595–603, 1992.

94. TR Coté, M Dosemeci, N Rothman, RB Banks, RJ Biggar. Non–Hodgkin's lymphoma and occupational exposure to hair dyes among people with AIDS. Am J Public Health 83:598–599, 1993.

95. TR Coté, RJ Biggar. Does zidovudine cause non–Hodgkin's lymphoma? AIDS 9:404–405, 1995.

96. AM Levine, L Bernstein, J Sullivan-Halley, D Shibata, SB Mahterian, BN Nathwani. Role of zidovudine therapy in the pathogenesis of acquired immunodeficiency-related lymphoma. Blood 86:4612–4616, 1995.

97. EME MacMahon, JD Glass, SD Hayward, RB Mann, PS Becker, H Charache,

JC McArthur, RF Ambinder. Epstein–Barr virus in AIDS-related primary central nervous system lymphoma. Lancet 338:969–974, 1991.

98. JA Arribas, DB Clifford, CJ Fichtenbaum, RL Roberts, WG Powderly, GA Storch. Detection of Epstein–Barr virus DNA in cerebrospinal fluid for diagnosis of AIDS-related central nervous system lymphoma. J Clin Microbiol 33:1580–1583, 1995.

99. I Ernberg. Epstein–Barr virus and acquired immunodeficiency syndrome. In: Advances in Viral Oncology. New York: Raven Press, 1989:203–217.

100. D Shibata, LM Weiss, BN Nathwani, RK Brynes, AM Levine. Epstein–Barr virus in benign lymph node biopsies from individuals infected with the human immunodeficiency virus is associated with concurrent or subsequent development of non-Hodgkin's lymphoma. Blood 77:1527–1533, 1991.

101. DL Birx, RR Redfield, G Tosato. Defective regulation of Epstein–Barr virus infection in patients with acquired immunodeficiency syndrome (AIDS) or AIDS-related disorders. N Engl J Med 314:874–879, 1986.

102. A Neri, F Barriga, G Inghirami, DM Knowles, J Neequaye, IT Magrath, R Dalla-Favera. Epstein–Barr virus infection precedes clonal expansion in Burkitt's and acquired immunodeficiency syndrome-associated lymphoma. Blood 77:1092–1095, 1991.

103. P Ballerini, G Gaidano, JZ Gong, V Tassi, G Saglio, DM Knowles, R Della-Favera. Multiple genetic lesions in acquired immunodeficiency syndrome-related non-Hodgkin's lymphoma. Blood 81:166–176, 1993.

104. DM Knowles, G Inghirami, A Ubiaco, R Della-Favera. Molecular genetic analysis of three AIDS-associated neoplasms of uncertain lineage demonstrates their B-cell derivation and possible pathogenetic role of Epstein–Barr virus. Blood 73:792–799, 1989.

105. J Soulier, L Grollet, E Oksenhendler, P Cacoub, D Cazals-Hatem, P Babinet, M d'Agay, J Clauvel, M Raphael, L Degos, F Sigaux. Kaposi's sarcoma-associated herpesvirus-like DNA sequences in multicentric Castleman's disease. Blood 86:1276–1280, 1995.

106. CA Presant, K Gala, C Wiseman, P Kennedy, D Blayney, K Sheibani, CD Winberg, S Rasheed. Human immunodeficiency virus-associated T-cell lymphoblastic lymphoma in AIDS. Cancer 60:1459–1461, 1987.

107. B Herndier, B Shiramizu, N Jewett, L Young, G Reyes, M McGrath. AIDS-associated T-cell lymphoma: evidence for HIV-1 associated T-cell transformation. Blood 79:1768–1774, 1992.

108. B Shiramizu, B Herndier, MS McGrath. Identification of a common clonal human immunodeficiency virus integration site in human immunodeficiency virus-associated lymphomas. Cancer Res 54:2069–2072, 1994.

109. RJ Biggar, RE Curtis, TR Coté, CS Rabkin, M Melbye. Risk of other cancers following Kaposi's sarcoma: relation to acquired immunodeficiency syndrome. Am J Epidemiol 139:362–368, 1994.

110. JS Mandelblatt, M Fahs, K Garibaldi, RT Senie, HB Peterson. Association between HIV infection and cervical neoplasia: implications for clinical care of women at risk for both conditions. AIDS 6:173–178, 1992.

111. JK Kreiss, NB Kiviat, FA Plummer, PL Roberts, P Waiyaki, E Ngugi, KK Holmes.

Human immunodeficiency virus, human papillomavirus, and cervical intraepithelial neoplasia in Nairobi prostitutes. Sex Transm Dis 19:54–59, 1992.

112. FD Johnstone, E McGoogan, GE Smart, RP Brettle, RJ Prescott. A population-based, controlled study of the relation between HIV infection and cervical neoplasia. Br J Obstet Gynaecol 101:986–991, 1994.

113. LK Schrager, GH Friedland, D Maude, K Schreiber, A Adachi, DJ Pizzuti, LG Koss, RS Klein. Cervical and vaginal squamous cell abnormalities in women infected with human immunodeficiency virus. J Acquir Immune Defic Syndr 2:570–575, 1989.

114. M Maiman, N Tarricone, J Vieira, J Suarez, E Serur, JG Boyce. Colposcopic evaluation of human immunodeficiency virus-seropositive women. Obstet Gynecol 78: 84–88, 1991.

115. GYF Ho, RD Burk, I Fleming, RS Klein. Risk of genital human papillomavirus infection in women with human immunodeficiency virus-induced immunosuppression. Int J Cancer 56:788–792, 1994.

116. AB Williams, TM Darragh, K Vranizan, C Ochia, AR Moss, JM Palefsky. Anal and cervical human papillomavirus infection and risk of anal and cervical epithelial abnormalities in human immunodeficiency virus-infected women. Obstet Gynecol 83:205–211, 1994.

117. XW Sun, JP Koulos, JC Felix, A Ferenczy, RM Richart, TW Park, TO Wright Jr. Human papillomavirus testing in primary cervical screening. Lancet 346:636 1995.

118. M Laga, JP Icenogle, R Marsella, AT Manoka, N Nzila, RW Ryder, SH Vermund, WL Heyward, A Nelson, WC Reeves. Genital papillomavirus infection and cervical dysplasia—opportunistic complications of HIV infection. Int J Cancer 50:45–48, 1992.

119. CS Rabkin, WA Blattner. HIV infection and cancers other than non-Hodgkin's lymphoma and Kaposi's sarcoma. Cancer Surv 10:151–160, 1991.

120. R Newton, A Grulich, V Beral, B Sindikubwabo, PJ Ngilimana, A Nganyira, DM Parkin. Cancer and HIV infection in Rwanda. Lancet 345:1378–1379, 1995.

121. RG Fruchter, M Maiman, CD Arrastia, R Matthews, EJ Gates, K Holcomb. Is HIV infection a risk factor for advanced cervical cancer. J Acquir Immune Def Syndr Hum Retrovirol 18:241–45, 1998.

122. RJ Biggar, CS Rabkin. The epidemiology of AIDS-related neoplasms. Hematol Oncol Clin North Am 10:997–1010, 1996.

123. JM Palefsky. Anal human papillomavirus infection and anal cancer in HIV-positive individuals: an emerging problem. AIDS 8:283–295, 1994.

124. M Melbye, CS Rabkin, M Frisch, RJ Biggar. Changing patterns of anal cancer incidence in the United States, 1940–1989. Am J Epidemiol 139:772–780, 1994.

125. M Frisch, M Melbye, H Moller. Trends in incidence of anal cancer in Denmark. Br Med J 306:419–422, 1993.

126. M Melbye, TR Coté, L Kessler, M Gail, RJ Biggar. High incidence of anal cancer among AIDS patients. Lancet 343:636–639, 1994.

127. NB Kiviat, CW Critchlow, KK Holmes, J Kuypers, J Sayer, C Dunphy, C Surawicz, P Kirby, R Wood, JR Daling. Association of anal dysplasia and human papillomavirus with immunosuppression and HIV infection among homosexual men. AIDS 7:43–50, 1993.

128. D Caussy, JJ Goedert, J Palefsky, J Gonzales, CS Rabkin, R DiGioia, WC Sanchez, RJ Grossman, G Colclough, SZ Wiktor, A Krämer, RJ Biggar, WA Blattner. Interaction of human immunodeficiency and papilloma viruses: association with anal epithelial abnormality in homosexual men. Int J Cancer 46:214–219, 1990.
129. M Melbye, J Palefsky, J Gonzales, LP Ryder, H Nielsen, O Bergmann, J Pindborg, RJ Biggar. Immune status as a determinant of human papillomavirus detection and its association with anal epithelial abnormalities. Int J Cancer 46:203–206, 1990.
130. JP Allain, W Hodges, MH Einstein, J Geisler, C Neilly, S Delaney, B Hodges, H Lee. Antibody to HIV-1, HTLV-I, and HCV in three populations of rural Haitians. J Acquir Immune Defic Syndr 5:1230–1236, 1992.
131. RJ Biggar, W Burnett, J Mikl, PC Nasca. Cancer among New York men at risk of acquired immunodeficiency syndrome. Int J Cancer 43:979–985, 1989.
132. NA Hessol, MH Katz, JY Liu, SP Buchbinder, CJ Rubino, SD Holmberg. Increased incidence of Hodgkin disease in homosexual men with HIV infection. Ann Intern Med 117:309–311, 1992.
133. P Reynolds, LD Saunders, ME Layefsky, GF Lemp. The spectrum of acquired immunodeficiency syndrome (AIDS)-associated malignancies in San Francisco, 1980–1987. Am J Epidemiol 137:19–30, 1993.
134. SL Glaser, WG Swartz. Time trends in Hodgkin's disease incidence. The role of diagnostic accuracy. Cancer 66:2196–2204, 1990.
135. R Rubio. Hodgkin's disease associated with human immunodeficiency virus infection. A clinical study of 46 cases. Cooperative Study Group of Malignancies Associated with HIV Infection of Madrid. Cancer 73:2400–2407, 1994.
136. LJ Medeiros, TC Greiner. Hodgkin's disease. Cancer 75:357–369, 1995.
137. U Tirelli, D Errante, R Dolcetti, A Gloghini, D Serraino, E Vaccher, S Franceschi, M Boiocchi, A Carbone. Hodgkin's disease and human immunodeficiency virus infection: clinicopathologic and virologic features of 114 patients from the Italian Cooperative Group on AIDS and Tumors. J Clin Oncol 13:1758–1767, 1995.
138. CA Moran, S Tuur, P Angritt, AH Reid, TJ O'Leary. Epstein–Barr virus in Hodgkin's disease from patients with human immunodeficiency virus infection. Mod Pathol 5:85–88, 1992.
139. FJJ DiCarlo, VV Joshi, JM Oleske, EM Connor. Neoplastic diseases in children with acquired immunodeficiency syndrome. Prog AIDS Pathol 2:163–185, 1990.
140. KL McClain, CT Leach, HB Jenson, VV Joshi, BH Pollock, RT Parmley, FJ DiCarlo, EG Chadwick, SB Murphy. Association of Epstein–Barr virus with leiomyosarcomas in children with AIDS. N Engl J Med 332:12–18, 1995.
141. ES Lee, J Locker, M Nalesnik, J Reyes, R Jaffe, M Alashari, B Nour, A Tzakis, PS Dickman. The association of Epstein–Barr virus with smooth-muscle tumors occurring after organ transplantation. N Engl J Med 332:19–25, 1995.
142. HB Jenson, CT Leach, EA Montalvo, JC Lin, SB Murphy. Absence of herpes virus in AIDS-associated smooth-muscle tumors. N Engl J Med 335:1690 1996.
143. C Ateeny-Agaba. Conjunctival squamous-cell carcinoma associated with HIV infection in Kampala, Uganda. Lancet 345:695–696, 1995.
144. JJ Goedert, TR Coté. Conjunctival malignant disease with AIDS in USA. Lancet 346:257–258, 1995.
145. CL Karp, IU Scott, TS Chang, SC Pflugfelder. Conjunctival intraepithelial neopla-

sia. A possible marker for human immunodeficiency virus infection? Arch Ophthalmol 114:257–261, 1996.

146. F Buzelin, G Karam, A Moreau, O Wetzel, F Gaillard. Testicular tumor and the acquired immunodeficiency syndrome. Eur Urol 26:71–76, 1994.

147. JM Timmerman, DM Northfelt, EJ Small. Malignant germ cell tumors in men infected with human immunodeficiency virus: natural history and results of therapy. J Clin Oncol 13:1391–1397, 1995.

148. DW Lyter, J Bryant, R Thackeray, CR Rinaldo, LA Kingsley. Incidence of human immunodeficiency virus-related and nonrelated malignancies in a large cohort of homosexual men. J Clin Oncol 13:2540–2546, 1995.

149. JJ Goedert, TR Coté, P Virgo, S Scoppa, D Kingma, MH Gail, E Jaffe, RJ Biggar. The spectrum of AIDS malignancies. The AIDS-Cancer Match Study Group. Lancet 351:1833–39, 1998.

150. M Melbye, TR Coté, D West, L Kessler, RJ Biggar. Nasopharyngeal carcinoma: an EBV-associated tumour not significantly influenced by HIV-induced immunosuppression. The AIDS/Cancer Working Group. Br J Cancer 73:995–997, 1996.

151. SBM Gaya, AJ Rees, RI Lechler, G Williams, PD Mason. Malignant disease in patients with long-term renal transplants. Transplantation 59:1705–1709, 1995.

152. I Penn. Neoplastic complications of transplantation. Semin Respir Infect 8:233–239, 1993.

153. SD Holmberg, SP Buckbinder, LJ Conley, LC Wong, MH Katz, KA Penley, RC Hershow, FN Judson. The spectrum of medical conditions and symptoms before acquired immunodeficiency syndrome in homosexual and bisexual men infected with the human immunodeficiency virus. Am J Epidemiol 141:395–404, 1995.

154. KA Sepkowitz. Effect of HAART on natural history of AIDS-related opportunistic disorders. Lancet 351:228–230, 1998.

155. SB Lucas, KM De Cock, C Peacock, M Diomande, A Kadio. Effect of HIV infection on the incidence of lymphoma in Africa. East Afr Med J 73:S29–S30, 1996.

156. SB Lucas, M Diomande, A Hounnou, A Beaumel, C Giordano, A Kadio, CS Peacock, M Honde, KM De Cock. HIV-associated lymphoma in Africa: an autopsy study in Cote d'Ivoire. Int J Cancer 59:20–24, 1994.

157. FR Cleghorn, A Manns, R Falk, P Hartge, B Hanchard, N Jack, E Williams, E Jaffe, F White, C Bartholomew. Effect of human T-lymphotropic virus type I infection on non-Hodgkin's lymphoma incidence. J Natl Cancer Inst 87:1009–1014, 1995.

158. A Manns, FR Cleghorn, RT Falk, B Hanchard, E Jaffe, C Bartholomew, P Hartge, J Benichou, WA Blattner, HTLV Lymphoma Study Group. Role of HTLV-I in development of non–Hodgkin lymphoma in Jamaica and Trinidad and Tobago. Lancet 342:1447–1450, 1993.

4

Diagnosis and Treatment of AIDS-Associated Kaposi's Sarcoma

Susan E. Krown
Memorial Sloan-Kettering Cancer Center and Cornell University Medical College, New York, New York

I. INTRODUCTION

Kaposi's sarcoma (KS), the most common acquired immunodeficiency syndrome (AIDS)-associated cancer, was one of the first conditions recognized as an opportunistic complication of human immunodeficiency virus type-1 (HIV) infection (1). Unlike many of the infectious sequelae of HIV infection, which occur primarily in patients with severe immune impairment and CD4+ lymphocyte depletion, KS can occur at almost any stage of HIV infection, but its incidence rises as immune function declines (4–6).

Kaposi's sarcoma in the setting of HIV infection presents several diagnostic and therapeutic challenges that will be discussed in this chapter. Whereas in most instances the diagnosis of cutaneous KS lesions is quite straightforward, atypical skin or subcutaneous lesions sometimes occur, and other pigmented lesions may be confused with KS. On the other hand, the symptoms and radiographic findings of visceral KS lesions are often difficult to distinguish from those of a variety of other neoplastic and infectious diseases, and invasive techniques are often required for their definitive diagnosis. The conventions used to stage KS and the methods used to evaluate the benefits of KS therapy have been evolving over more than a decade, in response to changes in HIV therapy and recognition of deficiencies in standard tumor assessments. The clinical course of KS and the selection of and response to the wide variety of available treatments are strongly influenced by the severity of the underlying HIV infection and its nonneoplastic complications. Finally, the recent discovery of a new human herpesvirus (HHV-8) associated with KS (5–8) may permit the identification of patients at risk for subsequent KS, and allow the development of preventive strategies.

II. EVALUATION OF KAPOSI'S SARCOMA

A. Clinical Features of KS

1. Skin

The skin is the site of initial KS presentation in the vast majority of patients, and a periodic (every 6–12 month) skin examination should be performed in all HIV-infected individuals as a screening procedure. Although KS can, and does, occur any place on the skin surface, lesions on the soles of the feet, between the toes, behind the ears, and in the perirectal and genital areas are quite frequent, although often missed on cursory examination. Other characteristic, but more obvious, sites of involvement include the nose and eyelids. Cutaneous KS lesions that have recently developed may be difficult to recognize, and may appear as small, faint, pink to reddish-violet macules. More typically, however, KS lesions are raised above the skin surface and may develop into frank nodules. In some cases, KS occurs as large, diffusely indurated plaques; this type of presentation is common on the soles of the feet, and may also occur on the legs, particularly the upper medial thighs, often in association with lymphedema. Whereas some patients may present with only a few lesions confined to one, or a few, anatomical sites, in others dozens or even hundreds of widespread lesions may appear concurrently (Fig. 1). Lesion color may be pink, red, purple, or brown (or intermediate shades), and some lesions, particularly those that are rapidly growing, may be surrounded by a yellowish discoloration (a so-called ''halo''). Lesion color typically darkens with time. In black or olive-skinned people, even new lesions often appear dark brown or black. Occasionally, lesions may be subcutaneous, without pigment changes in the overlying skin, or with an overlying ecchymotic appearance.

2. Lymph Nodes

Although lymph node involvement with KS is common and may occur in the absence of KS elsewhere, involved lymph nodes are often only minimally enlarged and are generally soft and nontender. Massive or asymmetrical lymph node involvement sometimes occurs, but is relatively unusual.

3. Edema

Edema is a frequent complication of KS, is usually nonpitting (lymphedema), and most commonly occurs in the lower extremities (Fig. 2), but is not uncommon

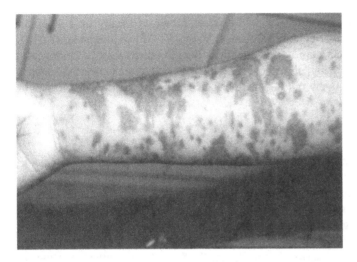

Figure 1   KS lesions on the arm: Multiple lesions are present and are difficult to accurately count. Many of the lesions are irregularly shaped and difficult to measure precisely.

in the periorbital tissues and the external genitalia, and may also affect the upper extremities and chest or abdominal wall. The severity of edema may be disproportionate to the number of skin lesions. Edema generally occurs in the absence of significant proximal lymph node enlargement. The precise cause of KS-associated edema is not known, but it may be a consequence of either KS involvement

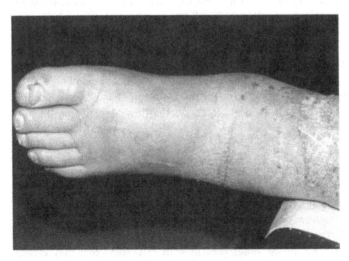

Figure 2   Severe tumor-related edema of the foot in a patient with KS.

of dermal lymphatic vessels, or of cytokines produced locally by KS spindle cells, such as vascular endothelial growth factor (VEGF) or interleukin-1 (IL-1; 9). Extremity edema may be asymmetrical. Severe edema may be complicated by diffuse serous oozing, ulceration, and superinfection, often with gram-negative bacteria. Even relatively mild KS-associated edema is frequently complicated by bacterial cellulitis.

4. Oral Cavity

The oral cavity may be the initial site of presentation of KS in a few patients, but oral KS often occurs in conjunction with KS elsewhere in the body. It has been estimated that about one-third of patients with KS have some oral lesions (10). Oral KS lesions are most common on the hard and soft palate, and are often observed on the gingival margins where they may present as purple plaques or large, grape-like nodules. KS lesions may also be observed on the tongue, the uvula, the posterior pharynx, the tonsils, and the floor of the mouth (11). Although lesions of the hard and soft palate may be flat and asymptomatic, nodular oral lesions may become very large, exophytic, develop ulcerations and bleeding, cause pain, interfere with speech and food intake, and lead to tooth loss or upper airway obstruction.

5. Gastrointestinal Tract

Involvement of the gastrointestinal (GI) tract with KS has been reported in approximately 40% of patients at the time of the initial KS diagnosis, and in up to 80% of patients at autopsy, and may sometimes occur in the absence of cutaneous disease (12–14). KS may occur throughout the gastrointestinal tract, including the esophagus, stomach, duodenum, the small and large intestine, and the anorectum. For many patients (probably the majority), GI tract involvement is asymptomatic. In some patients, however, GI tract KS causes symptoms, which may include abdominal pain, signs of obstruction (e.g., bloating, nausea, and vomiting), and gross or occult GI bleeding. Weight loss may accompany GI KS, but it is rarely an isolated symptom of GI tract involvement. Diarrhea may occur in patients who have GI KS, but whether KS causes diarrhea per se is questionable.

6. Lungs

Pulmonary KS is common, particularly in patients with a long-standing diagnosis of KS in other sites, but occasionally may also be the initial or only site of KS. KS may involve the lung parenchyma, the pleural surfaces, and the bronchial tree. Although asymptomatic pulmonary KS is sometimes diagnosed after evaluation of abnormal chest radiographic findings on routine screening, more commonly patients with KS of the lungs present with symptoms that may include cough, dyspnea, or blood-streaked sputum, occasionally accompanied by chest pain. Gross hemoptysis is uncommon, but may occur with ulcerated endobronchial lesions. These symptoms may occur with or without physical findings, which may include wheezing, decreased breath sounds, and dullness to percussion. Fever sometimes accompanies pulmonary KS in the absence of clear evidence for pulmonary infection, but it is probably most often caused by coexisting bronchial infection.

B. Evaluation by Anatomical Site, Signs, and Symptoms

Table 1 summarizes evaluations for KS.

1. Skin

In addition to a careful examination of the skin surface to document the extent and character of the skin lesions, biopsy of at least one lesion is essential to confirm the diagnosis of KS. Although a diagnosis of KS may appear obvious to the experienced observer, a biopsy is particularly important in patients considering investigational therapy or when atypical lesions are present. A biopsy is particularly important for rapidly growing lesions associated with systemic symptoms (fever, chills, headache, anorexia, and malaise), which may be signs of bacillary angiomatosis (15).

2. Lymph Nodes

Biopsies of small, palpable lymph nodes in patients with confirmed KS are probably not warranted, as lymph node involvement with KS has not been associated with a worse prognosis than disease confined to the skin (16), and moderate lymph node enlargement is a common, but nonspecific finding in HIV-infected individuals. Although KS may completely replace lymphoid tissue, it is more typical for affected lymph nodes to show only focal KS involvement. Massively or asymmetrically enlarged lymph nodes merit biopsy to exclude other infectious or neoplastic conditions.

3. Edema

In the presence of extremity lymphedema, scans (e.g., computed tomography [CT] scans of the pelvis) rarely provide diagnostically or therapeutically useful information. Asymmetrical extremity edema frequently prompts investigation for deep venous thrombosis. In the absence of other signs of thrombosis (e.g., erythema, venous cords, or pain), such tests infrequently yield useful information. Foul-smelling drainage requires culture and empiric broad-spectrum antibiotic coverage. Measurement of limb circumference at fixed anatomical landmarks is

Table 1 Evaluation for Kaposi's Sarcoma

I. Skin/oral cavity
  A. Physical examination: include feet, ears, perianal, genitals, scalp, gingiva
    1. Biopsy suspicious or representative lesion
      a. Histological confirmation of KS
      b. Exclude other skin conditions (e.g., bacillary angiomatosis)
II. Lymph nodes
  A. Enlarged ($\geq$ 2 cm), or asymmetrical, or tender
    1. Consider biopsy to confirm KS and, especially, to rule out NHL or tuberculosis
  B. Small, symmetrical, nontender or nonpalpable
    1. No further evaluation required
III. Gastrointestinal tract
  A. Rectal examination: digital and occult blood
    1. Mass or visible lesion
      a. Colonoscopy and biopsy
        i. Positive biopsy: definitive KS
        ii. Negative biopsy, typical red lesion(s): presumptive KS
    2. Positive stool occult blood test
      a. Colonoscopy ($\pm$ UGI endoscopy): definitive or presumptive KS as above
  B. Signs/symptoms
    1. None
      a. No further GI evaluation
    2. Obstructive signs, pain, bleeding (gross or occult)
      a. Colonoscopy or UGI endoscopy: definitive or presumptive KS as above
IV. Lungs
  A. Chest x-ray films abnormal
    1. Effusion
      a. Diagnostic thoracentesis: cultures, cytology, cell count, chemistry
        i. Serous or serosanguinous exudate: presumptive KS
        ii. Exclude infection (e.g. tuberculosis), NHL
        iii. Evaluate for parenchymal pulmonary KS
    2. Diffuse interstitial or alveolar infiltrates (especially perihilar) or nodules
      a. Bronchoscopy
        i. Red endobronchial lesions: presumptive KS
        ii. No endobronchial lesions
          (1) Transbronchial biopsy: often nondiagnostic
        iii. Bronchial washings/lavage for culture and cytology: rule out infection, other neoplasms
      b. Supplemental tests
        i. Nodiagnostic test
          (1) CT (?MRI): nodules, masses, bronchovascular thickening
          (2) Gallium scan: typically negative in KS

Table 1 Continued

(3) Thallium scan: reportedly positive in KS (?sensitivity, ?specificity)
(4) Pulmonary function tests
(i) $\downarrow$ Diffusing capacity
(ii) $\downarrow$ PO$_2$
(iii) $\downarrow$ FEV$_1$/FVC
ii. Diagnostic
(1) Open or CT-guided biopsy
B. Signs and symptoms (e.g., cough, hemoptysis, dyspnea, wheezing, chest pain)
1. Chest x-ray film
a. Abnormal: proceed as above
b. Normal
i. Sputum (spontaneous or induced) culture; treat infection
ii. Nondiagnostic supplemental tests (e.g., gallium scan, PFTs)
iii. Consider bronchoscopy for unexplained persistent symptoms

useful for following the progress of edema and for assessing the response to treatment.

4. Oral Cavity

A careful examination of the oral cavity, with particular attention to the palate and the gingival margins, often discloses KS, which is frequently first observed during a routine dental examination. When physical examination discloses no evidence of KS elsewhere in the body, a biopsy of an oral lesion may be required to confirm the diagnosis. In patients with proven KS elsewhere, however, the characteristic appearance of oral KS lesions is usually sufficient for presumptive diagnosis.

5. Gastrointestinal Tract

There is no convincing evidence that the presence of asymptomatic GI lesions affects prognosis or mandates treatment modification. Therefore, routine endoscopic evaluations are not currently recommended in asymptomatic individuals, although in the past they were performed as screening tests for many patients who had KS diagnosed in other sites. Rectal examination should be performed on a routine basis and may identify lesions in the anorectal area or disclose occult blood in the stool, which requires evaluation. In addition, formal evaluation of the GI tract is required for clinically apparent signs and symptoms of GI tract KS, such as abdominal pain, signs of obstruction, and gross or occult GI bleeding. Although KS lesions in the GI tract may be discovered during the course of evaluation for diarrhea, other potential causes of diarrhea are often diagnosed, and it is likely that KS is an incidental finding in most such cases.

Endoscopic evaluation is the diagnostic method of choice, together with digital rectal examination to evaluate anorectal lesions. GI lesions are often submucosal and may be small, making contrast radiographic studies of limited usefulness. Upper and lower GI endoscopy allows direct visualization and biopsy of the typical raised, red lesions. Although superficial biopsies of nonulcerated lesions sometimes fail to yield diagnostic tissue, in such cases a presumptive diagnosis of gastrointestinal KS can be made on the basis of the typical lesion appearance in a patient with biopsy-confirmed KS elsewhere in the body.

6. Lungs

In the presence of pleural effusion, thoracentesis is used diagnostically and, sometimes, therapeutically. Pleural involvement with KS is generally a diagnosis of exclusion, after other neoplasms (e.g., lymphomas) or infections that may be associated with effusions have been ruled out with appropriate cytological and microbiological studies. In over 90% of patients with pleural effusions from KS, parenchymal lung disease is also present (17). Pleural effusions associated with KS are typically serous or serosanguinous exudates with nondiagnostic cytological findings; pleural biopsy is generally avoided because of concerns about morbidity (bleeding, pneumothorax) and the poor diagnostic yield (18).

Frequent radiographic findings include pleural effusions, ill-defined nodules, or diffuse interstitial or alveolar infiltrates, the latter often in a predominantly perihilar distribution (Fig. 3). Interstitial infiltrates caused by KS may appear indistinguishable from those associated with *Pneumocystis carinii* pneumonia (PCP). Less commonly, mediastinal or hilar adenopathy, or an isolated pulmonary nodule may be observed (17).

Bronchoscopy is the diagnostic procedure of choice to evaluate unexplained pulmonary symptoms or parenchymal radiographic findings; supplemental but nondiagnostic information may also be gained from scans (CT, gallium, and possibly, thallium and magnetic resonance imaging (MRI)) and pulmonary function testing. Some patients with endobronchial KS may have a normal plain chest radiograph, but symptoms, such as chronic cough, may prompt diagnostic bronchoscopy.

Figure 3   Chest x-ray films of a patient with pulmonary KS: (A) before therapy; note diffuse increase in interstitial markings and patchy, ill-defined nodular infiltrates; (B) after eight cycles of paclitaxel at a dose of 135 mg/m^2 every 3 weeks. Reticulonodular densities are still present, but considerable improvement has occurred.

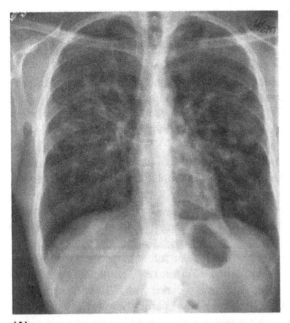

(A)

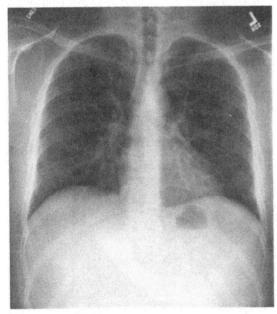

(B)

Endobronchial KS can generally be visualized as red, slightly raised or flat lesions, and a presumptive diagnosis of KS is usually made on this basis. Endobronchial lesions are most commonly observed at branching points or carinas of the lower airways, but are sometimes present in the trachea (17). When endobronchial lesions are absent, however, a diagnosis of pulmonary KS may be more difficult, because transbronchial biopsy often fails to yield diagnostic tissue (18).

In the absence of typical endobronchial lesions or a tissue diagnosis, gallium–thallium scanning has been suggested (19), KS having been described as gallium-negative and thallium-avid, and the reverse pattern holding for most infectious or inflammatory causes of similar radiographic abnormalities. In practice, few physicians use thallium scanning. However a negative gallium scan in a patient with proved KS, a negative bronchoscopy (for both KS and infection), and compatible radiographs may permit a presumptive diagnosis of pulmonary KS.

Typical CT scan findings (Fig. 4) include nodules, masses, and bronchovascular thickening, with or without pleural effusion (20); preliminary studies of MRI have suggested characteristic patterns associated with KS, but these findings require confirmation (21). A CT scan may be of particular value in monitoring the response to treatment in patients with poorly defined lesions on plain radiographs. In some patients in whom the diagnosis was in question, open-lung biopsy or transthoracic CT-guided needle biopsy have been used to distinguish pulmo-

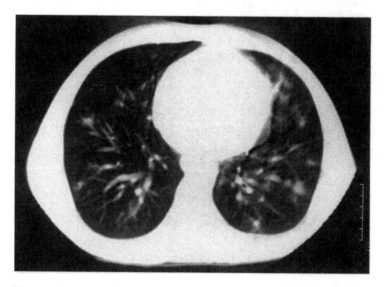

Figure 4 Chest CT image of a patient with pulmonary KS. Note peribronchial thickening and multiple, ill-defined nodular infiltrates.

nary KS from other neoplasms or infectious diseases. It should be remembered that KS and pulmonary infection may be present concurrently, together with symptoms and radiographic findings of both processes. Although pulmonary function tests may be useful in monitoring the response to treatment, they are not specific enough to be used diagnostically. Patients with pulmonary KS typically show a reduced diffusing capacity. In the presence of endobronchial disease, there is also often a reduced forced expiratory volume in 1 sec over forced vital capacity ratio (FEV_1/FVC; 17).

C. Laboratory Evaluation

There are no specific, established laboratory tests for evaluating patients with AIDS-associated KS save for diagnostic biopsies. The standard laboratory evaluation includes an assessment of immune function (CD4+ T-lymphocyte count) and HIV viral load, which are generally performed every 3–4 months for routine HIV monitoring, but may be required more frequently if changes in KS (or HIV) therapy are contemplated. The role of human herpesvirus 8 (HHV-8; KSHV) monitoring is not yet established in patients with a confirmed KS diagnosis, but it is conceivable that quantitative measurement of HHV-8 viral load may some day prove useful in monitoring the course of the disease and its response to treatment. In the near future, however, it is likely that serological assays to detect infection with HHV-8 will be used to identify patients at high risk for subsequent KS development. Such tests may be used to identify patients who require more careful and frequent screening for KS, and to select subjects who might benefit from KS prevention strategies. HHV-8 infection is probably a prerequisite for KS development, as the virus is almost invariably found in KS lesions, but patients with KS are not always seropositive for antibodies to the virus and HHV-8 DNA is not invariably detected in the peripheral blood mononuclear cells of affected patients (5–7). In addition, some individuals considered to be at low risk for the development of KS show serological evidence for HHV-8 infection (6,7). Thus, the specificity and sensitivity of assays for HHV-8 infection need to be refined, and cofactors that increase the risk of developing KS need to be identified.

Additional laboratory tests are geared to the type of therapy being contemplated for patients with KS. These include a complete blood count and white blood cell count differential in all patients in whom chemotherapy or interferon alfa (IFN-α) therapy is being considered, liver function tests in patients for whom interferon alfa, anthracycline, or vinca alkaloid therapy is under consideration, and tests to ensure adequate renal function in patients for whom bleomycin therapy is a consideration. Patients with a history of cardiac disease, or those who have received prior therapy with anthracyclines, should have cardiac ejection fraction (EF) tested before treatment with liposomal anthracyclines; a minimum EF of 50% is the standard for such treatment. The carbon monoxide diffusion capacity (DLco) should probably be tested before treatment with bleomycin; a value of at least 70% of predicted is generally considered safe. As part of the physical examination, patients in whom treatment with vinca alkaloids, etoposide, or paclitaxel is considered should be specifically assessed for signs and symptoms of distal sensory peripheral neuropathy.

III. PROGNOSTIC FACTORS AND STAGING

Multiple KS lesions often appear concurrently in anatomically separated areas of the body, without a defined "primary" lesion that subsequently spreads to regional and distant sites. A standard tumor–node–metastasis (TNM) classification is, therefore, not appropriate for classification of the tumor. Several staging systems have been proposed for KS. The most frequently applied classification was proposed in 1989 by the AIDS Clinical Trials Group (ACTG; 22). This staging system divided patients into good- or poor-risk groups according to extent of tumor (T), immune system status measured by CD4+ T-lymphocyte count (I), and severity of systemic HIV-associated illness (S). A subsequent prospective analysis of 294 patients entered into ACTG therapeutic trials for KS between 1989 and 1995 showed that each of the TIS variables was independently associated with survival (23). Multivariate analysis showed that immune system impairment was the most important single predictor of survival, but tumor stage added to its predictive value in patients with relatively high CD4+ T-lymphocyte counts (23). A CD4 cell count cutpoint of 150/μL provided better discrimination between prognostic groups than the previously proposed cutpoint of 200/μL. A revised staging system for KS suggested by this analysis is shown in Table 2. A study is in development to determine if viral load measurements add predictive information to this staging system. Although in this analysis the presence of

Table 2 Proposed Revised Staging System for AIDS-Associated Kaposi's Sarcoma

Stage	CD4 count	Tumor risk group	Median survival (mo)
I	≥ 150/μL (I_0)	Good (T_0): KS confined to skin, lymph nodes, or flat palate lesions; no tumor-associated edema or visceral KS.	NR[a]
II	≥ 150/μL (I_0)	Poor (T_1): Any visceral KS, nodular oral KS or tumor-associated edema.	35
III	< 150/μL (I_1)	Any	13

[a] NR, median not reached
Source: Ref. 23.

symptoms of HIV-associated illness (S) did not add significant prognostic information to the CD4 count (I) and tumor stage (T), the presence of HIV-associated signs and symptoms is a factor in the choice of therapy.

In an earlier analysis (24), tumor burden was not associated with survival. There were, however, distinct survival distributions for KS patients, depending on their history of opportunistic infection (OI), CD4+ count, and the presence of systemic HIV-associated symptoms. Median survivals were 31,20,15, and 7 months, respectively, for patients with (1) no prior OI and CD4 $\geq$ 300/μL; (2) no prior OI, no systemic symptoms, and CD4 < 300/μL; (3) systemic symptoms, but no prior OI; and (4) prior OI.

A retrospective study (25) of 688 patients with KS diagnosed between 1981 and 1990 identified four baseline variables that correlated best with survival: CD4+ T-lymphocyte count, hematocrit, number of KS lesions, and body mass index. When survival was adjusted for these factors, a time-dependent decrease in mortality was observed (25), corresponding to improvements in survival observed during this period among other patients with AIDS. At the same time, however, the median CD4 cell count at the time of KS presentation fell, from 161/μL in 1981–1983, to 100/μL in 1986, and to 56/μL in 1988–1990, so crude survival did not improve with time.

It is important to note that none of the studies cited was conducted at a time when highly active antiretroviral regimens were available. It will require considerable time to determine the specific effect of such therapy on survival in KS patients. Even less information exists about the factors predicting response to KS therapy. With the exception of interferon alfa trials (see Section IV.C.3), in which the range of CD4+ T-lymphocyte counts was wide and in which pretreatment CD4+ counts were associated with the probability of tumor regression, most large therapeutic trials of chemotherapy have been performed in patients with homogeneously low CD4+ counts. Tumor stage or location has also not been clearly associated with response, although the results of some studies have suggested lower response rates in patients with pulmonary KS. It remains to be seen whether other factors, such as control of HIV viral burden, or the HHV-8 viral burden, will permit better prediction of therapeutic outcome in the future.

IV. MANAGEMENT AND THERAPY

A. Management of Underlying HIV Disease

Delivery of optimal antiretroviral therapy for the stage of HIV infection, prophylaxis for OIs, and prompt recognition and treatment of intercurrent infections are essential components of a successful KS management strategy. KS progression is influenced by inflammatory cytokines (9,26), the production of which is increased in the setting of acute OIs and unchecked HIV replication, and may also be stimulated by the HIV Tat protein, which acts synergistically with autocrine and paracrine growth factors to stimulate KS cell growth in vitro (27,28). The observation that KS sometimes regresses after initiation of protease inhibitor-containing antiretroviral regimens suggests that, in some cases, reversal of immunosuppression and control of HIV replication may be sufficient to control KS. Therefore, modification of the antiviral regimen to achieve viral load suppression should be considered in all patients presenting with KS who show a high viral load; in patients with relatively low tumor burden and the absence of symptomatic lesions, a trial period of antiretroviral therapy can be considered before specific anti-KS therapy is instituted. It must be cautioned, however, that the potential exists for adverse interactions between drugs used to treat HIV infection and specific therapies directed against KS. Sudden progression of KS occurs frequently in the setting of acute OIs, so prevention of such infections is important. In addition, the occurrence of intercurrent infections often leads to interruptions in KS therapy, during which lesions may progress.

B. Assessment of Response to Therapy

Accurate assessment of tumor response during treatment for KS has proved difficult. Standard criteria for evaluating response of other solid tumors generally rely on defined changes in the products of bidimensionally measured lesion diameters, which are commonly measured on radiographs or scans and subject to independent confirmation. In contrast, the KS lesions most accessible for response evaluation are usually on the skin (see Fig. 1). Often, when an elevated or frankly nodular KS lesion decreases in volume, it becomes flat and sometimes shows central clearing, but there is usually measurable residual pigment and the product of the two-dimensional diameters of the lesion may not decrease by 50%. KS-specific response criteria, proposed in 1989 (22), included lesion flattening, in addition to defined changes in the total number of lesions and measured diameters of selected indicator lesions, as criteria for response. These evaluation criteria have been applied with varying rigor, however, and many earlier studies were conducted using other, sometimes poorly defined, response criteria that make assessment of reported response rates difficult and direct comparisons between studies unreliable.

Additional problems have arisen because rigorous quantitative response criteria were not established for mucosal or viceral KS or for KS-associated edema. KS in these sites is also often difficult to measure: edema may wax and wane with walking or leg elevation; oral lesions may be irregularly shaped and lack distinct margins; gastrointestinal lesions usually require endoscopy for serial assessment; and chest radiographs or scans often show ill-defined infiltrates.

Moreover, because survival in most HIV-infected patients with KS is more strongly influenced by the course of the underlying HIV infection than by the outcome of KS treatment, assessments of clinical benefit are needed to fully evaluate the value of treatment-induced tumor regression. This has led to an ongoing collaborative effort between the U.S. Food and Drug Administration (FDA), the National Cancer Institute (NCI), and the AIDS Malignancy Consortium to develop more rigorously defined tumor response criteria that will be supplemented by quantitative scales of clinical benefit (e.g., pain relief and functional assessments) that can be correlated with objective changes in tumor burden (29).

C. Standard Therapies

1. Local Therapy

Several treatments can achieve local control of individual KS lesions. The most commonly used conventional approaches are liquid nitrogen cryotherapy (30) and intralesional injections of vinblastine (31). In addition, several other locally injected agents have been tested in small clinical trials and induced KS regression. These include recombinant interferon alfa (IFN-α; 32), recombinant granulocyte–macrophage colony-stimulating factor (GM–CSF; 33), recombinant platelet factor 4 (34), and human chorionic gonadotropin (hCG; 35), but the data supporting their superiority over the more commonly used local agents are scant. One exception may be hCG, which has been reported to induce apoptotic death of KS spindle cells (35). The available data suggest, however, that the active moiety in hCG is not the intact hormone, but rather, a breakdown product that is not uniformly present in all hCG preparations.

Local approaches to lesion control may be most appropriate in patients with slowly progressing cutaneous KS who have relatively few, small lesions, or in patients with contraindications to available systemic therapies who desire control of certain lesions for cosmetic reasons. In addition, local injections of both vinblastine and the sclerosing agent, sotradecol (36), have been reported to induce local regression of oral KS lesions. Local treatments induce minimal or no systemic side effects and can often be completed over a short time, yielding acceptable cosmetic results in many patients. It must be recognized, however, that the benefits of local treatment are confined to the treated lesions. Lesions may recur at treated sites, and treatment may be complicated by pain, local eschar formation, and residual hyper- or hypopigmentation. Occasionally, surgical removal of isolated lesions, for example pedunculated lesions on the toes that interfere with walking and wearing shoes, may be appropriate.

2. Radiation Therapy

Radiation therapy (RT) has often been used to treat localized areas of KS involvement of the skin and oral cavity, and less frequently to control pulmonary, GI, or other sites of KS lesions. Although it is beyond the scope of this chapter to give full details of the technical aspects of radiation to different sites of KS involvement, several generalizations can be offered.

For cutaneous KS lesions, the type of RT should be individualized based on the intent of treatment and the overall health status of the patient. A prospectively randomized trial (37) compared the results of treatment of individual lesions with 6-MeV electrons, given either as 800 cGy in one fraction (a frequently recommended regimen; 38), 2000 cGy in ten fractions over 2 weeks, or 4000 cGy in 20 fractions over 4 weeks to fields that included the palpable tumor with a 2-cm margin. Complete resolution of the palpable lesion was significantly better for the fractionated (2000-cGy or 4000-cGy) regimens (79 and 83%, respectively) than for the single-dose (800 cGy) regimen (50%), and complete resolution of residual pigmentation was significantly better for the 4000-cGy regimen (43%) than for either 2000- or 800-cGy regimens (8% each). In addition, the 4000-cGy regimen led to a significantly longer median duration of lesion control before regrowth (43 weeks) than the 2000-cGy (26 weeks) or 800-cGy (13 weeks) regimens. Although acute toxicity was somewhat higher in the 4000-cGy–treated lesions, this did not exceed mild erythema, dry desquamation, local alopecia, and hyperpigmentation. However, the 4000-cGy regimen was reported, in one patient, to be associated with a subsequent radiation recall reaction (i.e., recurrence of acute toxicity in a previously quiescent radiation field) when bleomycin was administered, whereas no recall reaction occurred in other lesions in the same patient who had been treated with 800 or 2000 cGy (39).

These data suggest that if cosmetic improvement is the primary aim of therapy, a 4000-cGy regimen over a protracted course is optimal. However, for lesions that are of lesser cosmetic importance (e.g., on unexposed body parts) or for treatment of lesions in very ill or symptomatic patients with limited mobility or a short overall life expectancy, a more rapid fractionation regimen may produce acceptable local results and may be more compatible with immediate quality-of-life concerns than a regimen that requires repeated treatment visits over many weeks. In addition, in patients who are likely to need subsequent systemic chemotherapy for control of disseminated KS, the more rapid fractionation regimens may offer a lower risk of recall reactions.

For treatment of diffusely involved extremities, with or without edema, larger fields requiring penetrating photons are generally required. Chak et al. (40) described intense skin erythema, pain, and desquamation of skin on the sole of the foot in five of seven patients who received 2000 cGy to the feet over 2 weeks. Berson et al. (38), however, used a single 800-cGy fraction to treat KS of the foot, and by virtue of the low total dose induced a lower incidence of high-grade local reactions. Lower doses per fraction and a planned rest period may allow delivery of higher total doses without severe acute reactions, and may avoid later radiation-induced edema from subcutaneous fibrosis (K. Stelzer, personal communication). Although reduction in edema often occurs with RT, resolution of edema is rarely complete (38,40).

Oral KS has also been treated successfully with RT. Patients with HIV infection have been noted, however, to sometimes have unusual or idiosyncratic sensitivity of normal tissues to RT. Oral radiation in patients with AIDS-associated KS using 4-MeV photons at 180 cGy daily for 9 days (total, 1620 cGy) was reported (40) to be associated with severe mucositis, mouth dryness, and altered sense of taste, which was decreased, but not eliminated, by lowering the total dose to 1400 cGy. Similarly, a high incidence of severe mucositis was reported (38) when the oropharynx was treated with high-dose fractions (180–400 cGy) to total doses of 2000–2400 cGy. Mucositis was decreased significantly by using 150-cGy fractions to a total dose of 1500 cGy (38). Stelzer (personal communication) has advocated using 150-cGy fractions, 5 days a week for ten doses, to the oral cavity, followed by a 1-week–scheduled break in therapy to reduce the risk of mucositis. Patients are then given as many as five additional fractions, depending on tolerance. Tumor shrinkage is rapid with oral RT, and may be most appropriate in cases where very rapid relief of symptoms from bulky lesions is required. However, systemic therapy (e.g., chemotherapy, and in some cases, interferon therapy) is also effective for many patients with oral KS, so the decision between local RT or systemic therapy may depend on whether or not extraoral indications for systemic KS treatment coexist with the oral disease.

Radiation therapy has also been used occasionally in selected patients with lung or GI KS. Berson et al. (38) reported responses in 88% of patients treated with involved field photons to GI lesions, which were mainly located in the anorectum; relief of obstructive symptoms in two preterminal patients with upper GI lesions was also described. Both Berson et al. (38) and Meyer (41) have described rapid subjective improvement in patients with pulmonary KS who received whole-lung radiation, generally in 150-cGy fractions to total doses between 900 and 1500 cGy. In addition, Meyer (41) reported a significant reduction in hemoptysis and the requirement for supplemental oxygen, although only 28% of patients with radiographic abnormalities showed a 50% or greater reduction in measurable lesions.

3. Interferon Therapy

Interferons are multifunctional cytokines with a variety of effects on cell growth and function as well as antiviral effects that may influence the complex processes involved in the growth of KS (9,42). Recombinant interferons $\alpha 2a$ (Roferon-A) and $\alpha 2b$ (Intron-A) are both FDA approved for the treatment of certain patients with AIDS-associated KS. Approval of these agents was obtained on the basis of studies performed in the early- and mid-1980s, before the development of active antiretroviral drugs. Thus, the approved (i.e., labeled) doses are based on single-agent studies, which generally demonstrated a requirement for very high interferon (IFN) doses (e.g., 36 million U daily, or 30 million U/m^2 three times a week). In studies of high-dose IFN monotherapy, objective tumor regression was documented in approximately 30% of patients overall. Responses were usually observed in patients with CD4+ lymphocyte counts of 200/μL or more, who had no history of opportunistic infection, and who lacked other signs and symptoms of advanced HIV infection. In these good-risk patients, tumor regression was observed even in some patients who had extensive cutaneous, oral or gastrointestinal KS (43). Median response durations were 6–12 months for partial responders and up to 2 years for those showing a complete response. High-dose IFN monotherapy was also often complicated by fatigue, malaise, anorexia, and hepatotoxicity.

High-dose IFN monotherapy is rarely used today. Instead, IFN is now generally used to treat KS in combination with other agents used to treat HIV infection. When IFN was combined with chemotherapy, responses were poor from the standpoint of both efficacy and tolerance (44–46). However results superior to those obtained with IFN monotherapy were obtained when IFN-α was combined, at lower doses than those used for monotherapy, with nucleoside reverse transcriptase inhibitors. The results of several phase I studies of combined IFN-α and zidovudine demonstrated KS response rates exceeding 40% in patients treated with IFN-α doses ranging from 4 to 18 million IU/day (47–49), and the high response rates were confirmed in a phase II trial of the combination, which used a daily IFN dose of 18 million IU and a zidovudine dose of 100 mg every 4 h (50). Significantly, the IFN-α and zidovudine combination induced KS regression in 25–30% of patients with CD4+ lymphocyte counts of fewer than 200/μL (47,50), whereas less than 10% of such patients responded to high-dose IFN-α monotherapy (51).

A high rate of dose-limiting neutropenia was observed with the combination of IFN-α and zidovudine, and some patients developed hepatotoxicity, particularly at the higher IFN doses (47–50). Although neutropenia could be prevented or reversed by administration of GM-CSF (52,53), the development of less myelosuppressive nucleoside reverse transcriptase inhibitors led to a trial of IFN-α with didanosine. In this trial, which is undergoing analysis, patients have been randomly assigned to receive either 1 million or 10 million IU/day of IFN-α together with standard doses of didanosine. Although the final results of this trial are not available, objective tumor regression has been observed in some patients in each dosage group, and significant hematological toxicity has been uncommon.

With the development of more powerful antiretroviral drug combinations, a new phase I study was initiated by the NCI-sponsored AIDS Malignancy Consortium to evaluate the combination of recombinant IFN-α2b with protease inhibitor-containing combination antiretroviral regimens. One objective of the study is to evaluate the pharmacological interactions of these agents, for IFNs may inhibit hepatic cytochrome P-450 enzymes involved in the metabolism of protease inhibitors (54).

The response to IFN-α, whether as monotherapy or as part of combinations with antiretroviral therapy, tends to occur slowly. Maximal responses are generally achieved after 6 or more months of treatment. Thus, despite documented activity in some patients with visceral disease, IFN probably should not be considered for treatment of patients with very rapidly progressive, symptomatic KS, particularly those with symptomatic visceral (i.e., lung or GI tract) involvement. For patients with less aggressive mucocutaneous or asymptomatic GI disease in whom rapid relief of symptoms is not required, however, IFN therapy should be considered, particularly because responses may persist for several years.

4. Chemotherapy

Systemic chemotherapy is indicated for patients with KS who have extensive or rapidly progressive lesions that cause medical or functional impairment. The major goals of therapy are to induce durable regression of disfiguring or disabling skin lesions, to control life-threatening or symptomatic visceral KS, and to reduce functional impairments caused by KS lesions or tumor-associated edema. Although a wide variety of single- and combination-drug regimens have activity against KS, current usage favors one of the liposomal anthracyclines as the initial chemotherapeutic agents of choice. For second-line therapy, most investigators agree that paclitaxel is the most active available agent. However, other active single agents or drug combinations maybe used in certain circumstances, for example, third-line chemotherapy or when one desires to avoid specific adverse reactions associated with liposomal anthracyclines or paclitaxel.

Single Agent Chemotherapy. Etoposide was one of the first drugs to be tested for activity in AIDS-associated KS. With an intravenous dose of 150 mg/m^2 per day for 3 consecutive days, every 4 weeks, Laubenstein et al. (55) described a response rate of 76%. Another study, which used the same dose, schedule, and route of etoposide, described no objective responses (56), however, although the patients in both studies had similar characteristics, including limited KS and no prior treatment. In a more recent phase I study, a single oral weekly dose of etoposide was evaluated over a dose range of 150–400 mg/week (57). In 25 evaluable patients, many of whom had advanced or previously treated KS, a response rate of 36% was reported and responses lasted a median of 20 weeks; objective tumor regression was observed across the full range of doses tested (57). In another study of orally administered etoposide, a daily dose of 25 mg/m^2 twice daily for 7 consecutive days, every 2 weeks induced a response rate of 32% in patients who had received no prior chemotherapy (58), and a third study, in which oral etoposide was administered at a dose of 50 mg daily for 21 days, yielded a response rate of 21% (59). In a single study of another topoisomerase II inhibitor, teniposide, administered at a dose of 360 mg/m^2 intravenously every 3 weeks, an objective tumor response rate of 40% was reported (60), with a median duration of 9 weeks and frequent leukopenia and thrombocytopenia.

Several vinca alkaloids have also shown activity against KS. Vinblastine administered at a dose of 4 mg weekly, with weekly increments of 2 mg, as tolerated, induced a response in 30% of patients, at a median weekly tolerated dose of 6 mg (61). The major toxicity of vinblastine was neutropenia. Vincristine, at a weekly dose of 2 mg for the first 2–5 weeks, and then every 2 weeks, induced partial responses in 61% of patients, and reversed thrombocytopenia in several patients (62), but was associated with frequent peripheral neuropathy. A preliminary report described the use of vinorelbine, a semisynthetic vinca alkaloid, at a dose of 30 mg/m^2 every 2 weeks. An overall response rate of 44% was achieved, with 11% complete and 33% partial responses. Of note, all patients had previously received vincristine. Although grade 3 or 4 neutropenia occurred in about half the patients, it was controlled with G-CSF, and no patient experienced peripheral neuropathy (63).

Several routes and schedules of bleomycin administration have also been reported to induce KS regression. In one study, intramuscular bleomycin at a dose of 5 mg/day for 3 days every 3 weeks was reported to have induced a response in 71% of patients (64). As a continuous intravenous infusion, bleomycin induced a 48% response rate in patients treated at a dose of 6 mg/m^2 per day for 4 days every 4 weeks (65), and a 65% response rate in patients treated at a dose of 20 mg/m^2 per day for 3 days every 3 weeks (66). Bleomycin treatment has sometimes been associated with cutaneous toxicity and Raynaud's phenomenon, which occasionally progresses to digital necrosis.

Anthracyclines, including doxorubicin and liposomally encapsulated formulations of both doxorubicin and daunorubicin, also have activity against KS. At a weekly dose of 15 mg/m^2, doxorubicin was reported to induce an objective response rate of only 10%, which was associated with dose-limiting neutropenia in 18% of patients (67). However, this study used standard oncological criteria that excluded flattening of nodular skin lesions as an indicator of tumor response. In another study that used KS-specific response criteria, doxorubicin at a dose of 20 mg/m^2 every 2 weeks induced a response rate of 48% (68). In a separate study evaluating the same dose and schedule of doxorubicin in patients with pulmonary KS, however, only a 14% response rate was demonstrated (69).

The first chemotherapeutic agents approved by the U.S. FDA specifically for treatment of KS were liposomal doxorubicin (Doxil) and liposomal daunorubicin (DaunoXome); these are now considered by most experts in the field to be the initial therapies of choice in KS patients who require chemotherapy. Liposomal encapsulation prolongs the circulating half-life of the anthracyclines (measured in hours, compared with minutes for the unencapsulated drugs), leads to much higher drug concentrations within tumor tissue, and modifies the toxicity profile (70–72). Although neutropenia is frequently induced by these agents (73–76), alopecia, nausea, and vomiting, which are common after administration of free anthracyclines, are uncommon with the liposomal preparations (74,77,78). Anthracycline-induced cardiac toxicity has been observed rarely after administration of high cumulative doses to patients with KS (71,79,80), but maximum safe cumulative doses have not been defined. Treatment with Doxil, which consists of doxorubicin enclosed within a polyethylene glycol-coated liposome that markedly increases drug circulation time, has sometimes been associated with the hand–foot syndrome (81), possibly by simulating a continuous drug infusion, and both Doxil and DaunoXome administration have, on occasion, been complicated by acute infusional reactions characterized by back pain, a sensation of choking, and intense flushing (82). The latter reaction usually occurs within minutes of starting treatment and generally subsides quickly after stopping the drug infusion.

The recommended dose and treatment schedule for Doxil is 20 mg/m^2 as a slow (30- to 60-min) intravenous infusion every 3 weeks. For DaunoXome, the approved dose is 40 mg/m^2 every 2 weeks, but escalation to 60 mg/m^2 has sometimes induced responses in patients who did not respond, or who relapsed, after treatment at the lower dose. Reported objective response rates with these agents have varied tremendously. Although some initial reports, often of single-center studies in relatively small numbers of patients, suggested that response rates might be as high as 70–90% (71,73,75,83–87) even in previously treated patients, some multicenter trials that strictly applied response criteria have documented response rates of only 25–43% (74,76,88). It is likely that the percentage of patients in whom palliation of KS lesions and associated symptoms is achieved falls somewhere between these extremes. Significantly, the lesions of some patients whose tumors had progressed on regimens containing unencapsulated doxorubicin responded subsequently to one of the liposomal anthracyclines.

More recently, several studies which showed that paclitaxel is also an active agent for treatment of KS (see Fig. 3) led, in 1997, to FDA approval of this agent for second-line therapy. Paclitaxel, a mitotic spindle poison, promotes microtubulin formation (89), leading to mitotic arrest (90). In addition, paclitaxel inhibits cell chemotaxis and invasion induced by angiogenic factors (91) and induces *bcl-2* phosphorylation and apoptosis in hormone resistant, *bcl-2*-positive, prostate cancer cells (92). Pertinently, HHV-8 encodes a homologue of cellular *bcl-2*, and both viral and cellular *bcl-2* mRNAs have been identified in KS biopsies (93). Two studies using different doses and schedules of paclitaxel administration, but almost identical dose intensity, have been performed in patients with advanced KS, many of whom had visceral disease and KS-associated edema (94,95). Most patients had previously received treatment for KS, had very low CD4+ T-lymphocyte counts (median $\leq 20/\mu L$), and had symptomatic KS lesions. Using dosing regimens of either 135 mg/m^2 every 3 weeks, or 100 mg/m^2 every 2 weeks, both administered as 3-h infusions, objective response rates of 69 and 59% were documented in a total of 85 patients, with median response durations of 7–10 months. Lesion regression was accompanied by improvements in KS-associated edema, pain, and performance status, but treatment was complicated by significant myalgias, neutropenia, and alopecia in a high proportion of patients. Acute hypersensitivity reactions to paclitaxel have not been observed in immunosuppressed patients with AIDS-associated KS who were given standard dexamethasone, diphenhydramine, and cimetidine (or ranitidine) pretreatment. A randomized phase III trial is in progress that will compare the efficacy, toxicity, and clinical benefits of paclitaxel and liposomal doxorubicin (Doxil) as first-line therapy for KS.

Combination Chemotherapy. Before the development and approval of liposomal anthracyclines, the general consensus was that combination chemotherapy regimens induced higher objective response rates than single agents, but with few exceptions, this was not prospectively tested. A weekly regimen of vinblastine 0.1 mg/kg alternating with vincristine 2 mg was reported to induce a response rate of 43% (96); the alternating schedule was intended to minimize vinblastine-associated neutropenia and vincristine-associated neuropathy. Several variations of a bleomycin and vincristine combination induced relatively little myelosuppression and alopecia. In one such study (97), bleomycin was given at a dose of 30 mg with vincristine at a dose of 2 mg, every 3–4 weeks. Vinblastine at a dose of 2.5–5 mg was substituted for vincristine if neuropathy developed. A partial response rate of 57% was reported, and 28% of patients developed neuropathy (97). A more commonly used regimen has combined bleomycin 10 U/m^2 with vincristine at a dose of 1–2 mg, every 2 weeks. This regimen reportedly induced a 72% response rate in a single, small trial (98). A similar response rate (64%) was reported for a regimen of bleomycin (15 mg/m^2) and vincristine (1.4 mg/m^2) every 2 weeks for a total of six cycles (99), with a mean response duration of 86 days. However, a response rate of only 23% was reported for a combination of bleomycin (15 U/m^2) and vincristine (2 mg) every 3 weeks (100); it is unclear whether the lower response rate in this study can be explained by the less frequent dosing schedule (every 3 weeks, rather than every 2 weeks) or a more rigorous application of response criteria. Bleomycin-containing regimens often induce fever, chills, nausea, and vomiting, which can generally be ameliorated or prevented by premedication with dexamethasone. However, there is concern about the potential of corticosteroids to stimulate the growth of KS and some clinicians advise omitting dexamethasone premedication, whereas others routinely use it.

Laubenstein et al. (55) reported a 90% response rate using doxorubicin, 40 mg/m^2 on day 1; vinblastine, 6 mg/m^2 on day 1; and bleomycin, 15 U on days

1 and 15, every 28 days. Building on this regimen, Gelmann et al. (101) described a 72% response rate with a regimen of doxorubicin 20 mg/m^2, vinblastine 4 mg/m^2, and bleomycin 15 U/m^2 on day 1; actinomycin D 1 mg/m^2, vincristine 1.4 mg/m^2, and dacarbazine 375 mg/m^2 on day 8, and bleomycin 15 U/m^2 on day 15, every 28 days. Response durations were short, however, and the frequency of opportunistic infection was high. A similar intensive regimen (102) in patients with pulmonary KS also induced a high response rate (82%), but despite concomitant use of antiretroviral therapy, *P. carinii* prophylaxis, and G-CSF support, responses persisted only 2–3 months.

The regimen that has been the most frequent subject of published reports is a combination of doxorubicin, bleomycin, and vincristine (ABV). A regimen combining doxorubicin 20 mg/m^2, bleomycin 10 U/m^2, and vincristine 1.4 mg/m^2 (maximum 2 mg) was originally reported (68) to induce an overall response rate of 88%, and in a separate study in patients with pulmonary KS, to induce a response rate of 80% (69). Both were randomized trials that compared ABV to doxorubicin alone; the single agent induced responses in 48% and 14% of patients, respectively (68,69). Other ABV regimens using both higher and lower doxorubicin doses have been described. These include a study that demonstrated a 64% partial response rate in patients with pulmonary KS who received doxorubicin 30 mg/m^2, bleomycin 10 U/m^2, and vincristine 2 mg every 4 weeks (103), and another small trial, in which a 90% response rate was reported in patients treated with an ABV regimen that included a doxorubicin dose of only 10 mg/m^2 every 2 weeks (104).

Many of the earliest studies of chemotherapy for KS were performed without the concomitant use of antiretroviral therapy, and before the routine use of *P. carinii* prophylaxis, or the availability of hematopoietic colony-stimulating factors. As the use of these agents became more routine, and as the types of available antiretroviral therapy increased, several combination studies were conducted. In one such study, successive patient cohorts received bleomycin 10 U/m^2, vincristine 1.4 mg/m^2 (maximum 2 mg), and doxorubicin (either 0, 10, or 15 mg/m^2) every 2 weeks with zidovudine 100 mg every 4 h and standard *P. carinii* prophylaxis, without concomitant use of hematopoietic colony-stimulating factors (105). The maximum tolerated doxorubicin dose was 10 mg/m^2, and an overall response rate of 71% was observed, along with a lower incidence of opportunistic infections than observed historically when similar chemotherapy was administered in the absence of zidovudine and *P. carinii* prophylaxis (105). Although higher doxorubicin doses were tolerated with zidovudine when recombinant GM–CSF was used either to treat or prevent neutropenia (106,107), these studies did not show superior response rates or survival duration. The ABV regimen, with a doxorubicin dose of 20 mg/m^2, has also been tested with nucleoside analogues that are less myelotoxic than zidovudine, but that are more likely to be associated with peripheral neuropathy. In a randomized trial, patients with advanced KS who had not received prior chemotherapy received ABV with either didanosine or zalcitabine. Respective response rates of 58 and 60% were observed, and the incidence of peripheral neuropathy and opportunistic infection was low (108).

Recently, the results of several randomized studies were reported in which liposomal anthracyclines were compared prospectively with conventional combination chemotherapy regimens. A study that compared Doxil, 20 mg/m^2, with ABV (at a doxorubicin dose of 20 mg/m^2 every 2 weeks, yielded a significantly higher response rate (43%) for Doxil than for ABV (25%) (76). A comparison of DaunoXome, 40 mg/m^2, with ABV (at a doxorubicin dose of 10 mg/m^2) every 2 weeks, yielded equivalent response rates of 25 and 28%, respectively (74). A third study compared Doxil, 20 mg/m^2, with the combination of bleomycin (15 U/m^2) and vincristine (2 mg), each regimen given every 3 weeks; this study also demonstrated a significantly higher response rate among patients who received Doxil (59%) than among those who received bleomycin and vincristine (23%) (100). In each study, patients who received the liposomal anthracycline showed a significantly lower incidence of peripheral neuropathy and nausea and vomiting than those who received combination therapy that included vincristine. Doxil induced more neutropenia than bleomycin and vincristine, and more mucositis than ABV, but was less likely than ABV to cause significant alopecia and severe neutropenia. An unexplained observation is that the response rates documented in each of these randomized trials were considerably lower than those reported previously for both the liposomal anthracyclines (in uncontrolled trials), and for the standard combination regimens (in both single-arm and randomized studies).

To determine if Doxil might be more effective as part of a combination chemotherapy regimen, a randomized multicenter trial was conducted by the AIDS Clinical Trials Group to compare biweekly Doxil alone (at a dose of 20 mg/m^2) and Doxil (at the same dose and schedule) in combination with bleomycin (10 U/m^2) and vincristine (1 mg) in patients with advanced KS who had received no prior chemotherapy. The two regimens induced almost identical response rates of similar duration, but the combination regimen proved significantly more toxic than Doxil alone and was associated with a more rapid decline in quality of life (109).

5.   Monitoring During Systemic Therapy

Patients require frequent laboratory monitoring for toxicity during systemic therapy with IFN-α or chemotherapy. A complete blood count with white blood cell differential is required immediately before each chemotherapy cycle, and at least monthly during IFN-α therapy. More frequent blood counts may be required during the first few weeks of IFN-α therapy, and 7–14 days after chemotherapy, to assess the need for hematopoietic growth factor support in patients with marginal neutrophil counts. More intensive blood count monitoring may be required when new antiretroviral agents or drugs used to treat specific opportunistic infections are added to a stable KS treatment regimen. Some of these drugs (e.g., ganciclovir or trimethoprim–sulfamethoxazole) are known to cause neutropenia. In other cases, anecdotal evidence suggests that some antiretroviral drugs may alter the metabolism of chemotherapeutic agents, leading to greater toxicity.

Blood tests to assess liver and kidney function are generally performed every 4–8 weeks during therapy; liver enzymes should be checked more frequently during the first 1–2 months of IFN-α therapy, when acutely elevated enzymes are most commonly observed.

Patients receiving anthracycline chemotherapy should have the cardiac ejection fraction monitored when the cumulative anthracycline dose reaches 450–500 mg/m^2 body surface area. Patients receiving liposomal anthracycline therapy who have a normal ejection fraction may continue to receive treatment, but cardiac function should be formally assessed after each 100 mg/m^2 increment in dose. The major toxicity of bleomycin is pulmonary fibrosis, which increases in frequency with cumulative doses above 300 U. Although bleomycin is not currently used frequently as first-line therapy for KS, when it is used, patients should be monitored with carbon monoxide diffusing capacity and measurement of vital capacity and total lung volume to detect restrictive ventilatory defects.

Patients receiving paclitaxel, vinca alkaloids, or etoposide require regular questioning about peripheral neuropathic symptoms (numbness, tingling, pain, or dysesthesias in the hands and feet), and should have a neurological examination approximately every-other chemotherapy cycle to detect diminished light touch, vibration, and position sense.

Patients undergoing treatment for AIDS-associated KS also require standard monitoring of their HIV infection with measurement of the HIV viral load and peripheral blood CD4 cell counts. The frequency of such monitoring is usually every 3–4 months, but more frequent tests may be required under certain circumstances; for example, when the antiretroviral drug regimen has recently been changed.

Monitoring for response to therapy is generally performed every 4–6 weeks, depending upon the length of each treatment cycle. Standardized response assessments generally include measurement of the perpendicular diameters of five designated "marker lesions," enumeration of the total number of raised and flat lesions (either total body or on selected anatomical areas in the case of large numbers of lesions; e.g., > 50), assessment of oral lesions, and evaluation of edema (which may include measurement of extremity circumference). Evaluation of visceral KS generally is performed less frequently, particularly when invasive procedures, such as bronchoscopy or GI endoscopy, are required for disease assessment.

6. Supportive Care

In addition to therapy directed specifically against KS lesions and against HIV infection and its nonneoplastic sequelae, successful management of the patient with KS also requires attention to supportive care. Nutritional deficiencies, mucositis, pain, disease- or drug-induced myelosuppression, neuropathy, and tumor-associated edema may all complicate therapy and adversely influence quality of life in patients with KS. Patients may benefit from nutritional counseling, high-calorie, high-protein, liquid nutritional supplements, appetite stimulants and, when testosterone deficiency is documented, anabolic steroids. Poor intake because of painful chemotherapy- or radiation-induced mucositis may be ameliorated by topical agents; for example, a mouthwash prepared with equal volumes of Kaopectate or Mylanta, diphenhydramine elixir, and viscous lidocaine. Most of the chemotherapeutic agents used to treat KS have a relatively low emetogenic potential. Prophylactic antiemetics are not generally required before administration of the most commonly used regimens; if nausea occurs after therapy, oral prochlorperazine or metoclopramide are usually sufficient to control symptoms, but the occasional patient may benefit from pretreatment with a serotonin antagonist (e.g., ondansetron or granisetron), with or without dexamethasone.

Although pain is not often emphasized as a complication of KS, individual lesions near joints or pressure points can cause discomfort and may require non-narcotic analgesics. Moderate to severe pain, frequently requiring narcotic analgesics, often complicates limb edema, particularly when joint mobility is reduced or when lesions ulcerate and become infected.

Supportive management of edema is a difficult problem, particularly because edema may persist, even after successful therapy of other KS lesions. Lower extremity edema generally worsens with dependency (i.e., walking, standing, or sitting), and is lessened with leg elevation. Similarly, periorbital edema is generally worse after sleeping, but may be ameliorated by keeping the head elevated. Genital edema is a particularly difficult problem, but discomfort may be alleviated with athletic support garments; careful local hygiene is extremely important, particularly in uncircumcised men. Daily foot care is important in the presence of edema, and patients should be instructed to clean and dry carefully between the toes to prevent infection. When edema is complicated by skin breakdown and serous drainage, secondary infection is a common complication. Frequent cleansing with bacteriostatic agents (e.g., dilute hydrogen peroxide or dilute [1:10,000] potassium permanganate solutions) may be helpful for cleansing and drying oozing areas. We recommend that patients follow local cleansing of draining areas with antibiotic ointments (e.g., mupirocin) and dry, nonstick dressings. Discolored or foul-smelling drainage requires culture and appropriate antibiotic treatment. Local cleansing with metronidazole solution may be helpful in some cases with foul-smelling drainage. Severe infections or those caused by resistant organisms frequently require intravenous antibiotic therapy for control. Intertriginous fungal infections are common and require treatment with topical or systemic antimycotic drugs. Diuretics and elastic support garments are rarely very helpful in alleviating KS-associated edema. Patients with ulcerated or draining lesions or large KS nodules are not suitable candidates for restrictive stockings, although some patients with relatively mild edema find support stockings helpful when they are physically active.

Neuropathy frequently complicates HIV infection, may be a side effect of some antiretroviral drugs, and is often exacerbated by chemotherapeutic agents used to treat KS. Although vinca alkaloids and etoposide are not used as frequently as they once were, paclitaxel is being used more commonly, and may cause or exacerbate distal sensory peripheral neuropathy. For severe neuropathy, discontinuation of the offending drug may be necessary, but, in some cases, a reduction in the dose may provide relief. For some patients, treatment with drugs, such as amitriptyline, may alleviate neuropathic symptoms. It is not yet known whether recombinant nerve growth factor will alleviate chemotherapy-induced neuropathy in patients with AIDS-associated KS.

Myelosuppression, particularly neutropenia, frequently complicates HIV infection and is often exacerbated by KS treatment with interferon and, especially, chemotherapy. G-CSF (less often, GM-CSF) has been used successfully to treat HIV and KS therapy-associated neutropenia, and is eventually required in the majority of patients who receive standard chemotherapy for KS, even those with normal neutrophil counts at baseline. Neutropenic patients often respond rapidly to fairly low doses of G-CSF, and the neutrophil count can often be maintained at adequate levels on an intermittent (e.g., three times a week or less) schedule. The dose and schedule of G-CSF can be titrated to maintain adequate neutrophil counts to permit continued KS therapy. Mild anemia often accompanies HIV infection and may increase with KS treatment. In some patients, particularly those with severe debilitation or chronic infection, moderate to severe anemia may occur. Specific nutrient deficiencies need to be identified and treated. In patients with inappropriately low serum erythropoietin levels, administration of recombinant erythropoietin may alleviate anemia.

7. Investigational Therapy

Many investigational agents for KS are being tested, or are considered potential candidates for future study, and are discussed in detail in Chapter 8. Among the chemotherapeutic agents, the camptothecins are of interest because of their dual functions as cellular topoisomerase I inhibitors and as inhibitors of HIV integrase, an enzyme that facilitates integration of proviral DNA into the host genome (110). Various agents, acting by different mechanisms, may inhibit angiogenesis, an integral histological feature of the KS lesion. These include several synthetic retinoids administered topically, orally, and intravenously (111–113); thalidomide (which may affect KS growth through inhibition of tumor necrosis factor [TNF] and through various TNF-independent mechanisms; 9,114,115); inhibitors of endothelial cell proliferation, such as TNP-470 (116,117); and inhibitors of matrix metalloproteinases, enzymes that facilitate capillary budding and invasion by disrupting the integrity of the extracellular matrix. Other potential therapeutic targets and approaches include agents that abrogate tyrosine kinase-mediated transmembrane receptor signals for various angiogenic growth factors, antisense oligonucleotides directed against these growth factors (118), and agents directed against distinctive endothelial cell surface molecules expressed preferentially on proliferating vasculature; for example, the integrin, $\alpha_v\beta_3$ (119). In addition, there is considerable interest in evaluating antiherpesvirus drugs as therapeutic agents for KS, and particularly as potential prophylactic agents for patients identified as high-risk for subsequent KS development (see following section). The role of more effective anti-HIV therapy in the treatment and prevention of KS also requires better definition, and the safety and efficacy of many regimens combining two or more active single agents remains to be evaluated.

8. Prophylactic Strategies for Kaposi's Sarcoma

The role of HHV-8 in the development of KS is discussed in detail in another chapter, but it is clear that the virus is intimately involved in KS pathogenesis and that infection and seroconversion precede the development of clinical KS (7). The ability to screen HIV-infected persons without KS for evidence of HHV-8 infection (7), and the identification of several drugs with inhibitory activity against HHV-8, raises the possibility that preventive strategies can be developed for a targeted group of HHV-8–seropositive individuals who are likely to develop KS within a short time. Because the likelihood that an HHV-8–seropositive individual without KS will develop KS may be affected by the degree to which HIV is suppressed and immune function is restored, placebo-controlled studies will be required to assess the efficacy of prophylaxis. In addition, because not all HHV-8–infected individuals will develop KS, and because long-term prophylaxis will probably be required, a desirable agent would have a good safety and tolerance profile and activity when administered orally.

9. Development of a KS Treatment Strategy

Many drugs and techniques can effect KS regression and provide symptom palliation, but treatment for KS is not curative. The choice of therapy needs to be based on several factors that must be carefully weighed for each individual. Table 3 outlines therapeutic options for various clinical scenarios. Among the considerations in the choice of therapy are the overall severity of the KS, the presence of specific KS-associated symptoms (e.g., edema, pain, or dyspnea), the rate of

Table 3 Therapeutic Options for AIDS-Associated Kaposi's Sarcoma[a]

KS presentation	HIV Viral load	First-line therapy[b]	Second-line therapy	Other options/comments
Skin				
Limited, asymptomatic, cosmetically acceptable	Low	IFNα + ARV Tx Local therapy Radiation therapy		Choice depends on number and location of lesions, personal preference; IFN-α best in patients with CD4 ≥ 100/μL, but some response seen at lower CD4 counts.
Limited, cosmetically unacceptable	High Any	Optimize ARV Tx Radiation therapy Local therapy	As for low viral load Systemic chemo I	Systemic chemo II
Extensive or bulky ± cosmetically unacceptable	Any	Systemic chemo I	Systemic chemo II Radiation therapy to local bulky sites	IFNα + ARV Tx may be used in selected cases with extensive, but nonbulky lesions, good PS, few tumor-related symptoms and good HIV control.
Oral				
Limited, asymptomatic	Any	Optimize ARV Tx	IFNα + ARV Tx	IFNAα + ARV Tx has been effective in selected patients with good PS and relatively high CD4 counts.
Bulky or symptomatic	Any	Systemic chemo I; radiation therapy; local therapy		
Edema				
Tumor-associated, symptomatic	Any	Systemic chemo I	Systemic chemo II; radiation therapy	
Visceral				
Symptomatic GI; any pulmonary	Any	Systemic chemo I	Systemic chemo II	Radiation therapy may palliate selected cases of end-stage KS Other chemo, (e.g., VP-16, Bleo + Vcr)

[a] Abbreviations: ARV Tx, antiretroviral treatment; Systemic chemo I, liposomal doxorubicin (Doxil) or liposomal daunorubicin (DaunoXome); Systemic chemo II, paclitaxel; VP-16, etoposide; Bleo, bleomycin; Vcr, vincristine; PS, performance status.
[b] Whenever possible, optimization of antiretroviral therapy should be part of the KS treatment strategy.

KS progression, and the patient's prior treatment history. Individual patient goals are also important. For example, the choice of treatment may be influenced by specific cosmetic issues or concerns about treatment side effects such as alopecia. The severity of the underlying HIV infection and its nonneoplastic complications also requires consideration. Overall life expectancy, control of the underlying HIV infection, performance status, and the presence of concomitant conditions (e.g., neuropathy, wasting, chronic infections requiring ongoing treatment, abnormal cardiac, hepatic, or pulmonary function), all may influence the therapeutic approach. However, most chemotherapy trials have been conducted in patients with very low CD4 counts, and a low CD4 count alone should not preclude systemic therapy when its use is otherwise warranted. Finally, a successful treatment strategy requires attention to supportive care, including nutritional support, pain control, and adjunctive therapy for myelosuppression, in addition to standard infection prophylaxis and effective HIV suppression.

REFERENCES

1. Centers for Disease Control. Kaposi's sarcoma and *Pneumocystis* pneumonia among homosexual men—New York City and California. MMWR Morbid Mortal Wkly Rep 30:305–308, 1981.
2. Jacobson LP, Munoz AP, Fox R, et al. Incidence of Kaposi's sarcoma in a cohort of homosexual men infected with the human immunodeficiency virus type 1. The Multicenter AIDS Cohort Study Group. J Acquir Immune Defic Syndr 3(suppl 1): S24–S31, 1990.
3. Lyter DW, Bryant J, Thackeray R, et al. Incidence of human immunodeficiency virus-related and nonrelated malignancies in a large cohort of homosexual men. J Clin Oncol 13:2540–2546, 1995.
4. Schwartlander B, Horsburgh CR Jr, Hamouda O, et al. Changes in the spectrum of AIDS-defining conditions and decrease in CD4+ lymphocyte counts as AIDS manifestations in Germany from 1986 to 1991. AIDS 6:413–420, 1992.
5. Whitby D, Howard MR, Tenant-Flowers M, et al. Detection of Kaposi sarcoma associated herpesvirus in peripheral blood of HIV-infected individuals and progression to Kaposi's sarcoma. Lancet 346:799–802, 1995.
6. Simpson GR, Schulz TF, Whitby D, et al. Prevalence of Kaposi's sarcoma associated herpesvirus infection measured by antibodies to recombinant capsid protein and latent immunofluorescence antigen. Lancet 348:1133–1138, 1996.
7. Gao SJ, Kingsley L, Hoover DR, et al. Seroconversion to antibodies against Kaposi's sarcoma-associated herpesvirus-related latent nuclear antigens before the development of Kaposi's sarcoma. N Engl J Med 335:233–241, 1996.
8. Gao SJ, Kingsley L, Li M, et al. KSHV antibodies among Americans, Italians and Ugandans with and without Kaposi's sarcoma. Nat Med 2:925–928, 1996.
9. Karp JE, Pluda JM, Yarchoan R. AIDS-related Kaposi's sarcoma: a template for the

translation of molecular pathogenesis into targeted therapeutic approaches. Hematol Oncol Clin North Am 10:1031–1049, 1996.

10. Dezube BJ. Clinical presentation and natural history of AIDS-related Kaposi's sarcoma. Hematol Oncol Clin North Am 10:1023–1029, 1996.
11. Nichols CM, Flaitz CM, Hicks MJ. Treating Kaposi's lesions in the HIV-infected patient. J Am Dent Assoc 124:78, 1993.
12. Barrison IG, Foster S, Harris JW, et al. Upper gastrointestinal Kaposi's sarcoma in patients positive for HIV antibody without cutaneous disease. Br Med J 296: 92–93, 1988.
13. Danzig JB, Brandt LJ, Reinus JF, et al. Gastrointestinal malignancy in patients with AIDS. Am J Gastroenterol 8:715–718, 1991.
14. Laine L, Amerian J, Rarick M, et al. The response of symptomatic gastrointestinal Kaposi's sarcoma to chemotherapy: a prospective evaluation using an endoscopic method of disease quantification. Am J Gastroenterol 85:959–961, 1990.
15. Adal KA, Cockerell CJ, Petri WA Jr, et al. Cat scratch disease, bacillary angiomatosis, and other infections due to *Rochalimaea*. N Engl J Med 330:1509, 1994.
16. Myskowski PL, Niedzwiecki D, Shurgot BA, et al. AIDS-associated Kaposi's sarcoma: variables associated with increased survival. J Am Acad Dermatol 18:1299–1306, 1988.
17. White DA. Pulmonary complications of HIV-associated malignancies. Clin Chest Med 17:755–761, 1996.
18. Meduri G, Stover D, Lee M, et al. Pulmonary Kaposi's sarcoma in the acquired immune deficiency syndrome: clinical, radiographic, and pathologic manifestations. Am J Med 81:11–18, 1986.
19. Lee V, Fuller J, O'Brien M, et al. Pulmonary Kaposi sarcoma in patients with AIDS: scintigraphic diagnosis with sequential thallium and gallium scanning. Radiology 180:409–412, 1991.
20. Wolff SD, Kuhlman JE, Fishman EK. Thoracic Kaposi's sarcoma in AIDS: CT findings. J Comput Assist Tomogr 17:60–62, 1993.
21. Khalil AM, Carette MF, Cadranel JL, et al. Magnetic resonance imaging findings in pulmonary Kaposi's sarcoma: a series of 10 cases. Eur Respir J 7:1285–1289, 1995.
22. Krown SE, Metroka C, Wernz JC. Kaposi's sarcoma in the acquired immune deficiency syndrome: a proposal for uniform evaluation, response and staging criteria. J Clin Oncol 7:1201–1207, 1989.
23. Krown SE, Testa MA, Huang J. AIDS-related Kaposi's sarcoma: prospective validation of the AIDS Clinical Trials Group staging classification. J Clin Oncol 15: 3085–3092, 1997.
24. Chachoua A, Krigel R, Lafleur F, et al. Prognostic factors and staging classifications of patients with epidemic Kaposi's sarcoma. J Clin Oncol 7:774, 1989.
25. Miles SA, Wang H, Elashoff R, et al. Improved survival for patients with AIDS-related Kaposi's sarcoma. J Clin Oncol 12:1910–1916, 1994.
26. Miles SA. Pathogenesis of AIDS-related Kaposi's sarcoma. Evidence of a viral etiology. Hematol Oncol Clin North Am 10:1011–1021, 1996.
27. Ensoli B, Barillari G, Salahuddin SZ, et al. Tat protein of HIV-1 stimulates growth of cells derived from Kaposi's sarcoma lesions of AIDS patients. Nature 345:84–86, 1990.

28. Ensoli B, Gendelman R, Markham P, et al. Synergy between basic fibroblast growth factor and HIV-1 Tat protein in induction of Kaposi's sarcoma. Nature 371:674–680, 1994.

29. Little RF, Pluda JM, Feigal E, et al. The challenge of designing clinical trials for AIDS-related Kaposi's sarcoma. Oncology 12:871–883, 1998.

30. Tappero JW, Berger, TG, Kaplan LD, et al. Cryotherapy for cutaneous Kaposi's sarcoma (KS) associated with acquired immune deficiency syndrome (AIDS): a phase II trial. J Acquir Immune Defic Syndr 4:839–846, 1991.

31. Boudreaux AA, Smith LL, Cosby CD, et al. Intralesional vinblastine for cutaneous Kaposi's sarcoma associated with acquired immunodeficiency syndrome. A clinical trial to evaluate efficacy and discomfort associated with injection. J Am Acad Dermatol 28:61–65, 1993.

32. Depuy J, Price M, Lynch G, et al. Intralesional interferon-alpha and zidovudine in epidemic Kaposi's sarcoma. J Am Acad Dermatol 28:966–972, 1993.

33. Boente P, Sampaio C, Brandáo MA, et al. Local perilesional therapy with rhGM-CSF for Kaposi's sarcoma. Lancet 341:1154, 1993.

34. Staddon A, Henry D, Bonnem E. A randomized dose finding study of recombinant platelet factor 4 (rPF4) in cutaneous AIDS-related Kaposi's sarcoma [abstract]. Proc Am Soc Clin Oncol 13:50, 1994.

35. Gill PS, Lunardi-Iskandar Y, Louie S, et al. The effects of preparations of human chorionic gonadotropin on AIDS-related Kaposi's sarcoma. N Engl J Med 335:1261–1269, 1996.

36. Lucatoro FM, Sapp JP. Treatment of oral Kaposi's sarcoma with a sclerosing agent in AIDS patients. A preliminary study. Oral Surg Oral Med Oral Pathol, 75:192–198, 1993.

37. Stelzer KJ, Griffin TW. A randomized prospective trial of radiation therapy for AIDS-associated Kaposi's sarcoma. Int J Radiat Oncol Biol Phys 27:1057–1061, 1993.

38. Berson AM, Quivey JM, Harris JW, Wara WM. Radiation therapy for AIDS-related Kaposi's sarcoma. Int J Radiat Oncol Biol Phys 19:569–575, 1990.

39. Stelzer KJ, Griffin TW, Koh WJ. Radiation recall skin toxicity with bleomycin in a patient with Kaposi sarcoma related to acquired immune deficiency syndrome. Cancer 71:1322–1325, 1993.

40. Chak LY, Gill PS, Levine AM, et al. Radiation therapy for acquired immunodeficiency syndrome-related Kaposi's sarcoma. J Clin Oncol 6:863–867, 1988.

41. Meyer JL. Whole-lung irradiation for Kaposi's sarcoma. Am J Clin Oncol 16:372–376, 1993.

42. Krown SE. Acquired immunodeficiency syndrome-associated Kaposi's sarcoma. Biology and management. Med Clin North Am 81:471–494, 1997.

43. Real FX, Krown SE, Oettgen HF. Kaposi's sarcoma and the acquired immunodeficiency syndrome: treatment with high and low doses of recombinant leukocyte A interferon. J Clin Oncol 4:544–551, 1986.

44. Evans LM, Itri LM, Campion M, et al. Interferon-alpha 2a in the treatment of acquired immunodeficiency syndrome-related Kaposi's sarcoma. J Immunother 10:39–50, 1991.

45. Krigel RL, Slywotzky CM, Lonberg M, et al. Treatment of epidemic Kaposi's sar-

coma with a combination of interferon-α2b and etoposide. J Biol Respir Med 7: 359–364, 1988.

46. Shepherd FA, Evans WK, Garvey B, et al. Combination chemotherapy and α-interferon in the treatment of Kaposi's sarcoma associated with acquired immune deficiency syndrome. Can Med Assoc J 139:635–639, 1988.

47. Krown SE, Gold JWM, Niedzwiecki D, et al. Interferon-α with zidovudine: safety, tolerance, and clinical and virologic effects in patients with Kaposi's sarcoma associated with the acquired immunodeficiency syndrome (AIDS). Ann Intern Med 112: 812–821, 1990.

48. Fischl MA, Uttamchandani R, Resnick L, et al. A phase I study of recombinant human interferon alfa-nl and concomitant zidovudine in patients with AIDS-related Kaposi's sarcoma. J Acquir Immune Defic Syndr 4:1–10, 1991.

49. Kovacs JA, Deyton L, Davey R, et al. Combined zidovudine and interferon-α therapy in patients with Kaposi's sarcoma and the acquired immunodeficiency syndrome (AIDS). Ann Intern Med 111:280–287, 1989.

50. Fischl MA, Finkelstein DM, He W, et al. A phase II study of recombinant human interferon-α2a and zidovudine in patients with AIDS-related Kaposi's sarcoma. J Acquir Immune Defic Syndr Hum Retrovirol 11:379–384, 1996.

51. Evans LM, Itri LM, Campion M, et al. Interferon-alpha 2a in the treatment of acquired immunodeficiency syndrome-related Kaposi's sarcoma. J Immunother 10: 39–50, 1991.

52. Krown SE, Paredes J, Bundow D, et al. Interferon-α, zidovudine and granulocyte–macrophage colony-stimulating factor: a phase I trial in patients with Kaposi's sarcoma associated with the acquired immunodeficiency syndrome (AIDS). J Clin Oncol 10:1344–1351, 1992.

53. Scadden DT, Bering HA, Levine JD, et al. Granulocyte–macrophage colony-stimulating factor mitigates the neutropenia of combined interferon alfa and zidovudine treatment of acquired immune deficiency syndrome-associated Kaposi's sarcoma. J Clin Oncol 9:802–808, 1991.

54. Mannering GJ, Renton KW, El Azhary R, et al. Effect of interferon-inducing agents on hepatic cytochrome P-450 drug metabolizing systems. Ann NY Acad Sci 350: 314–331, 1980.

55. Laubenstein LJ, Krigel RL, Odajnyk CM, et al. Treatment of epidemic Kaposi's sarcoma with etoposide or a combination of doxorubicin, bleomycin and vinblastine. J Clin Oncol 2:1115–1120, 1984.

56. Bakker PJM, Danner SA, Lange JMA, Veenhof KHN. Etoposide for epidemic Kaposi's sarcoma: a phase II study. Eur J Cancer Clin Oncol 24:1047–1048, 1988.

57. Paredes J, Kahn JO, Tong WP, et al. Weekly oral etoposide in patients with Kaposi's sarcoma associated with human immunodeficiency virus infection: a phase I multicenter trial of the AIDS Clinical Trials Group. J Acquir Immune Defic Syndr Hum Retrovirol 9:138–144, 1995.

58. Schwartsmann G, Sprinz E, Kromfield M, et al. Clinical and pharmacokinetic study of oral etoposide in patients with AIDS-related Kaposi's sarcoma with no prior exposure to cytotoxic therapy. J Clin Oncol 15:2118–2124, 1997.

59. Bufill JA, Grace WR, Astrow AB. Phase II trial of prolonged, low-dose, oral VP-

16 in AIDS-related Kaposi's sarcoma (KS) [abstract]. Proc Am Soc Clin Oncol 11:47, 1992.

60. Schwartzmann G, Sprinz E, Kronfeld M, et al. Phase II study of teniposide in patients with AIDS-related Kaposi's sarcoma. Eur J Cancer 27:1637–1639, 1991.
61. Volberding PA, Abrams DI, Conant M, et al. Vinblastine therapy for Kaposi's sarcoma in the acquired immunodeficiency syndrome. Ann Intern Med 103:335–338, 1985.
62. Mintzer DM, Real FX, Jovino L, et al. Treatment of Kaposi's sarcoma and thrombocytopenia with vincristine in patients with acquired immunodeficiency syndrome. Ann Intern Med 102:200–202, 1985.
63. Errante D, Spina M, Nasti G, et al. Evidence of activity of vinorelbine (VNR) in patients (pts) with previously treated epidemic Kaposi's sarcoma (KS). J Acquir Immune Defic Syndr Hum Retrovirol 14:A36, 1997. [Abstracts of the National AIDS Malignancy Conference, Bethesda, MD, April 28–30, 1997, abstract 80].
64. Caumes E, Guermonprez G, Katlama C, et al. AIDS-associated mucocutaneous Kaposi's sarcoma treated with bleomycin. AIDS 6:1483–1487, 1992.
65. Lassoued K, Clauvel JP, Katlama C, et al. Treatment of the acquired immune deficiency syndrome-related Kaposi's sarcoma with bleomycin as a single agent. Cancer 66:1869–1872, 1990.
66. Remick SC, Reddy M, Herman D, et al. Continuous infusion bleomycin in AIDS-related Kaposi's sarcoma. J Clin Oncol 12:1130–1136, 1994.
67. Fischl MA, Krown SE, O'Boyle KP, et al. Weekly doxorubicin in the treatment of patients with AIDS-related Kaposi's sarcoma: J Acquir Immune Defic Syndr 6:259–264, 1993.
68. Gill PS, Rarick M, McCutchan JA, et al. Systemic treatment of AIDS-related Kaposi's sarcoma: results of a randomized trial. Am J Med 90:427–433, 1991.
69. Gill PS, Akil B, Colletti P, et al. Pulmonary Kaposi's sarcoma: clinical-findings and results of therapy. Am J Med 87:57–61, 1989.
70. Brenner DC. Liposomal encapsulation: making old and new drugs do new tricks. J Natl Cancer Inst 81:13–15, 1989.
71. Gill PS, Espina BM, Muggia F, et al. Phase I/II clinical and pharmacokinetic evaluation of liposomal daunorubicin. J Clin Oncol 13:996–1003, 1995.
72. Northfelt DW, Martin FJ, Working P, et al. Doxorubicin encapsulated in liposomes containing surface-bound polyethylene glycol: pharmacokinetics, tumor localization, and safety in patients with AIDS-related Kaposi's sarcoma. J Clin Pharmacol 36:55–63, 1996.
73. Bogner JR, Kronawitter U, Rolinski B, et al. Liposomal doxorubicin in the treatment of advanced AIDS-related Kaposi's sarcoma. J Acquir Immune Defic Syndr 7:463–468, 1994.
74. Gill PS, Wernz J, Scadden DT, et al. Randomized phase II trial of liposomal daunorubicin (DaunoXome) versus doxorubicin, bleomycin, vincristine (ABV) in AIDS-related Kaposi's sarcoma. J Clin Oncol 14:2353–2364, 1996.
75. Harrison M, Tomlinson D, Stewart S. Liposomal-entrapped doxorubicin: an active agent in AIDS-related Kaposi's sarcoma. J Clin Oncol 13:914–920, 1995.
76. Northfelt DW, Dezube B, Miller B, et al. Randomized comparative trial of Doxil

vs. Adriamycin, bleomycin, and vincristine (ABV) in the treatment of severe AIDS-related Kaposi's sarcoma [abstract]. Blood 86:382a, 1995.

77. Cowens JW, Creaven PJ, Greco WR, at al. Initial clinical (phase I) trial of TLC D-99 (doxorubicin encapsulated in liposomes). Cancer Res 53:2796–2808, 1993.

78. Wagner D, Kern WV, Kern P. Liposomal doxorubicin in AIDS-related Kaposi's sarcoma: long term experiences. Clin Invest 72:417–423, 1994.

79. Berry G, Billingham M, Alderman E, et al. Reduced cardiotoxicity of Doxil (pegylated liposomal doxorubicin) in AIDS Kaposi's sarcoma patients compared to a matched control group of cancer patients given doxorubicin [abstract] Proc Am Soc Clin Oncol 15:303, 1996.

80. Ross M, Gill PS, Espina BM, et al. Liposomal daunorubicin (DaunoXome) in the treatment of advanced AIDS-related Kaposi's sarcoma: Results of a phase II study [abstr PoB 3123]. Int Conf AIDS 8:B107, 1992.

81. Gordon KB, Tajuddin A, Guitart J, et al. Hand–foot syndrome associated with liposome-encapculated doxorubicin therapy. Cancer 75:2169–2173, 1995.

82. Uziely B, Jeffers S, Isaacson R, et al. Liposomal doxorubicin: antitumor activity and unique toxicities during two complementary phase I studies. J Clin Oncol 13: 1777–1785, 1995.

83. Chew T, Jacobs M, Huckabee M, et al. A phase II clinical trial of DaunoXome (VS103, liposomal daunorubicin) in Kaposi's sarcoma of AIDS patients [abstr WS-B15-3]. Int Conf AIDS 9:58, 1993.

84. Dupont B, Pialoux G, Gonzalez G, et al. Phase II study of liposomal daunorubicin (DaunoXome) in AIDS-related Kaposi's sarcoma [abstr PoB 3119]. Int Conf AIDS 8:B106, 1992.

85. James ND, Coker RJ, Tomlinson D, et al. Liposomal doxorubicin (Doxil): an effective new treatment for Kaposi's sarcoma in AIDS. Clin Oncol 6:294–296, 1994.

86. Money-Kyrle JF, Bates F, Ready J, et al. Liposomal daunorubicin in advanced Kaposi's sarcoma: a phase II study. Clin Oncol (R Coll Radiol) 5:367–371, 1993.

87. Sturzl M, Zeitz C, Eisenburg B, et al. Liposomal doxorubicin in the treatment of AIDS-associated Kaposi's sarcoma: Clinical, histological, and cell biological evaluation. Res Virol 145:261–269, 1994.

88. Northfelt DW, Dezube BJ, Thommes JA, et al. Efficacy of pegylated-liposomal doxorubicin in the treatment of AIDS-related Kaposi's sarcoma after failure of standard chemotherapy. J Clin Oncol 15:653–659, 1997.

89. Schiff PB, Fant J, Horwitz SB. Promotion of microtubule assembly in vitro by Taxol. Nature 277:665–667, 1979.

90. Schiff PB, Horwitz SB. Taxol stabilizes microtubules in mouse fibroblast cells. Proc Natl Acad Sci USA 77:1561–1565, 1980.

91. Belotti D, Vergani V, Drudis T, et al. The microtubule-affecting drug paclitaxel has antiangiogenic activity. Clin Cancer Res 2:1843–1849, 1996.

92. Haldar S, Chintapalli J, Croce CM. Taxol induces *bcl*-2 phosphorylation and death of prostate cancer cells. Cancer Res 56:1253–1255, 1996.

93. Opalenik SR, Browning PJ. Human herpesvirus 8 (HHV-8) encodes a *bcl*-2 homologue that is expressed in Kaposi's sarcoma. J Acquir Immune Defic Syndr Hum Retrovirol 14:A26, 1997. [Abstr Natl AIDS Malign Conf, Bethesda, MD, April 28–30, 1997, abstr 42].

94. Saville MW, Lietzau J, Pluda JM, et al. Treatment of HIV-associated Kaposi's sarcoma with paclitaxel. Lancet 346:26–28, 1995.
95. Gill PS, Tulpule A, Reynolds T, et al. Paclitaxel (Taxol) in the treatment of relapsed or refractory advanced AIDS-related Kaposi's sarcoma [abstr]. Proc Am Soc Clin Oncol 15:306, 1996.
96. Kaplan L, Abrams D, Volberding P. Treatment of Kaposi's sarcoma in acquired immunodeficiency syndrome with an alternating vincristine–vinblastine regimen. Cancer Treat Rep 70:1121–1122, 1986.
97. Gompels MM, Hill A, Jenkins P, et al. Kaposi's sarcoma in HIV infection treated with vincristine and bleomycin. AIDS 6:1175–1180, 1992.
98. Gill PS, Rarick M, Bernstein-Singer M. Treatment of advanced Kaposi's sarcoma using a combination of bleomycin and vincristine. Am J Oncol 13:315–319, 1990.
99. Rizzardini G, Pastecchia C, Vigevani GM, et al. Stealth liposomal doxorubicin or bleomycin/vincristine for the treatment of AIDS-related Kaposi's sarcoma. J Acquir Immune Defic Syndr Hum Retrovirol 14:A20, 1997. [Abstr Natil AIDS Malign Conf, Bethesda, MD, April 28–30, 1997, abstract 17].
100. Stewart S, Jablonowski H, Goebel FD, et al. Randomized comparative trial of pegylated liposomal doxorubicin versus bleomycin and vincristine in the treatment of AIDS-related Kaposi's sarcoma. International Pegylated Liposomal Doxorubicin Study Group. J Clin Oncol 16:683–691, 1998.
101. Gelmann EP, Longo D, Lane HC, et al. Combination chemotherapy of disseminated Kaposi's sarcoma in patients with the acquired immune deficiency syndrome. Am J Med 82:456–462, 1987.
102. Sloand E, Kumar PN, Pierce PF. Chemotherapy for patients with pulmonary Kaposi's sarcoma: benefit of filgrastim (G-CSF) in supporting dose administration. South Med J 86:1219–1224, 1993.
103. Cadranel JL, Kammoun S, Chevret S, et al. Results of chemotherapy in 30 AIDS patients with symptomatic pulmonary Kaposi's sarcoma. Thorax 49:958–960, 1994.
104. Gill PS, Rarick MU, Espina B, et al. Advanced acquired immune deficiency syndrome-related Kaposi's sarcoma: results of pilot studies using combination chemotherapy. Cancer 65:1074–1078, 1990.
105. Gill PS, Miles SA, Mitsuyasu RT, et al. Phase I AIDS Clinical Trials Group (075) study of Adriamycin, bleomycin and vincristine in the treatment of AIDS-related Kaposi's sarcoma. AIDS 8:1695–1699, 1994.
106. Bakker PJM, Danner SA, Napel CH, et al. Treatment of poor prognosis epidemic Kaposi's sarcoma with doxorubicin, bleomycin, vindesine and recombinant human granulocyte–monocyte colony stimulating factor (rh GM-CSF). Eur J Cancer 31A: 188–192, 1995.
107. Gill PS, Bernstein-Singer M, Espina BM, et al. Adriamycin, bleomycin and vincristine chemotherapy with recombinant granulocyte–macrophage colony-stimulating factor in the treatment of AIDS-related Kaposi's sarcoma. AIDS 6:1477–1481, 1992.
108. Mitsuyasu RT, Gill P, Paredes J, et al. Combination chemotherapy, Adriamycin, bleomycin, vincristine (ABV) with dideoxyinosine (ddI) or dideoxycytidine (ddC) in advanced AIDS-related Kaposi's sarcoma (ACTG 163) [abstr. 822]. Proc Am Soc Clin Oncol 14:289, 1995.

109. Mitsuyasu R, von Roenn J, Krown S, et al. Comparison study of liposomal doxorubicin (Dox) alone or with bleomycin and vincristine (DBV) for treatment of advanced AIDS-associated Kaposi's sarcoma (AIDS-KS): AIDS Clinical Trial Group (ACTG) protocol 286 [abstr 191]. Proc Am Soc Clin Oncol 16:55a, 1997.

110. Li CJ, Dezube BJ, Biswas DK, et al. Inhibitors of HIV-1 transcription. Trends in Microbiol 2:164, 1994.

111. Bonhomme L, Fredj G, Averous S, et al. Topical treatment of epidemic Kaposi's sarcoma with all-*trans* retinoic acid. Ann Oncol 2:234–235, 1991.

112. Bernstein ZP, Cohen P, Rios A, et al. A multicenter, phase II/III study of Atragen (tretinoin liposomal) in patients with AIDS-associated Kaposi's sarcoma. J Acquir Immune Defic Syndr Hum Retrovirol 14:A19, 1997. [Abstr Natl AIDS Malign Conf, Bethesda, MD, April 28–30, 1997, abstr. 14].

113. Duvic M. Friedman-Kien AE, Miles SA, et al. Phase I-II evaluation of Panretin (ALRT1057; LGD1057; AGN192013; 9-*cis*-retinoic acid) topical gel for AIDS-related cutaneous Kaposi's sarcoma [abstr 160]. Proc Am Soc Clin Oncol 16:46a, 1997.

114. Welles L, Little R, Wyvill K, et al. Preliminary results of a phase II study of oral thalidomide in patients with HIV infection and Kaposi's sarcoma (KS). J Acquir Immune Defic Syndr Hum Retrovirol 14:A21, 1997. [Abstr Natl AIDS Malign Conf, Bethesda, MD, April 28–30, 1997, abstr 20].

115. Bower M, Howard M, Gracie F, et al. A phase II study of thalidomide for Kaposi's sarcoma: activity and correlation with KSHV DNA load. J Acquir Immune Defic Syndr Hum Retrovirol 14:A35, 1997. [Abstr Natl AIDS Malign Conf, Bethesda, MD, April 28–30, 1997, abstr 76].

116. Dezube BJ, vonRoenn JH, Holden-Wiltse J, et al. Fumagillin analog in the treatment of Kaposi's sarcoma: a phase I AIDS clinical trial group study. AIDS Clinical Trial Group No. 215 Team. J Clin Oncol 16:1444–1449, 1998.

117. Pluda JM, Wyvill KK, Lietzau J, et al. A phase I trial administering the angiogenesis inhibitor TNP-470 (AGM-1470) to patients (pts) with HIV-associated Kaposi's sarcoma (KS). J Acquir Immune Defic Syndr Hum Retrovirol 14:A19, 1997. [Abstr Natl AIDS Malign Conf, Bethesda, MD, April 28–30, 1997, abstr 13].

118. Ensoli B, Markham P, Kao V, et al. Block of AIDS–Kaposi's sarcoma (KS) cell growth, angiogenesis and lesion formation in nude mice by antisense oligonucleotide targeting basic fibroblast growth factor. J Clin Invest 94:1736–1746, 1994.

119. Brooks PC, Montgomery AMP, Rosenfeld M, et al. Integrin $\alpha_v\beta_3$ antagonists promote tumor regression by inducing apoptosis of angiogenic blood vessels. Cell 79:1157, 1994.

5
Diagnosis and Treatment of Non–Hodgkin's Lymphoma in the Patient with AIDS

Alexandra M. Levine
University of Southern California School of Medicine and USC/Norris Cancer Center, Los Angeles, California

I. GENERAL CONCEPTS: COMPARISON BETWEEN AIDS LYMPHOMA AND LYMPHOMA ARISING IN ALTERNATIVE SETTINGS

A. "De Novo" Versus AIDS Lymphoma

1. Pathological Spectrum of Disease

The de novo lymphomas, which may occur in human immunodeficiency virus (HIV)-noninfected individuals, are clearly distinct from those occurring in the setting of underlying HIV infection. Pathologically, acquired immunodeficiency syndrome (AIDS)-related lymphomas comprise a rather narrow spectrum of histological types, consisting almost exclusively of B-cell tumors, of high-grade or large cell type (1). These include diffuse large cell lymphoma, B-immunoblastic and small-noncleaved lymphomas, the latter of which may represent either Burkitt's or Burkitt-like subtypes. All three of these pathological types appear equally distributed in patients with AIDS lymphoma (2), so that approximately two-thirds of AIDS lymphomas are of the high-grade, B-cell type. This pathological spectrum of disease is in sharp contrast with that expected in the usual setting, in which only approximately 10% of patients have a diagnosis of high-grade lymphomas (1). Recently, several additional pathological entities have been described in HIV-infected patients with lymphoma, including body–cavity-based lymphoma (BCBL; also termed primary effusion lymphomas), associated with coinfection by the newly discovered human herpes virus type 8 (HHV-8; 3–5); and anaplastic large cell lymphoma (6). Although primary effusion lymphoma appears more common in HIV-infected individuals, the entity has also been described without underlying HIV infection, and appears to be clinically similar in both settings (7). Likewise, anaplastic large cell lymphoma has also been well-described in de novo lymphoma, with similar clinical and pathological characteristics in both HIV-infected and noninfected individuals (8).

2. Clinical Characteristics

The AIDS lymphomas are distinct clinically from those which arise de novo, and are much more likely to be associated with widespread, extranodal disease at initial presentation. Thus, approximately 80–90% of patients with AIDS lymphoma present with extranodal involvement (9–15), whereas such extranodal disease is described in only 40% of patients with de novo lymphoma (16). The specific sites of visceral involvement may be similar, with the exception of central nervous system (CNS) lymphoma, described in approximately one-third of HIV-infected patients at diagnosis, and in as many as 60% throughout the course of disease (9). This is in sharp contrast with de novo lymphoma, where CNS involvement is quite unusual, except in certain settings, such as maxillary sinus or testicular lymphoma, small noncleaved lymphoma with marrow involvement, or in the T-lymphoblastic lymphomas (17). Even in these latter circumstances, however, the prevalence of CNS involvement is far less than is expected in patients with AIDS-related lymphoma. AIDS lymphomas are also distinct in terms of systemic "B" symptoms, including fever, night sweats, or weight loss, occurring in approximately 80–90% of HIV-infected patients with lymphoma, and in approximately 17–31% of those with de novo disease (16).

3. Response to Therapy and Survival

The efficacy of dose-intensive therapy has been explored extensively in patients with de novo lymphoma, with evidence suggesting the value of such dose intensity (18). Recently, a large national trial compared the less intensive CHOP regimen (cyclophosphamide, doxorubicin [hydroxydaunomycin], vincristine, prednisone) with alternate regimens of theoretically greater dose intensity (19). Although rates of complete remission and disease-free survival appeared similar in all treatment groups, the actual dose intensity of CHOP was higher than that achieved in the other regimens, owing to the higher incidence of marrow toxicity and intercurrent infection in the more complex regimens, leading to delays in the next scheduled cycles of treatment (19). Preliminary results from recent trials of dose-escalated CHOP, used with hematopoietic growth factor support would indicate that the concept of high-dose therapy, administered within specific intervals of time is, in fact, valid in patients with de novo lymphoma, and may be associated with greater efficacy (20). As will be discussed later, the value of dose-intensive therapy has not been validated in patients with AIDS-related lymphoma, in whom low-dose chemotherapy is now considered the treatment of choice (21).

Long-term, disease-free survival has been documented in approximately 25–75% of patients with de novo lymphoma, according to baseline prognostic indicators, as described within the guidelines of the International Prognostic Index for large cell lymphoma (22). In contrast, long-term survival is unusual in patients with AIDS lymphoma, with only 10–20% of all patients still alive beyond 2 years from initial diagnosis and treatment (23). This decreased survival in the setting of underlying HIV infection is due to several factors, including decreased rates of complete remission when compared with patients with de novo lymphoma; increased rates of intercurrent infection while receiving chemotherapy; and death of other, AIDS-related complications while still in remission from lymphoma. In addition, although several salvage regimens have demonstrated efficacy in patients with relapsed de novo lymphoma (24), such is not true in patients with AIDS-related lymphomatous disease.

B. Organ Transplant-Associated Versus AIDS-Related Lymphoma

As with HIV-induced immune compromise, patients with iatrogenic immunodeficiency related to organ transplantation also have an increased incidence of lymphoma. Thus, the incidence of lymphoma in the setting of transplantation is approximately 25- to 50-fold increased when compared with that expected in the general population, with an average latent period of approximately 3 years between transplantation and development of lymphomatous disease (25). Although approximately 2% of all organ transplant recipients develop posttransplant lymphoproliferative disease, the chance of lymphoma appears to be related to the extent of immunosuppressive therapy employed, with higher prevalence and shorter latent periods observed, for example, after cyclosporine or monoclonal antibody-induced T-cell depletion (26).

The pathological spectrum of lymphomatous disease is quite complex in the setting of organ transplantation, with a variety of disorders described, ranging from polyclonal, atypical polymorphic lymphoproliferations, to frank monoclonal lymphomas of high-grade immunoblastic B-cell type (27). Immunoglobulin gene rearrangements have been described in these cases, demonstrating the B-cell nature of the process, and the genotypic monoclonality that may occur (28). Epstein–Barr virus (EBV) is etiologically related to these transplant-associated lymphomas, with demonstration of EBV genome within the vast majority of lymphoma tissues (29,30).

Similar to the AIDS-related lymphomas, patients with transplantation-associated lymphoma tend to present with extranodal disease, which may involve the CNS in 30% of cases (29). Furthermore, in a group of 182 patients who underwent cardiac transplantation at Stanford University, 9 developed lymphoma over a follow-up period ranging from 2 to 14 years. All cases presented with extranodal lymphoma, which included the brain in 5 (31). It is thus apparent that AIDS lymphoma and transplant-associated lymphomas are similar in terms of presentation, with widespread, extranodal disease, which often involves the CNS.

Interestingly, the initial treatment of patients with transplant-associated lymphoma usually consists of a reduction or discontinuation of immunosuppressive therapy. Thus, in a group of 17 patients with lymphoproliferative disorders developing from 2 to 68 months after cadaveric organ transplantation, 10 experienced a complete resolution of lymphomatous disease after decrease or cessation of immunosuppressive therapy, and 3 additional patients responded to reduction of immunosuppression in addition to use of attenuated chemotherapy or radiation (32). Although discontinuation of HIV-induced immunosuppression has not been feasible in the past, recent combinations of antiretroviral agents have had a major influence on HIV-viral load, associated with significant increases in CD4 cells (33). It will be of great interest to determine if use of these newer combinations may be effective in ameliorating lymphomatous disease in patients with AIDS, similar to that described in the setting of organ transplantation.

II. EVALUATION AND DIAGNOSTIC WORKUP OF THE PATIENT WITH AIDS-LYMPHOMA

A. Evaluation According to Symptoms and Signs of Disease

Almost all patients with AIDS-related lymphoma present with systemic B symptoms, including fever, night sweats, or weight loss in excess of 10% of normal body weight. Thus, as many as 82% of patients with systemic lymphoma, and 91% of those with primary CNS lymphoma first present with systemic symptoms (9–15,34). The importance of this mode of presentation relates to the fact that many opportunistic infections may also present similarly. Thus, infection with cytomegalovirus (CMV), *Mycobacterium avium* complex (MAC), *Cryptococcus,* and other organisms may be rather occult, without localizing findings, and with fever, night sweats, or weight loss as the only clinical complaints for which the patient has sought medical attention. Although oncologists may recognize the importance of such symptoms in terms of the possibility of underlying lymphoma, this may not be true of the generalists who provide primary care to HIV-infected patients. It is important, therefore, to recognize that systemic B symptoms may be indicative of lymphoma, mandating careful physical examination, a computed tomography (CT) scan of chest, abdomen, and pelvis, or bone marrow examination, in addition to workup for infection in an attempt to clarify the etiology of these symptoms.

Because AIDS-related lymphoma frequently presents in extranodal sites, a wide array of symptoms may occur, related to the specific site(s) of lymphomatous involvement. Symptoms of bone marrow failure, with fatigue related to anemia, bleeding related to thrombocytopenia, or infection related to neutropenia may be seen in patients with lymphomatous involvement of the bone marrow. Lymphoma in the gastrointestinal tract may present with abdominal pain, anorexia, nausea, and vomiting, or change in bowel habits. Abdominal distention or an abdominal mass may be noted. AIDS lymphoma may present in the oral cavity, with involvement of maxilla, mandible, or gums (9,35). In these cases, patients often first seek dental care, and may then be referred for medical evaluation after discovery of mass lesions, necrotic tissue around what appears to be an abscessed tooth, or other similar abnormalities. Lymphomatous involvement of the skin or soft tissues may present with nodules or larger mass lesions, which may be tender or painful. Cough, shortness of breath, or hemostasis may occur in patients who have lymphomatous involvement of the lung. Development of jaundice may prompt medical attention in patients who present with lymphoma in the liver or hepatobiliary tree, or in those with involvement of the pancreas, or peripancreatic lymph nodes, leading to bile duct obstruction. In general, almost any symptom may occur in patients with AIDS-related lymphoma, depending on the specific site of lymphomatous disease.

B. Evaluation According to Anatomical Presentation

1. Lymphadenopathy

The appropriate evaluation of lymphadenopathy in patients with HIV infection can be quite problematic, because reactive lymphadenopathy, termed *persistent, generalized lymphadenopathy* (PGL) is quite common in the setting of HIV, representing an exuberant immune response to the virus. Enlarged reactive lymph nodes in the setting of HIV are firm and rubbery, similar to the physical findings in lymphoma. Furthermore, although axillary, cervical, and inguinal adenopathy may be present in most patients with PGL, rather unusual sites of reactive lymphadenopathy have also been described, including epitrochlear and supraclavicular adenopathy in 9 and 6% of cases, respectively. Reactive splenomegaly may be seen in as many as 6% of HIV-infected patients (36). Of further difficulty in terms of differentiating enlarged reactive nodes from those of lymphoma is the fact that patients with PGL may also experience systemic B symptoms, with fever in 47%, night sweats in 35%, and weight loss in 24% (36). The factors that might suggest that lymph node enlargement is due to lymphoma, as opposed to reactive

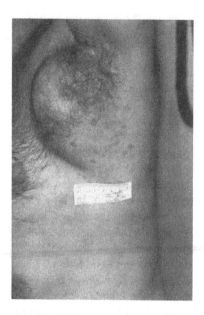

Figure 1   Example of asymmetrical lymphadenopathy in a patient with newly diagnosed AIDS lymphoma.

PGL, include rapidity of growth and asymmetry of enlarged nodes in the former (Fig. 1), whereas fluctuation of lymph node size over time is quite characteristic of the latter (36). Ultimately, however, lymph node biopsy is the only truly definitive method by which PGL can be distinguished from lymphoma (37). An alternative to excisional biopsy may be performance of fine-needle aspiration, with evaluation of aspirated cells both morphologically and by monoclonal antibodies, to determine the clonality of the lesion (38). If monoclonal immunophenotype is present, one may conclude that the process is consistent with malignant lymphoma. Conversely, a polyclonal immunophenotype would still mandate further evaluation, for some AIDS-related lymphomas may be polyclonal (39). Furthermore, pathological processes other than PGL may present with lymphadenopathy, including Kaposi's sarcoma, tuberculosis, atypical mycobacterial infection, and others. In these conditions, a polyclonal immunophenotype would be expected. Despite polyclonality, however, further evaluation would be required to diagnose the underlying condition causing the enlarged lymph nodes (37).

2.   Abdominal and Gastrointestinal Involvement

Patients with AIDS lymphoma frequently present with gastrointestinal (GI) involvement, reported in 4–28% of large series (9). Any site within the GI tract may be involved, and lymphomatous involvement of the entire GI tract has also been observed. Patients may present with abdominal pain, anorexia, weight loss, change in bowel habits, pain on defecation, hematemesis, hematochezia, or melena. Abdominal CT scan reveals evidence of focal lymphomatous involvement in almost all patients who present with symptoms or signs related to the abdomen, documented in 58 of 59 (98%) such patients described by Radin et al. (40). In a series of 112 patients with AIDS lymphoma, undergoing abdominal CT scan as part of routine-staging evaluation, evidence of intra-abdominal lymphoma was seen in 64%, with abnormalities within the GI tract in 54%, liver in 29%, kidney and adrenal in 11% each, pancreas in 5%, and peritoneum and omentum in 7% (40). Abdominal lymph node enlargement (over 1 cm) was present in 56% of 72 patients with evidence of abdominal lymphoma on the initial CT scans.

In patients with GI involvement by lymphoma, stomach and small intestine are the sites most frequently involved, although any site is possible. Involvement of rectum or perianal region is not uncommon, occurring more frequently in homosexual or bisexual men than in other population groups at risk for HIV (41).

Definitive diagnosis of lymphoma within the abdomen or GI tract usually requires endoscopic evaluation, with biopsy. Percutaneous or fine-needle aspirates may also be useful, in an attempt to avoid full diagnostic celiotomy.

3. Liver Involvement

The liver is involved by lymphoma in 9–26% of reported series (9). The most common abnormality on CT scan of the abdomen is focal hepatic lesions, varying from solitary to innumerable. The lesions range from relatively small 1-cm nodules to huge masses, larger than 15 cm in diameter. Lesions are typically less dense than the adjacent liver parenchyma. Larger masses are often heterogeneous in density, with areas of necrosis. In the absence of specific hepatic lesions, hepatomegaly, if present, is only mild and infrequent, occurring in 9 of 72 patients (13%) with abdominal CT evidence of focal lymphomatous involvement (40). All patients with moderate or marked hepatomegaly also had focal hypodense hepatic lesions. Definitive diagnosis of liver involvement requires liver biopsy, although presence of intrahepatic lesions on a CT scan, which are also avid on gallium-67 scanning, would be highly suggestive of lymphoma within the liver. In the absence of biopsy-confirmed lymphoma in another more accessible site, liver biopsy would be mandatory to confirm the etiology of such hepatic lesions.

4. Bone Marrow or Bony Involvement

Bone marrow is involved in approximately 21–33% of patients with AIDS lymphoma (9–15) and may present with generalized bony ache or pain, or with anemia, thrombocytopenia, or neutropenia in the peripheral blood. Anemia is the most common of these cytopenias, but is clearly nonspecific for the diagnosis of marrow involvement by lymphoma. Lymphomatous infiltration of marrow may also present in the absence of significant abnormalities in the peripheral blood; this is why bone marrow aspirate and biopsy is routinely performed as part of the staging evaluation of any patient with newly diagnosed AIDS lymphoma.

In the presence of bony involvement by lymphoma, pain is the most common method of presentation. Intractable headache has been described in a patient whose AIDS-related lymphoma was confined to the frontal and temporal regions of the skull (42). Although a CT scan of brain and lumbar puncture results were normal, a bone scan confirmed abnormal uptake, which led to open biopsy and the appropriate diagnosis. Alternatively, a gallium scan, done routinely in the staging evaluation of AIDS lymphoma, may also demonstrate abnormal uptake in bony sites involved by lymphoma.

5. Pulmonary Involvement

Involvement of the lung by lymphoma may present with shortness of breath, chest pain, or hemostasis. Occasional patients may also be asymptomatic. Findings on a chest x-ray film or CT scan may be extremely varied, with presence of pleural effusions or parenchymal abnormalities the most commonly encountered (43). Of the abnormalities within lung parenchyma, no predominant pattern of involvement has been reported, although interstitial infiltrates, pulmonary nodules, and alveolar lung disease all have been described. In contrast with de novo lymphoma, in which mediastinal or hilar adenopathy are the most frequent sites of disease within the chest (44), these sites are abnormal in the minority of HIV-infected patients with chest disease, seen in only 1 of 11 cases of intrathoracic AIDS lymphoma (43). In fact, the presence of such adenopathy in an HIV-infected patient may be more likely a result of fungal or acid-fast organisms, rather than lymphoma (45). The definitive diagnosis of lymphoma in the setting of intrathoracic abnormalities requires bronchoscopy and biopsy, evaluation of pleural fluid by cytological and monoclonal antibody staining, fine-needle aspiration, or open lung biopsy.

6. Primary Central Nervous System Lymphoma

Patients with primary CNS lymphoma usually present with headache and other symptoms of increased intracranial pressure (14%); seizures (27%); focal neurological deficit (51%); or altered mental status (53%) (46). In the latter circumstance, although profound abnormalities of mental status are common, very subtle changes in behavior or personality may also serve as the only symptoms of AIDS-related primary CNS lymphoma. These patients tend to have far-advanced HIV-induced immunocompromise, with CD4 cell counts well below $50/mm^3$. Presence of any of these symptoms would mandate an immediate workup for the presence of CNS lymphoma.

Magnetic resonance imaging (MRI) studies with use of gadolinium contrast may be the most useful initial diagnostic tool in this setting, as other disorders that must be considered, including cerebral toxoplasmosis, or progressive multifocal leukoencephalopathy (PML), may be more easily differentiated from lymphoma employing the MRI technique, as opposed to CT scans (47). Lymphoma tends to present with relatively large lesions on CT or MRI scan (2–5 cm or more). Usually, relatively few lesions are seen (less than five), which are enhanced by contrast or gadolinium. Ring enhancement may be seen in as many as 52% of cases (46). In cerebral toxoplasmosis, ring enhancement is quite common, lesions tend to be smaller than those seen in primary CNS lymphoma, and multiple lesions are expected. No single finding on MRI scan, however, will prove that a given patient has lymphoma versus toxoplasmosis. Recently, use of positron-emission tomography (PET) scanning has demonstrated some increased ability to differentiate cerebral lymphoma from toxoplasmosis, with lymphoma demonstrating increased uptake on PET scan, whereas lesions of toxoplasmosis tend to be "cold" and metabolically inactive (48,49). Another tool that may be useful in differentiating primary CNS lymphoma from cerebral toxoplasmosis is an evaluation for IgG antibody against toxoplasmosis. Because the vast majority of cerebral toxoplasmosis occurs as a consequence of reactivation of a preexisting infection, the absence of IgG antibody against toxoplasma would indicate that the patient has probably never been exposed to the organism, making a diagnosis of cerebral toxoplasmosis highly unlikely. IgG antitoxoplasmosis titers less than 1:4 are also unlikely to be associated with cerebral toxoplasmosis (50).

Additional evaluations that may be of help in making the diagnosis of primary CNS lymphoma include performance of a diagnostic lumbar puncture, with material sent for pathological evaluation. Although involvement of the cerebrospinal fluid (CSF) is seen in only approximately 23% of patients with primary CNS lymphoma (46), the presence of malignant cells, in the setting of mass lesion(s) in the brain, would allow a definitive diagnosis of lymphoma to be made. Additional diagnostic information may be obtained by evaluating CSF for presence of EBV DNA, because EBV is present in almost 100% of AIDS-related primary CNS lymphomas (51). Additionally, the presence of EBV DNA in CSF is a rather specific finding in CNS lymphoma, not seen in other pathological processes within brain of HIV-infected patients (52). Despite all of these evaluations, however, in most cases, the ultimate diagnosis of primary CNS lymphoma depends on pathological evaluation, obtained after open or stereotaxic brain biopsy (53).

C. General Evaluation of the Patient with Newly Diagnosed AIDS Lymphoma

The routine evaluation of a patient with newly diagnosed AIDS-related lymphoma is summarized in Table 1, and consists of a CT scan of chest, abdo-

Table 1   Routine Evaluation of Patient with Newly Diagnosed
AIDS Lymphoma

General
    CT scan of chest, abdomen, pelvis
    Gallium-67 scan
    Bone marrow biopsy
    Lumbar puncture with cytological assessment
    Blood work: LDH, CBC, liver function, and enzyme studies
Other focused workup depending on symptoms and signs
    Upper GI series with small bowel follow-through
    Barium enema
    Upper endoscopy
    Colonoscopy
    Bronchoscopy
    MRI of brain or PET scan of brain
    EBV DNA within CSF

men, and pelvis; bone marrow biopsy; lumbar puncture; gallium scan; blood work
to include LDH level; and other tests as clinically indicated.

Gallium-67 scanning may be particularly useful, and may differentiate malignant lymphoma from reactive lymphadenopathy (54). High-grade lymphoma
is almost uniformly gallium-avid, and may be useful in identifying lesions that
have not yet caused specific organ or nodal enlargement on a CT scan. Aside
from its known sensitivity and specificity in lymphoma, gallium-67 scanning may
be particularly useful in the assessment of residual, stable masses after the completion of chemotherapy. As described by Kaplan et al. (55), residual masses
may be seen in as many as 40% of patients with lymphoma who have successfully
completed chemotherapy; the residual masses in these instances represent fibrosis, and are gallium-negative. In the presence of a residual mass which remains
gallium-avid at the conclusion of chemotherapy, one can assume that residual
active lymphomatous disease is still present, and that further therapy will be
required.

Lumbar puncture is an important staging tool in the patient with systemic
AIDS-related lymphoma, as approximately 20% of patients who are asymptomatic for CNS involvement may have malignant cells circulating in this site (56).
Other symptoms of CSF involvement include cranial neuropathy, or chin numbness (57).

Determination of serum lactic dehydrogenase (LDH) levels may be very
valuable in patients with AIDS-related lymphoma, because LDH is usually quite
elevated. Thus, the finding of a markedly elevated LDH in an HIV-infected patient would mandate consideration of the possibility of underlying lymphoma.

LDH values are also useful in predicting prognosis in both AIDS-related and de novo lymphoma (22,58,59).

III. PROGNOSTIC FACTORS FOR RESPONSE AND SURVIVAL

A. De Novo Lymphoma

In HIV-seronegative patients with de novo intermediate or high-grade lymphoma, several factors are of prognostic importance in terms of survival. Thus, as defined by the International Non–Hodgkin's Lymphoma Prognostic Factors Project, a model based on patient age, tumor stage, serum LDH, performance status, and number of extranodal sites identified four risk groups, which predicted 5-year survival rates ranging from 73 to 26% (22). Specific factors associated with poorer prognosis included age older than 60 years; serum LDH values higher than the upper limit of normal; Eastern Cooperative Group performance status of 2–4 (versus 0 or 1); stage III or IV; and more than one site of extranodal disease. If present, each factor was given a numeric value of 1. Low-risk patients, with no or one risk factor, experienced a complete remission rate of 87%, with 5-year survival of 73%. Patients with two risk factors (low-intermediate group) had a complete remission (CR) rate of 67%, with 5-year survival of 51%; whereas those with three risk factors experienced a 55% CR rate, and a 43% five-year survival. Finally, those with four or five factors, the "high-risk" group, demonstrated a CR rate of 44%, with 5-year survival of 26% (22). This index has proved quite useful in predicting which patients are expected to do well, and which patients may require alternative types of therapy, in an attempt to improve the predicted prognosis.

B. AIDS-Related Lymphoma

Similar to de novo lymphoma, patients with AIDS-related disease may also demonstrate differing prognosis, based on factors that may be identified at the time of initial diagnosis. Of interest, certain of these factors relate to the extent of tumor, some relate to the overall vigor of the patient (in terms of age and performance status), whereas additional factors are related to the state of the underlying HIV infection. These poor prognostic factors were identified rather early in the AIDS epidemic, and have been modified over time as the epidemic has advanced. Initially, Levine et al. performed a multivariate analysis on 49 patients, noting that history of another AIDS-defining diagnosis (before the diagnosis of lymphoma); lower CD4 cell counts on a continuous scale; Karnofsky performance status less than 70%; and bone marrow involvement by lymphoma, were each associated with shorter survival (34). Pathological type of disease, presence of leptomeningeal disease, presence of systemic B symptoms, or mass size did not appear to influence subsequent survival times. Kaplan and colleagues noted that, in addition to these factors, CD4 cell counts of fewer than $100/mm^3$, and use of more intensive regimens of chemotherapy were also associated with poor prognosis (11). More recently, prognostic factors were evaluated in a group of 192 patients with newly diagnosed AIDS-related lymphoma, who participated in a randomized trial comparing low-dose m-BACOD (methotrexate, bleomycin, doxorubicin [Adriamycin; hydroxydaunomycin], cyclophosphamide, vincristine, dexamethasone) with standard-dose m-BACOD and GM–CSF (21,60,61). On multivariate analysis, the factors associated with decreased survival included age older than 35 years; history of injection drug use; stage III or IV disease; and CD4 cell counts of fewer than $100/mm^3$ (61). The median overall survival for patients with one or none of these risk factors was 46 weeks, versus 44 weeks with two factors, and 18 weeks for those with three or more poor-risk factors (61). In a further analysis performed on 96 patients from a single institution in Italy, factors that were of prognostic significance on multivariate analysis included age older than 40 years, elevated LDH values, and CD4 cell counts of fewer than $100/mm^3$ (58). It is thus apparent from these studies that prognosis in patients with AIDS-related lymphoma will depend on HIV-related factors (history of AIDS before lymphoma; CD4 cell counts of fewer than $100/mm^3$); host factors (age older than 35 or 40; poor performance status); and factors that relate to the bulk of lymphoma (stage III or IV; elevated LDH value). Of further importance, when patients with primary CNS lymphoma are also considered, this group clearly stands out as associated with extremely poor prognosis and short survival, despite use of chemotherapy or radiation therapy (9,34,62).

IV. MANAGEMENT OF THE PATIENT WITH AIDS-RELATED LYMPHOMA

A. Standard Therapies for Patients with Newly Diagnosed Disease

1. Role of Dose Intensity

At the outset of the AIDS epidemic in the early 1980s, the use of dose-intensive therapy was considered important in achievement of complete remission and long-term survival in patients with de novo intermediate- or high-grade lymphoma. As shown on Table 2, regimens such as m-BACOD (63); ProMACE-MOPP (64), MACOP-B (65), and others were studied in single-institutional trials, and were more effective when compared with older, less intensive regimens, such as CHOP (66). It was appropriate, then, to consider use of similar regimens of high-dose intensity in patients with AIDS-related lymphoma, who commonly

Table 2 Summary of Reported Therapeutic Trials in Patients with Newly Diagnosed AIDS Lymphoma

Regimen	No. pts	% CR	% OIs	Comment	Median survival	Ref.
COMP	25	28%	100% grade 4 heme toxicity	1986	3 mo	67
ProMACE-MOPP	15	20%	27%	1986	5 mo	68
HD AraC, HDMTX, other agents	9	33%	78%	1987	6 mo	69
m-BACOD, standard	13	54%	8%	1987	11 mo	69
COMET-A	38	58%	28%	1989	5.2 mo	11
Low-dose m-BACOD	35	46%	20%	1991	6.5 mo	56
CCNU, etoposide, cytophosphamide, procarbazine orally ± C–GSF	38	20%	28% febrile neutropenia	1993 1997	7 mo	75,76
CDE, by CI, + ddI	46	57%	20%	1996, 1997	18 mo	73,74
Low-dose m-BACOD plus ddC	28	56%	12%	1996	8.1 mo	77
Low-dose m-BACOD	94	41% (p = ns)	22%	1997	8.8 mo (p = ns)	21
vs.						
Standard m-BACOD	81	52%	26%		7.8 mo	21
AZT + chemo	31	17%	44%	Poor prognosis	3.5 mo	79
MACOP-B	12	67%	N.D.	Good prognosis	20 mo	70
LNH-84	141	63%	9% Rx related death, incl. OI	Good prognosis	9 mo	71
ACVB	52	77% (p = ns)	34%	Good prognosis	Not given	72
vs.						
Standard CHOP	57	58%	34%		Not given	72

presented with widespread, bulky disease of a high-grade pathological type. Accordingly, the earliest published trials in patients with HIV-related lymphoma employed regimens such as COMP (67) or ProMACE-MOPP (68). Despite evidence of efficacy in patients with de novo lymphoma, however, these regimens were largely ineffective in the setting of HIV-related lymphoma, with complete remission achieved in 28 and 20%, respectively, and median survival of only 3–5 months (67,68). Acknowledging the high proclivity of CNS disease and the high-grade nature of lymphomatous disease, Gill and colleagues employed a novel regimen, consisting of high-dose cytarabine (cytosine arabinoside), high-dose methotrexate, and other agents in nine patients with AIDS lymphoma, noting a complete remission rate of 33%, median survival of 6 months, and development of intercurrent opportunistic infections in 78% (69). The trial was terminated early owing to these results, and consideration was given to the possibility that HIV-infected patients simply might not be able to tolerate such dose intensity. Similar conclusions were drawn by Kaplan et al., who employed a similar regimen, termed COMET-A, which resulted in complete remission in 58% of 38 patients; however, median survival was only 5.5 months, and 28% developed opportunistic infections that led to death (11). When outcome was compared with that achieved with various less intensive regimens, employed in 27 patients and retrospectively evaluated, the increased dose intensity of COMET-A was associated with significantly shorter survival. These early trials thus suggested that patients with AIDS-related lymphoma were distinct from those with de novo disease, experiencing undue toxicity, without real benefit after use of dose-intensive regimens of combination chemotherapy.

In an attempt to ascertain if lower doses of chemotherapy might be more effective in the setting of underlying HIV infection, Levine and colleagues employed a low-dose modification of the m-BACOD regimen, administered to a group of 35 patients, enrolled in the AIDS Clinical Trials Group (ACTG; 56). The low-dose m-BACOD regimen employed 50% doses of hydroxydaunomycin and cyclophosphamide, along with early institution of CNS prophylaxis, and attenuation in the number of cycles actually administered. Thus, patients were restaged after two cycles; if complete remission had been attained, two additional courses were given, with subsequent cessation of further chemotherapy, and institution of zidovudine (azidothymidine), the only antiretroviral agent licensed in the United States for HIV disease at that time. In patients who had attained partial remission after two cycles, an additional two cycles were administered. If subsequent restaging demonstrated CR status, these patients received two additional cycles, whereas those who failed to achieve CR were removed from protocol. Thus, most patients on this trial received four to six cycles of dose-reduced therapy. Of note, complete remission was attained in 46%, with clinical CR in an additional 5%, in whom bulky disease at diagnosis had regressed to smaller, but stable masses in sites that were inaccessible for repeat biopsy. Although the median survival was only 6.5 months, a median survival of 15 months was achieved in those who attained CR. Furthermore, 75% of complete responders remained in continuous complete remission. Because no patient experienced isolated CNS relapse, the use of intrathecal cytarabine (cytosine arabinoside) appeared effective in preventing recurrence in this site. It was thus apparent from this trial that low-dose chemotherapy could be associated with long-term, lymphoma-free survival. However, despite the use of dose-attenuated therapy, grade 4 hematological toxicity was observed in 21%, and 20% of patients developed opportunistic infections.

The value of dose intensity remained somewhat controversial, however, because other investigators reported evidence of efficacy with use of more intensive regimens. The MACOP-B regimen, for example, was employed in 12 patients, resulting in a complete remission rate of 67%, an overall median survival of 7 months, but a median survival of 20 months in those who achieved CR (70). Careful evaluation of the latter responders indicated that these individuals had good prognostic disease, with Karnofsky performance status of 100%, and no history of AIDS before the lymphoma (70). These results suggested the possibility that patients with good prognostic features might benefit from more dose-intensive therapy, whereas those with poor prognostic indicators were unable to tolerate these regimens, experiencing frequent development of intercurrent infections, and rapid death.

In an attempt to clarify the value of dose-intensive therapy in patients with AIDS lymphoma, the ACTG recently completed a prospective, multicenter trial (21), in which patients were stratified by baseline prognostic indicators, and randomized to receive either the low-dose m-BACOD regimen employed earlier (56), or standard-dose m-BACOD with hematopoietic growth factor support, employing GM–CSF. With 192 patients evaluable for response, no statistically significant difference was observed, with 41% attaining CR after low-dose therapy, versus 52% CR after standard-dose m-BACOD. Of note, 23% experienced recurrence after low-dose therapy, whereas 40% of those receiving standard-dose experienced relapse (p = 0.08). Median time to recurrence following CR was 106 weeks for those receiving standard-dose and in excess of 190 weeks in patients who received low-dose therapy (p = 0.06), whereas median overall survival was 31 weeks in the standard-dose group and 35 weeks in the low-dose group (21). In a multivariate analysis controlling for various prognostic factors, no statistically significant differences in survival were apparent in either treatment group, based on prognostic factors or on pathological type of disease. Although patients with CD4 cell counts of more than $100/mm^3$ lived longer than those with CD4 cell counts of fewer than $100/mm^3$, there were no significant differences in survival between treatment groups after controlling for CD4 cell count. Thus, this study did not confirm an advantage for standard-dose therapy among patients with good-risk disease. Although overall response and survival times were similar in the two treatment groups, toxicity was significantly greater in patients who received standard-dose m-BACOD, despite the use of GM–CSF. Thus, grade 3 or higher toxicity occurred in 70% of patients assigned to standard-dose, and 51% of those who received low-dose treatment (p = 0.008), consisting primarily of hematological toxicity. Opportunistic illnesses developed in 22% of those who received low-dose and 26% of patients receiving standard-dose treatment. This large prospective trial would thus seem to indicate that low-dose chemotherapy is the treatment of choice in patients with AIDS-related lymphoma, resulting in equivalent response rates, a trend toward longer overall and progression-free survival, and a statistically decreased risk of severe hematological toxicity in patients with either good-risk, or poor-risk disease (21).

2. Role of Dose Intensity in Patients with Good Prognosis AIDS-Related Lymphoma

Additional studies have been conducted to explore the use of dose-intensive therapy used specifically in patients with good-risk AIDS lymphoma. Gisselbrecht and colleagues (71) employed the intensive LNH 84 regimen in a group of 141 patients, whose median CD4 cell count was 227/μL, performance status was less than 3, and who had no active opportunistic infections. The regimen consisted of three cycles of doxorubicin (75 mg/m^2), cyclophosphamide (1200 mg/m^2); vindesine (2 mg/m^2 for 2 days); bleomycin (10 mg for 2 days); and prednisone (60 mg/m^2 for 5 days: ACVB). These three cycles were then followed by a consolidation phase of high-dose methotrexate plus leucovorin, ifosfamide, etoposide, asparaginase, and cytarabine. Intrathecal methotrexate was used in all patients as prophylaxis, and zidovudine maintenance therapy was employed after conclusion of chemotherapy. A complete remission rate of 63% was achieved, with 13% partial responders. Median survival was 9 months, whereas median disease-free survival for complete responders was 16 months. In multivariate analysis, the four factors associated with decreased survival were CD4 cell counts of fewer than 100/μL; performance status more than 1; immunoblastic lymphoma; and AIDS before the lymphoma. In the absence of all such factors, the 2-year survival was predicted to be 50%.

In an attempt to further clarify the optimal treatment regimens for patients with good-, intermediate-, or poor-risk AIDS lymphoma, the European Intergroup Study NHL–HIV began a randomized phase III study, in which patients have been stratified by prognostic categories and then treated with less or greater dose intensity, dependent on the underlying risk group (72). Patients with good-risk AIDS lymphoma included those with performance status ≤1 (WHO criteria), no prior diagnosis of AIDS, and CD4 cell count more than 100/μL. These patients were randomized to receive either the ACVB regimen (71), or standard dose CHOP, given every 3 weeks. All patients received intrathecal methotrexate at each treatment cycle, and all patients received G-CSF. Results in a total of 159 patients with good-prognosis AIDS lymphoma were recently reported (72). A complete remission was achieved in 66% of 80 patients randomized to ACVB, whereas a CR of 60% was observed in the 79 patients who received standard-dose CHOP (p = NS). Grade 4 hematological toxicity was observed more frequently in the ACVB-treated patients (36 versus 4%). Treatment-related death occurred in approximately 5% of patients in each treatment group, whereas approximately 34% from each group died of opportunistic infection. Overall survival in the two treatment groups was identical, at 50%. Although these results are still preliminary, it is clear that patients with good-prognosis AIDS lymphoma may be able to tolerate more dose-intensive therapy, although hematological toxicity remains common. Nonetheless, this trial demonstrated no advantage to the dose-intensive ACVB regimen when compared to standard dose CHOP.

3. Alternative Routes of Chemotherapy Administration: Infusional or Oral Regimens

Sparano and colleagues explored the feasibility of delivering a continuous infusion of chemotherapy, together with the antiretroviral didanosine in a group of 25 patients with newly diagnosed AIDS lymphoma (73). Employing a 96-h continuous intravenous infusion of cyclophosphamide (800 mg/m^2 for 96 h); doxorubicin (50 mg/m^2 for 96 h); and etoposide (240 mg/m^2 for 96 h), administered every 28 or more days, a complete remission rate of 58% was achieved (95% CI, 38–78%), with a median duration of CR in excess of 18 months, and a median survival of 18.4 months. In those patients who received didanosine, less bone marrow suppression was encountered, with significantly less neutropenia, thrombocytopenia, and need for fewer red cell transfusions during therapy. However, no significant change in CD4 cell counts was observed. These results were combined with an earlier study employing the same chemotherapeutic regimen, without addition of didanosine. Long-term follow-up of these total 46 patients was recently provided, with a minimum follow-up of 18 months (74). In the total group, a complete remission rate of 57% was achieved, with a median survival of 18 months. Median age in the group was 38 years, and median CD4 cell counts were 88/μL (range 2–1078/μL). Tumor-related mortality was 35%. In multivariate analysis, increased number of disease sites, and prior antiretroviral therapy were associated with significantly decreased overall survival, whereas increasing number of disease sites and poor performance status were associated with decreased lymphoma-specific survival times. Although patients with the small, noncleaved histological type had significantly higher CD4 cell counts at study entry, no significant differences in CR rate or survival were documented among patients with the various pathological types of lymphoma. The authors concluded that both lymphoma and AIDS contribute to mortality in these individuals.

In an attempt to provide an easier route of administration of chemotherapy, Remick and colleagues employed an oral regimen (75), administered on an outpatient basis to 18 patients with newly diagnosed AIDS lymphoma. The regimen consisted of lomustine (CCNU), 100 mg/m² on day 1; etoposide, 200 mg/m² on days 1 through 3; cyclophosphamide, 100 mg/m² on days 22 and 31; and procarbazine, 100 mg/m² on days 22 through 31, given at 6-week intervals. A complete remission rate of 39% was achieved, with 22% partial responders. The median duration of survival was 7 months (11 days to 36 months). Unfortunately, treatment-related mortality was 11%, nearly two-thirds of patients developed grade 3 or 4 leukopenia, and 28% of cycles were associated with febrile neutropenia. In an attempt to improve the therapeutic index of this regimen, Remick recently reported on the value of addition of G–CSF to the regimen (76). Twenty patients were treated, employing the same regimen of oral chemotherapy, with the addition of G–CSF, 300 μg (5 μg/kg) given subcutaneously on days 5–21 and days 33–42 of each cycle. The complete remission rate was 20%, with 40% partial remissions. Median survival was 7 months (0.5–24 months). Of the total combined patient group (38 patients), 1 (5%) developed CNS relapse, despite use of CCNU and procarbazine. Of interest, no difference in the incidence of grade 3 and 4 leukopenia was seen when G–CSF was employed (51 versus 64%). Moreover, there was no statistical difference in the episodes of febrile neutropenia or in the average number of days hospitalized for febrile neutropenia (16.4 versus 17.2), although the number of hospitalizations for febrile neutropenia was decreased in the G–CSF group (7 versus 13). It is apparent that although this regimen may be easier in terms of oral administration of chemotherapy, complete remission rates are somewhat less than those described with other regimens (21,56,71,73), and significant toxicity is encountered, even with the use of G–CSF.

4. Use of Chemotherapy in Combination with Antiretroviral Agents

It has become clear that the major challenge in treating patients with AIDS-related lymphoma is because underlying HIV infection must also be addressed, for patients are as likely to die of AIDS-related opportunistic infections as die of malignant lymphoma. With these considerations in mind, various investigators have explored the use of combined antiretroviral therapy along with multiagent chemotherapy. Levine et al. used zalcitabine (dideoxycytadine; ddC) along with the low-dose m-BACOD regimen in 28 patients with newly diagnosed AIDS lymphoma (77). Because both zalcitabine and vincristine may cause peripheral neuropathy, a phase I/II study design was employed, with initial withholding of vincristine, and subsequent addition of the drug at increasing doses. Complete remission was achieved in 14 of 25 evaluable patients (56%), with partial response in 5 (20%). Median survival of CR patients was 29.2 months, whereas median survival for the group as a whole was 8.1 months. No significant peripheral neuropathy was observed, even with full-dose vincristine and zalcitabine. Grade 4 neutropenia occurred in 16%, even though zalcitabine may itself be marrow-suppressive. Opportunistic infections developed in 12%. Of interest, serum immune complex-dissociated (ICD) p24 antigen levels either fell (7/14) or remained consistently negative (2/14) in 9 of 14 patients (64%), whereas 36% experienced an increase over time. Because IL-6 may function as a growth factor in the setting of AIDS lymphoma (78), serial IL-6 levels in serum were determined in this cohort receiving both chemotherapy and zalcitabine. Elevated serum IL-6 levels at diagnosis were associated with systemic B symptoms, whereas changes in IL-6 correlated with response to therapy over time (p = 0.006). This study would indicate that zalcitabine may be safely administered along with m-BACOD chemotherapy, and may be associated with smaller degrees of marrow compromise than reported in other series in which antiretroviral therapy was withheld (21,56).

Sparano has also noted less bone marrow compromise with the combined use of chemotherapy (the infusional CDE regimen) with the antiretroviral didanosine (73). In this prospective trial in which consecutive patients were assigned in an alternating fashion to receive didanosine during cycles 1, 2, 5, and 6; or during cycles 3, 4, 5, and 6, the use of didanosine was associated with smaller degrees of leukopenia, neutropenia, and thrombocytopenia, and less need for red blood cell transfusions. No substantial change in serum p24 antigen was observed during CDE chemotherapy, although the HIV blood culture converted from negative to positive in 64%, despite the use of didanosine. Likewise, didanosine had no effect on the CD4 cells, which significantly decreased from baseline in all. A total of 20% of patients died of opportunistic infection either during or soon after completion of chemotherapy. This study would indicate that didanosine may be administered safely with chemotherapy, may be associated with smaller degrees of hematological toxicity, but may not have the ability to decrease viral burden (as measured by p24 antigen levels), or to obviate the development of opportunistic infections.

Zidovudine (AZT) has also been employed along with chemotherapy in patients with AIDS lymphoma (79). However, zidovudine itself is associated with significant marrow suppression (80). Not surprisingly, use of zidovudine, even with low-dose chemotherapy, was associated with severe bone marrow suppression. Thus, only 20 of 31 patients actually received zidovudine, and only 12 of these were able to complete the planned therapy. Zidovudine was discontinued in 8 (40%) because of toxic effects on the marrow, and grade 4 leukopenia was documented in 50%. Of interest, aside from its association with severe marrow compromise, the use of chemotherapy with zidovudine was also ineffective in preventing opportunistic infections, which occurred in 44% of treated patients. These data would clearly indicate that use of zidovudine is not warranted in patients with AIDS lymphoma when used together with combination chemotherapy.

Although no data yet exist related to the use of protease inhibitors with combination chemotherapy, a prospective clinical trial has just been initiated within the AIDS Malignancy Consortium sponsored by the NCI to determine the effect of combination chemotherapy (a low-dose CHOP regimen) together with combination antiretroviral therapy (employing a protease inhibitor and two reverse transcriptase inhibitors) in patients with newly diagnosed AIDS lymphoma. Preliminary results suggest that CHOP chemotherapy may be given safely with a protease inhibitor (indinavir) and two reverse transcriptase inhibitors (stavudine and lamivudine).

5. HIV Viral Load (HIV RNA Levels) During Chemotherapy

Recent advances have led to the improved ability to measure HIV in blood, based on HIV RNA levels in plasma, as measured by polymerase chain reaction (PCR; 81). Even though current information is scanty, several small preliminary studies have indicated no significant increase in HIV RNA levels during chemotherapy for AIDS-related lymphoma. Employing the EPOCH regimen (etoposide, 200 mg/m^2; vincristine, 1.6 mg/m^2; doxorubicin, 40 mg/m^2) by continuous infusion for 96 h on days 1–4; with cyclophosphamide (750 mg) on day 5, and prednisone (60 mg on days 1–5), Little and colleagues (82) studied serial levels of HIV RNA in plasma, in ten patients. No antiretroviral therapy was employed during the first 6 weeks of therapy. Median plasma RNA before chemotherapy was 19,365 copies per microliter (range 0–730,000), whereas median RNA was 13,500 (range 0–28,000) 3 weeks posttherapy, and 5100 (range 1–15,000) 6 weeks postchemotherapy. The HIV RNA level was significantly decreased from baseline, when comparing the values obtained either 3 or 6 weeks postchemotherapy (p < 0.01). However, CD4 cell levels also significantly decreased during the course of chemotherapy.

Levine et al. studied serial HIV RNA levels during the first week of therapy with mitoguazone (83), used in patients with relapsed or refractory AIDS-related lymphoma. The median baseline HIV RNA level was 21,416 copies per milliliter, ranging from 1,354 to 1,280,315. At 24 h post mitoguazone, the median HIV RNA level was 21,979; at 48 h, the median was 16,005; and at 72 h, the median HIV RNA was 10,707 copies per milliliter (range 914–472,081). When comparing the initial and last HIV RNA levels, five patients experienced an increase (median 47%, range 10–150%), whereas five demonstrated a decrease from baseline (median 63%, range 47–71%). There was no relation between HIV RNA levels at baseline and stage of lymphomatous disease, age, risk factor for HIV disease, or subsequent response to therapy or survival.

Additional work will be required to ascertain the short- and long-term effect of chemotherapy on HIV vial load, and to determine the relation of viral burden to outcome in patients with newly diagnosed AIDS-related lymphoma.

B. Therapy for Patients with Relapsed or Refractory AIDS-Related Lymphoma

Unfortunately, options for patients with relapsed or refractory AIDS-related lymphoma have been quite limited. Tirelli (84) recently employed a regimen of etoposide (80 mg/m^2 orally days 1–5); prednimustine (80 mg/m^2 orally, days 1–5); and mitoxantrone (10 mg/m^2 IV, day 1) in 19 evaluable patients with relapsed AIDS lymphoma, all of whom had received only one prior regimen. A complete remission rate of 26% was achieved, occurring primarily in patients who had relapsed after achieving complete remission with primary therapy. Grade 4 neutropenia occurred in 42% of cycles, and 14% of patients were hospitalized with febrile neutropenia. Median survival for the group was 2 months, whereas that of complete responders was 13 months (range 6–13 months).

Recently (85), mitoguazone was explored in a group of 35 such patients, all of whom had failed one (51%) or multiple (two to six) prior regimens. Mitoguazone, as an inhibitor of polyamine biosynthesis, represents a new class of chemotherapeutic agents. An objective response rate of 23% was attained, with complete remission in half and partial response in the others. The regimen was exceptionally well-tolerated, with neutropenia documented in 20%, although only 1 (3%) experienced grade 4 neutropenia. Median survival was 21.5 months in complete responders, 5.6 months in partial responders, and 2.6 months for the group as a whole.

Use of zidovudine with methotrexate has been studied in 29 patients with either newly diagnosed or relapsed AIDS lymphoma (86). The regimen employed by Tosi and colleagues consisted of three weekly courses of methotrexate at 1 g/m^2 (days 1, 8, and 15), together with oral zidovudine (2 g/m^2, orally, on days 1, 2, and 3; 4 g/m^2 orally on days 8, 9, and 10; and 6 g/m^2 orally on days 15, 16, and 17), along with leucovorin rescue. Beginning with patient 11, all complete or partial responders continued with this regimen for three additional courses, using zidovudine at the 6 g/m^2 dose. In 26 evaluable patients, the complete remission rate was 46% (95% CI, 29–65%), with partial response in 31%. The median duration of CR was 12.8 months, and median survival for the group as a whole was 12 months. Hematological toxicity was significant, with grade 4 neutropenia in 52%, and grade 3 or 4 anemia in 31%. Neutropenia caused delay in administration of chemotherapy in 8 patients, with a median delay of 18.6 days. CD4 cell counts decreased significantly during treatment, whereas p24 antigen levels were not significantly changed. Although zidovudine was initially developed as an antineoplastic drug, its activity was only minimal, as it represents a poor substrate for human DNA polymerase, so that only small amounts can be incorporated into tumor cell DNA. However, inhibition of de novo thymidylate biosynthesis by methotrexate can markedly increase the phosphorylation of zidovudine, leading to increased incorporation into DNA, and to increased antineoplastic activity (87). This study is most interesting, and serves to validate the potential efficacy of zidovudine, used in combination with other agents in the treatment of patients with AIDS-related lymphoma.

Use of monoclonal antibodies, either alone or conjugated with various toxins has been explored by several investigators. However, such approaches still remain experimental, with results limited to phase I/II studies on small numbers of patients.

C. Alternative Therapeutic Options

Alternative targets for future therapeutic intervention in patients with AIDS-related lymphoma will be presented elsewhere (see Chapter 9). Of interest, several anecdotal reports of spontaneous remission of AIDS lymphoma have been documented (88,89), although such an occurrence is extremely unusual. Furthermore, several reports of successful remission of AIDS lymphoma after antiretroviral therapy alone have been described (90).

REFERENCES

1. Non-Hodgkin's Lymphoma Pathologic Classification Project. National Cancer Institute sponsored study of classifications of non-Hodgkin's lymphomas: summary and description of a working formulation for clinical usage. Cancer 49:2112–2135, 1982.
2. Raphael J, Gentihomme O, Tulliez M, Byron PA, Diebold J. Histopathologic features of high grade non-Hodgkin's lymphomas in acquired immunodeficiency syndrome. Arch Pathol Lab Med 115:15–20, 1991.
3. Chang Y, Cesarman E, Pessin MS, Lee F, Culpepper J, Knowles DM, Moore P. Identification of herpesvirus-like DNA sequences in AIDS-associated Kaposi's sarcoma. Science 266:1865–1869, 1994.
4. Nador RG, Cesarman E, Chadburn A, Dawson DB, Ansari MQ, Said J, Knowles DM. Primary effusion lymphoma: a distinct clinicopathologic entity associated with the Kaposi's sarcoma associated herpes virus. Blood 88:645–656, 1996.
5. Said L, Chien K, Takeuchi S, et al. KSHV in primary effusion lymphoma: ultrastructural demonstration of herpesvirus in lymphoma cells. Blood 87:4937–4943, 1996.
6. Chadburn A, Cesarman E, Jagirdar J, Subar M, Mir RN, Knowles DM. CD30 (Ki-1) positive anaplastic large cell lymphomas in individuals infected with the human immunodeficiency virus. Cancer 72:3078–3090, 1993.

7. Strauchen JA, Hauser D, Burstein D, Jimenez R, Moore PS, Chang Y. Body cavity-based malignant lymphoma containing Kaposi's sarcoma associated herpesvirus in an HIV negative man with previous Kaposi's sarcoma. Ann Intern Med 125:822–825, 1996.

8. Greer JP, Kinney MC, Collins RD, Salhany KE, Wolff SN, Hainsworth JD. Clinical features of 31 patients with Ki-1 anaplastic large cell lymphoma. J Clin Oncol 9: 539–547, 1991.

9. Levine AM. AIDS related lymphoma [review]. Blood 80:8–20, 1992.

10. Levine AM, Gill PS, Meyer PR, Burkes R, Dworsky RD, Krailo M, Parker JW, Taylor CR, Lukes RJ, Rasheed S. Retrovirus and malignant lymphoma in homosexual men. JAMA 254:1921–1925, 1985.

11. Kaplan LD, Abrams DI, Feigal E, McGrath M, Kahn J, Neville P, Ziegler J, Volberding PA. AIDS-associated non–Hodgkin's lymphoma in San Francisco. JAMA 261: 719–724, 1989.

12. Lowenthal DA, Straus DJ, Campbell SW, Gold JWM, Clarkson BD, Koziner B. AIDS-related lymphoid neoplasia: The Memorial Hospital experience. Cancer 61: 2325–2337, 1988.

13. Knowles DM, Chamulak GA, Subar M, Burke JS, Dugan M, Wernz J, Slywotzky C, Pelicci PG, Dalla-Favera R, Raphael B. Lymphoid neoplasia associated with the acquired immunodeficiency syndrome (AIDS). Ann Intern Med 108:744–753, 1988.

14. Levine AM, Meyer PR, Begandy MK, et al. Development of B cell lymphoma in homosexual men: clinical and immunologic findings. Ann Intern Med 100:7–13, 1984.

15. Ziegler JL, Beckstead JA, Volberding PA, et al. Non–Hodgkin's lymphoma in 90 homosexual men: relation to generalized lymphadenopathy and the acquired immunodeficiency syndrome. N Engl J Med 311:565–570, 1984.

16. Jones SE, Fuks Z, Bull M, Kadin ME, Dorfman RF, Kaplan HS, Rosenberg SA, Kim H. Non–Hodgkin's lymphomas IV: clinico-pathologic correlation in 405 cases. Cancer 31:806–823, 1973.

17. Mackintosh FR, Colby TV, et al. Central nervous system involvement in non–Hodgkin's lymphoma: an analysis of 105 cases. Cancer 49:586–595, 1982.

18. Goldie JH, Coldman AJ, Gudauskas GA. Rationale for the use of alternating non-cross resistant chemotherapy. Cancer Treat Rep 66:439–449, 1982.

19. Fisher RI, Gaynor ER, Dahlberg S, Oken MM, Grogan TM, Mize EM, Glick JH, Coltman CA, Miller TP. Comparison of a standard regimen (CHOP) with three intensive chemotherapy regimens for advanced non–Hodgkin's lymphoma. N Engl J Med 328:1002–1006, 1993.

20. Tanosaki R, Okamoto S, Akatsuka N, et al. Dose escalation of bi-weekly cyclophosphamide, doxorubicin, vincristine and prednisone using recombinant human granulocyte colony stimulating factor in non Hodgkin's lymphoma. Cancer 74:1939–1944, 1994.

21. Kaplan LD, Straus DJ, Testa MA, Von Roenn J, Dezube BJ, Cooley TP, Herndier B, Northfelt DW, Huang J, Tulpule A, Levine AM. Low dose compared with standard dose mBACOD chemotherapy for non-Hodgkin's lymphoma associated with human immunodeficiency virus infection. N Engl J Med 336:1641–1648, 1997.

22. International Non-Hodgkin's Lymphoma Prognostic Factors Project. A predictive

model for aggressive non-Hodgkin's lymphoma. N Engl J Med 329:987–994, 1993.

23. Mocharnuk RS, Ghadialy A, Tulpule A, Espina B, Levine AM. Long term, disease-free survival in AIDS-related lymphoma. Proc Am Soc Cancer Oncol 15:306, 1996.

24. Cabanillas F. Experience with salvage regimens at MD Anderson Hospital. Ann Oncol 2(supp 1):31–32, 1991.

25. Penn I. Cancers complicating organ transplantation. N Engl J Med 323:1767–1769, 1990.

26. Swinnen LJ, Costanzo-Nordin MR, Fisher SG, O'Sullivan EF, Johnson MR, Heroux AL, Dizikes GH, Pifarre R, Fisher RI. Increased incidence of lymphoproliferative disorders after immunosuppression with the monoclonal antibody OKT3 in cardiac transplant recipients. N Engl J Med 323:1723–1728, 1990.

27. Frizzera G, Hanto DW, Gajl-Peczalska KJ, Rosai J, McKenna RW, Sibley RK, Holahan KP, Lindquist LL. Polymorphic diffuse B cell hyperplasias and lymphomas in renal transplant recipients. Cancer Res 41:4262–4279, 1981.

28. Cleary ML, Warnke R, Sklar J. Monoclonality of lymphoproliferative lesions in cardiac transplant recipients: clinical analysis based on immunoglobulin gene rearrangements. N Engl J Med 30:477–482, 1984.

29. Hanto DW, Frizzera G, Purtile D, et al. Clinical spectrum of lymphoproliferative disorders in renal transplant recipients and evidence for the role of Epstein–Barr virus. Cancer Res 41:4253–4261, 1981.

30. Hanto DW, Gajl-Peczalkska KJ, Frizzera G, Arthur DC, Balfour HH, McClain K, Simmons RL, Najarian JS. Epstein Barr virus induced polyclonal and monoclonal B cell lymphoproliferative disease occurring after renal transplantation. Ann Surg 198:356–369, 1983.

31. Weintraub J, Warnke RA. Lymphoma in cardiac allotransplant recipients: clinical and histological features and immunological phenotype. Transplantation 33:347–351, 1982.

32. Starzl TE, Nalesnik MA, Porter KA, Ho M, Iwatsuki S, Griffith BP, Rosenthal JT, Hakala TR, Shaw BW Jr, Hardesty RL, Atchison RW, Jeffe R, Bahnson HT. Reversibility of lymphomas and lymphoproliferative lesions developing under cyclosporin-steroid therapy. Lancet 1:583–587, 1984.

33. Collier AC, Coombs RW, Shoenfeld DA, et al. Treatment of human immunodeficiency virus infection with saquinavir, zidovudine, and zalcitabine. N Engl J Med 334:1011–1017, 1996.

34. Levine AM, Sullivan-Halley J, Pike MC, Rarick MU, Loureiro C, Bernstein-Singer M, Willson E, Brynes R, Parker J, Rasheed S, Gill PS. HIV related lymphoma: prognostic factors predictive of survival. Cancer 68:2466–2472, 1991.

35. Delecluse HG, Anagnostopoulos I, Dallenbach F, Hummel M, Marafioti T, Schneider U, Huhn D, Schmidt-Westhausen A, Reichart PA, Gross U, Stein H. Plasmablastic lymphomas of the oral cavity: a new entity associated with the human immunodeficiency virus infection. Blood 89:1413–1420, 1997.

36. Levine AM, Gill PS, Rasheed S. Human retrovirus associated lymphoproliferative disorders in homosexual men. Prog Allergy 37:244–258, 1986.

37. Levine AM, Meyer PR, Gill PS, Burkes RL, Krailo M, Aguilar S, Parker JW. Results

of diagnostic lymph node biopsy in homosexual men with generalized lymphadenopathy. J Clin Oncol 4:165–169, 1985.

38. Strigle SM, Martin SE, Levine AM, Rarick MU. Use of fine needle aspiration cytology in the management of HIV related non-Hodgkin's lymphoma and Hodgkin's disease. J Acquir Immune Defic Syndr 6:1329–1334, 1993.

39. Shriamizu B, Herndier B, Meeker T, Kaplan L, McGrath M. Molecular and immunophenotypic characterization of AIDS-associated, Epstein–Barr virus negative, polyclonal lymphoma. J Clin Oncol 10:383–389, 1992.

40. Radin DR, Esplin JA, Levine AM, Ralls PW. AIDS-related non-Hodgkin's lymphoma: abdominal CT findings in 112 patients. AJR Am J Radiol 160:1133–1139, 1993.

41. Ioachim HL. Lymphoma: an opportunistic neoplasia of AIDS. Leukemia 6:(supp 3) 30S–33S, 1992.

42. Kelleher AD, Brew BJ, Milliken ST. Intractable headache as the presenting complaint of AIDS-related lymphoma confined to bone [letter]. J Acquir Immune Defic Syndr 7:629–630, 1994.

43. Sider LK, Weiss AJ, Smith MD, VonRoenn JH, Glassroth J. Varied appearance of AIDS-related lymphoma in the chest. Radiology 171:629–632, 1989.

44. Filly R, Blank N, Castellino RA. Radiographic distribution of intra thoracic disease in previously untreated patients with Hodgkin's disease and non-Hodgkin's lymphoma. Radiology 120:277–281, 1976.

45. Nyberg DA, Federle MP. AIDS-related Kaposi sarcoma and lymphomas. Semin Roentgenol 22:54–65, 1987.

46. Fine HA, Mayer RJ. Primary central nervous system lymphoma. Ann Intern Med 119:1093–1104, 1993.

47. Ciricillo SF, Rosenblum ML. Use of CT and MR imaging to distinguish intracranial lesions and to define the need for biopsy in AIDS patients. J Neurosurg 73:720–724, 1990.

48. Hoffman JM, Waskin HA, Schifter T, Hanson MW, Gray L, Rosenfeld S, Coleman RE. FDG-PET in differentiating lymphoma from nonmalignant central nervous system lesions in patients with AIDS. J Nucl Med 34:567–575, 1993.

49. Pierce MA, Johnson MD, Maciunas RJ, Murray MJ, Allen GS, Harbison MA, Creasy JL, Kessler RM. Evaluating contrast-enhancing brain lesions in patients with AIDS by using positron emission tomography. Ann Intern Med 123:594–598, 1995.

50. Cimino C, Lipton RB, Williams A, Ferau E, Harris C, Hirschfeld A. The evaluation of patients with human immunodeficiency virus-related disorders and brain mass lesions. Arch Intern Med 151:1381–1384, 1991.

51. MacMahon EME, Glass JD, Hayward SD, et al. Epstein–Barr virus in AIDS related primary central nervous system lymphoma. Lancet 338:969–973, 1991.

52. Cinque P, Brytting M, Vago L, Castagna A, Parravicini C, Zanchetta N, Monforte AD, Wahren B, Lazzarin A, Linde A. Epstein Barr virus DNA in cerebrospinal fluid from patients with AIDS related primary lymphoma of the central nervous system. Lancet 342:398–401, 1993.

53. Levy RM, Russell E, Yungbluth M, Frias Hidvegi D, Brody B, Dal Canto MC. The efficacy of image-guided stereotactic brain biopsy in neurologically symptomatic acquired immunodeficiency syndrome patients. Neurosurgery 30:186–190, 1992.

54. Podzamczer D, Ricart I, Bolao F, Romagosa V, Bonnin D, Guionnet N, Gudiol F. Gallium-67 scan for distinguishing follicular hyperplasia from other AIDS-associated diseases in lymph nodes. AIDS 4:683–685, 1990.

55. Kaplan WD, Jochelson M, Herman RS, Nadler LM, Stomper PC, Takvorian R, Anderson JW, Canellos GP. Gallium 67 imaging: a predictor of residual tumor viability and clinical outcome in patients with diffuse large cell lymphoma. J Clin Oncol 8: 1966–1970, 1990.

56. Levine AM, Wernz JC, Kaplan L, Rodman N, Cohen P, Metroka C, Bennett JM, Rarick MU, Walsh C, Kahn J, Miles S, Ehmann C, Feinberg J, Nathwani B, Gill PS, Mitsuyasu R. Low dose chemotherapy with central nervous system prophylaxis and azidothymidine maintenance in AIDS-related lymphoma: a prospective multiinstitutional trial. JAMA 266:84–88, 1991.

57. Lossos A, Siegal T. Numb chin syndrome in cancer: etiology, response to treatment, and prognostic significance. Neurology 42:1181–1184, 1992.

58. Vaccher E, Tirelli U, Spina M, Talamini R, Errante D, Simonelli C, Carbone A. Age and serum lactate dehydrogenase level are independent prognostic factors in HIV related non–Hodgkin's lymphomas: a single institution study of 96 patients. J Clin Oncol 14:2217–2223, 1996.

59. Silverman BA, Rubinstein A. Serum lactate dehydrogenase levels in adults and children with acquired immune deficiency syndrome and AIDS-related complex: possible indicator of B cell lymphoproliferation and disease activity. Am J Med 78:728–736, 1985.

60. Straus D, Huang J, Testa M, Levine AM, Kaplan L. Prognostic factors in the treatment of HIV associated non–Hodgkin's lymphoma: analysis of ACTG 142 (low dose versus standard-dose mBACOD with GM-CSF). Blood 86:604a, 1995.

61. Straus DJ, Huang J, Testa MA, Levine AM, Kaplan LD. Prognostic factors in the treatment of HIV associated non-Hodgkin's lymphoma: Analysis of ACTG 142 (low dose versus standard dose mBACOD + GM–CSF) [abstr 89], J Acquir Immune Defic Syndr Hum Retrovirol 14:38a, 1997.

62. Baumgartner JE, Rachlin JR, Beckstead JH, Meeker TC, Levy RM, Wara WM, Rosenblum ML. Primary central nervous system lymphomas: natural history and response to radiation therapy in 55 patients with acquired immunodeficiency syndrome. J Neurosurg 73:206–211, 1990.

63. Skarin AT, Canellos GP, Rosenthal DS, Case DC Jr, MacIntyre JM, Pinkus GS, Moloney WC, Frei E III. Improved prognosis of diffuse histiocytic and undifferentiated lymphoma by use of high dose methotrexate alternating with standard agents (M-BACOD). J Clin Oncol 1:91–98, 1983.

64. Longo DL, DeVita VT Jr, Duffey PL, et al. Superiority of PROMACE-CYTABOM over PROMACE-MOPP in the treatment of advanced diffuse aggressive lymphoma: results of a prospective randomized trial. J Clin Oncol 9:25–38, 1991.

65. Klimo P, Connors JM. MACOP-B chemotherapy for the treatment of diffuse large cell lymphoma. Ann Intern Med 102:596–602, 1985.

66. McKelvey EM, Gottlieb JA, Wilson HE, Haut A, Talley RW, Stephens R, Lane M, Gamble JF, Jones SE, Grozea PN, Butterman J, Coltman C, Moon TE. Hydroxydaunomycin (Adriamycin) combination chemotherapy in malignant lymphoma. Cancer 38:1484–1493, 1976.

67. Odajnyk C, Subar M, Dugan M, Knowles D, Dalla-Favera R, Pelicci P, Poiesz B, Lafleur F, Raphael B. Clinical features and correlates with immunopathology and molecular biology of a large group of patients with AIDS associated small non-cleaved lymphoma. Blood 68:131a, 1986.
68. Dugan M, Subar M, Odajnyk C, Walsh C, Lafleur F, Poiesz B, Knowles DM II, Raphael B. Intensive multiagent chemotherapy for AIDS related diffuse large cell lymphoma. Blood 68:124a, 1986.
69. Gill PS, Levine AM, Krailo M, Rarick MU, Loureiro C, Deyton L, Meyer P, Rasheed S. AIDS-related malignant lymphoma: results of prospective treatment trials. J Clin Oncol 5:1322–1328, 1987.
70. Bermudez M, Grant KM, Rodvien R, Mendes F. Non–Hodgkin's lymphoma in a population with or at risk for acquired immunodeficiency syndrome: indications for intensive chemotherapy. Am J Med 86:71–76, 1989.
71. Gisselbrecht C, Oksenhendler E, Tirelli U, Lepage E, Gabarre J, Farcet JP, Gastaldi R, Coiffier B, Thyss A, Raphael M, Monfardini S. Human immunodeficiency virus related lymphoma treatment with intensive combination chemotherapy. Am J Med 95:188–196, 1993.
72. Gisselbrecht C, Gabarre J, Spina M, Rizzardini G, Schlaifer D, Nigra E, Bouabdallah R, Schrappe M, Rapoport B, Carbone C, Raphael M, Tirelli U. Therapy of HIV related non–Hodgkin's lymphoma: an European multicentric randomized study in patients stratified according to their prognostic factors [abstr 55]. Proc ASCO 18: 16a, 1999.
73. Sparano JA, Wiernik PH, Hu X, Sarta C, Schwartz EL, Soeiro R, Henry DH, Mason B, Ratech H, Dutcher JP. Pilot trial of infusional cyclophosphamide, doxorubicin, and etoposide plus didanosine and filgrastim in patients with human immunodeficiency virus-associated non–Hodgkin's lymphoma. J Clin Oncol 14:3026–3035, 1996.
74. Sparano JA, Wiernik PH, Hu X, Sarta C, Domenech G, Cioczek H, Racevskis J. Infusional cyclophosphamide, doxorubicin and etoposide (CDE) for HIV associated non–Hodgkin's lymphoma (NHL): long term follow-up and analysis of prognostic factors [abstr 88]. J Acquir Immune Defic Syndr Hum Retrovirol 14:38a, 1997.
75. Remick SC, McSharry JJ, Wolf BC, Blanchard CG, Eastman AY, Wagner H, Portuese E, Wighton T, Powell D, Pearce T, Horton J, Ruckdeschel JC. Novel oral combination chemotherapy in the treatment of intermediate-grade and high-grade AIDS related non–Hodgkin's lymphoma. J Clin Oncol 11:1691–1702, 1993.
76. Remick SC, Bibighaus MR, Reddy M, Haase RF, Nazeer T, Kuman N, Anand PK, Rammes CR, Pearce TP, Mastrianni DM. Oral combination chemotherapy in conjunction with filgrastim (G-CSF) in the treatment of AIDS-related non–Hodgkin's lymphoma [abstr 86]. J Acquir Immune Defic Syndr Hum Retrovirol 14:37a, 1997.
77. Levine AM, Tulpule A, Espina B, Boswell W, Buckley J, Rasheed S, Stain S, Parker J, Nathwani B, Gill PS. Low dose methotrexate, bleomycin, doxorubicin, cyclophosphamide, vincristine and dexamethasone with zalcitabine in patients with acquired immunodeficiency syndrome related lymphoma: effect on HIV and serum interleukin-6 levels over time. Cancer 78:517–526, 1996.
78. Tohyama N, Karasuyama H, Tada T. Growth autonomy and tumorigenicity of in-

terleukin 6-dependent B cells transfected with interleukin 6 cDNA. J Exp Med 171: 389–400, 1990.

79.   Tirelli U, Errante D, Oksenhendler E, Vaccher E, Gastaldi R, Rizzardini G, Monfardini S, Gisselbrecht C. The treatment of AIDS-related lymphoma [letter]. JAMA 267:509–510, 1992.

80.   Gill PS, Rarick MU, Brynes RK, Causey D, Levine AM. Azidothymidine and bone marrow failure in AIDS. Ann Intern Med 107:502–505, 1987.

81.   Mulder J, McKinney N, Christopherson C, Sninsky J, Greenfield L, Swok S. Rapid and simple PCR assay for quantitation of human immunodeficiency virus type 1 RNA in plasma. J Clin Microbiol 32:292–300, 1994.

82.   Little R, Franchini G, Pearson D, Elwood P, Steinberg S, Yarchoan R, Wilson WH. HIV viral burden during EPOCH chemotherapy for HIV related lymphomas [abstr 104]. J Acquir Immune Defic Syndr Hum Retrovirol 14:42a, 1997.

83.   Levine AM, Tulpule A, Rochat R, Espina B, McPhee R, Tessman D, Von Hoff D. Short term impact of mitoguazone chemotherapy in HIV viral load in patients with relapsed/refractory AIDS lymphoma. Blood 88:503a, 1996.

84.   Tirelli U, Errante D, Spina M, Gastaldi R, Nigra E, Nosari AM, Magnani G, Vaccher E. Second line chemotherapy in human immunodeficiency virus related non–Hodgkin's lymphoma. Cancer 77:2127–2131, 1996.

85.   Levine AM, Tulpule A, Tessman D, Kaplan L, Giles F, Luskey BD, Scadden DT, Northfelt DW, Silverberg I, Wernz J, Espina B, Von Hoff D. Mitoguazone therapy in patients with refractory or relapsed AIDS-related lymphoma: results from a multicenter phase II trial. J Clin Oncol 15:1094–1103, 1997.

86.   Tosi P, Gherlinzoni F, Mazza P, Visani G, Coronado O, Costigliola P, Raise E, Mazzetti M, Gritti F, Chiodo F, Tura S. 3'-Azido 3'-deoxythymidine + methotrexate as a novel antineoplastic combination in the treatment of human immunodeficiency virus-related non–Hodgkin's lymphoma. Blood 89:419–425, 1997.

87.   Tosi P, Calabresi P, Goulette FA, Renaud CA, Darnowskij JW. Azidothymidine induced cytotoxicity and incorporation into DNA in the human colon tumor cell line HCT 8 is enhanced by methotrexate in vitro and in vivo. Cancer Res 52:4069, 1992.

88.   Daniels D, Lowdell CP, Glaser MG. The spontaneous regression of lymphoma in AIDS. Clin Oncol 4:196–197, 1992.

89.   Karnad AB, Jaffar A, Lands RH. Spontaneous regression of acquired immune deficiency syndrome-related high-grade extranodal non–Hodgkin's lymphoma. Cancer 69:1856–1857, 1992.

90.   Baselga J, Krown SE, Telzak EE, Filippa DA, Straus DJ. Acquired immune deficiency syndrome-related pulmonary non–Hodgkin's lymphoma regressing after zidovudine therapy. Cancer 71:2332–2334, 1993.

6
Anal Squamous Intraepithelial Lesions in HIV-Positive Men and Women

Joel Palefsky
*University of California, San Francisco,
San Francisco, California*

I. INTRODUCTION

Sexual activity has been the most important risk factor for genital human papillomavirus (HPV) infection in many previous studies (1). Likewise, sexual transmission has been the major form of acquisition of human immunodeficiency virus (HIV) infection. Because of shared risk factors, it is not surprising that anogenital HPV infection is common among HIV-positive men and women. In HIV-positive women, much attention has been devoted to cervical HPV infection and HPV-associated lesions, including cervical cancer and its precursor, cervical squamous intraepithelial lesion (CSIL). In HIV-positive men, most attention has focused on anal HPV infection and anal SIL (ASIL). Compared with cervical HPV infection and CSIL, our understanding of the natural history of anal HPV infection and ASIL is very limited. Only recently have methods developed for investigation of CSIL been applied to ASIL. However, recent data summarized in this chapter point to a high incidence and prevalence of ASIL in HIV-positive homosexual and bisexual (hereafter called homosexual) men. Although there are no direct data demonstrating that ASIL progresses to invasive anal cancer, the strong similarities with CSIL and the high incidence of anal cancer in populations known to have high rates of ASIL suggest that ASIL is likely to be the lesion from which anal cancer arises.

Anogenital HPV infection is a major source of morbidity in HIV-positive patients, but it is not a major source of mortality, as anogenital cancer is still relatively uncommon. However, several years may be required for ASIL to progress to invasive cancer, and the risk of progression of ASIL among HIV-positive men may have been mitigated in the past by mortality from other causes, such as opportunistic infections. Newer therapies that effectively suppress HIV replication, such as protease inhibitors, will probably prolong the survival of HIV-positive men (2) and if not accompanied by ASIL regression, these therapies may paradoxically increase the risk of developing invasive cancer.

There are two reasons why clinicians should be aware of HPV-related precancerous disease in HIV-positive as well as in high-risk HIV-negative individuals. First, unlike other cancers of HIV-positive men and women, such as Kaposi's sarcoma and non–Hodgkin's lymphoma, anal cancer may be preventable with treatment of anal high-grade squamous intraepithelial lesions (HSIL), analogous to treatment of cervical HSIL for prevention of cervical cancer. Second, several studies have addressed the role of sexually transmitted agents as cofactors for acquisition of HIV infection. *Chlamydia trachomatis, Neisseria gonorrhoeae*, and *Haemophilus ducreyi* have been identified as cofactors for HIV infection (3,4). HPV infection must also be considered a potential cofactor for HIV transmission, for HPV-related precancerous lesions are typically well-vascularized (5) and may bleed easily after sexual intercourse. HIV-negative men and women with ASIL, therefore, may be at increased risk of HIV infection compared with those with a normal anogenital mucosa. Conversely, HIV-positive men and women with ASIL may be at risk of acquiring new strains of HIV, an undesirable outcome that may potentiate progression of HIV-related disease or transmission of HIV to their sexual partners.

There are several biological and anatomical similarities between the cervix and the anus, including an association with HPV infection (6–8). The HPV types commonly found in the cervix are similar to those found in the anal canal (9), and evidence to date suggests that the oncogenic behavior of specific HPV types in the anal canal is similar to the behavior of the same HPV types in the cervix. As in the cervix, HPV-16 is the most common type found in association with anal cancer, and there are few or no cases in which the low-risk HPV types such as 6 or 11 are found alone (6,7).

In the cervix, the *transformation zone* (TZ), defined as the area where the squamous epithelium meets the columnar epithelium, is a common site of HPV infection, CSIL, and cancer. A similar TZ exists in the anal canal where the squamous epithelium of the anus meets the columnar epithelium of the rectum. Therefore, it is not surprising that ASIL and anal cancers often arise from the TZ. These lesions would not be visible on routine inspection of the perianal region, and must be visualized at anoscopy. Hyperpigmented perianal papules and plaques known as Bowen's disease may also progress to cancer.

II. ANAL CANCER IN HIV-POSITIVE MEN AND WOMEN

Before the onset of the HIV epidemic, anal cancer was found preponderantly among older persons, with a mean age of 61 years (10). In recent years, several epidemiological studies have documented the risk factors for this disease. Holly et al. have shown that, among men, the risk of anal cancer was elevated for those with a history of homosexual activity (relative risk of 12.4, with a relative risk of 2.7 after adjustment for other factors; 11). Other risk factors included a history of genital warts, anal fissure or fistula, and cigarette smoking. Daling et al. also reported that homosexuality and receptive anal intercourse were important risk factors for the development of anal cancer (12). These conclusions have been further supported in other studies, in which young, unmarried men, many of whom were presumably homosexual, had an elevated risk for the development of anal cancer (13–15). Likewise, in Washington State, the incidence of anorectal cancer among homosexual men was 25–50 times that of age-matched heterosexual controls (16).

The precise incidence of anal cancer among men with a history of receptive anal intercourse has been difficult to determine because cancer registries do not collect information on sexual orientation or behavior. However, Daling et al. estimated the incidence of anal cancer among homosexual men to be approximately 35:100,000 (12). This renders the incidence of anal cancer in this group several times higher than current rates of cervical cancer in women in the United States (17), and similar to rates of cervical cancer before the introduction of routine cervical cytological screening.

As described later, ASIL and anal HPV infection are more common in homosexual HIV-positive men than in homosexual HIV-negative men, raising the possibility that HIV-positive men may be at even higher risk of developing anal cancer than the latter. Thus far, data on the degree of excess incidence of anal cancer in HIV-positive homosexual compared with HIV-negative homosexual men are conflicting. Rabkin et al. reported little increased risk of anal cancer among single, never-married men aged 25–44 in the San Francisco Bay area since the onset of the HIV epidemic (18). However, linking HIV registries to the Surveillance, Epidemiology, and End Results database, Melbye et al. reported an increase in the observed/expected ratio of cases of anal cancer with increasing proximity to a diagnosis of AIDS (19).

There are still no data on the incidence of anal cancer among HIV-positive women, and it is not yet clear if HIV-positive women are at increased risk of anal cancer compared with HIV-negative women. In the general population, anal cancer is more common among women than among men. In the era before the HIV epidemic, anal cancer was found in women approximately four times more often than in men, with an incidence of 13:1 million per year in the United States (20). In the last 15 years, the incidence of anal cancer has increased over 35%

in women, and is currently rising at a rate of nearly 2% per year (A. Hauser, personal communication, Northern California Cancer Center). In Denmark, rates of anal cancer are lower than in the United States, but using a 50-year-old national cancer registry, Frisch et al. reported that between 1957 and 1987, the incidence of anal cancer among Danish women more than tripled to 7.4:1 million (21). Rates of anal cancer also increased among Danish men during this time, but less dramatically, increasing by 1.5-fold to 3.8:1 million.

Holmes et al. conducted a case–control study of 56 women with anal cancer and 56 matched controls (22). In that study, anal cancer was associated in univariate analysis with current cigarette smoking, positive herpes simplex virus type 2 (HSV-2) titers, and a history of a previously abnormal cervical Papanicolaou (Pap) smear, the latter suggesting a direct or indirect association with cervical HPV infection. Although the number of sexual partners was associated with anal cancer, history of receptive anal intercourse was not. Based on these data, it seems likely that, similar to men, anal cancer in women is related to sexual activity, and possibly to cervical HPV infection. It remains unclear if anal intercourse itself is required. One study reported that approximately 25% of American women have had at least one experience with receptive anal intercourse, and 8% practice it regularly (23). In a study of anal cancer among San Francisco Bay Area women, Holly et al. found that among women, chronic hemorrhoids and smoking were important risk factors in univariate analysis. In multivariate analysis, history of genital warts, anal fissures or fistulas, and hemorrhoids were significant (11). Similar findings were reported by Daling et al. (12).

III.   ANAL HPV INFECTION IN HIV-POSITIVE MEN AND WOMEN

By using a variety of methods, several studies have shown a higher prevalence of anal HPV infection among HIV-positive men compared with HIV-negative men (24–27). In one recent study of HIV-positive men with group IV HIV disease, 110 (93%) HIV-positive men were positive for at least one anal HPV type using polymerase chain reaction (PCR), and a wide variety of HPV types were detected (28). HPV-16 was the most commonly detected HPV type, followed by HPV-52 and HPV-33. Infection with more than one HPV type was detected in 97 of 118 (82%) of samples analyzed. These and earlier data suggest that most HIV-positive homosexual and bisexual men have anal HPV infection when using the highly sensitive PCR technique. Several earlier studies have also shown that among HIV-positive men, low CD4 cell counts were significantly associated with presence of HPV infection (29–31). Overall, the data indicate that anal HPV infection is very common among HIV-positive men, multiple types are frequently present, and HPV DNA is detectable at high levels, indicating active viral replication, particularly among the more immunosuppressed men.

Relatively little is known about anal HPV infection in HIV-positive or HIV-negative women. However, in one study, anal HPV infection was more frequent than cervical infection in both HIV-positive and high-risk HIV-negative women (9). In that study 76% of HIV-positive women had anal HPV infection measured by PCR. Analysis of the HPV types in the anal canal and the cervix in women infected at both sites showed little difference in the overall spectrum of types at these sites. Notably, however, the same types were found in the anus and cervix in only 50% of the women. These findings were confirmed in a study of HIV-positive women in Denmark (32).

The mode of acquisition of anal HPV infection in either men or women is currently unknown. The role of sexual behavior in acquisition of anal HPV infection has been difficult to ascertain in most of the study populations reported to date, for most studies were performed in subjects many years after initiation of sexual activity with many sexual partners. Receptive anal intercourse is probably the important route by which HPV infection is established in the anal canal. However, insertion of inert objects or fingers exposed to other HPV-infected tissues of the individual or their sexual partner may also result in anal HPV infection. The relation between anal and cervical infection is also not well understood. However, because many urinary tract infections in women are caused by fecal flora, it is possible that the cervix may be exposed to HPV from the anal canal on a regular basis. Conversely, HPV shed from the cervix may infect the perianal and intra-anal tissues.

IV. ASIL IN HIV-POSITIVE MEN AND WOMEN

Consistent with the data on anal HPV infection, ASIL is more common among HIV-positive homosexual men than among HIV-negative men in several studies (25,26,31). Furthermore, as with anal HPV infection, the prevalence of ASIL increases inversely with the CD4 level, suggesting that immunosuppression plays an important role in pathogenesis of the lesions. In a study of HIV-negative and HIV-positive men in San Francisco, the prevalence of anal cytological abnormalities was highest among those with CD4 cell counts of fewer than $250/mm^3$ (26), and similar findings were reported in two studies from Seattle (25,31). In a recent study of 129 HIV-positive men with group IV HIV disease in San Francisco, anal cytology was abnormal in 39% of the subjects (28). In that study, an abnormal cytological result was associated with detection of HPV by PCR and higher levels of HPV DNA, as indicated by higher HC relative light unit (RLU) ratios. Of interest was the observation that higher levels of group B types using HC (the oncogenic HPV group of types) were more strongly associated with anal cytological abnormalities than were elevated group A (the nononcogenic types) RLU ratios, suggesting that the oncogenic HPV types play a more important role in disease pathogenesis than nononcogenic HPV types. In logistic regression analyses of risk factors for abnormal cytological appearance, HPV infection, and history of intravenous drug use were the only independent risk factors. In another recent study of 346 HIV-positive men spanning a wider range of CD4 cell levels at the University of California, San Francisco, 23% of HIV-positive men with CD4 cell counts of more than 500/mm^3 had abnormal anal cytology, whereas 40 and 67% of those with counts between 200 and 500/mm^3 and fewer than 200/mm^3 had abnormal cytology, respectively (JM Palefsky, unpublished data). Together these data show a high prevalence of anal lesions in HIV-positive men and indicate that the prevalence increases with decreasing CD4 cell levels. HPV infection is strongly associated with anal disease in HIV-positive men, with the strongest association found with high levels of oncogenic HPV types. Immunosuppression as measured by CD4 cell levels and HPV infection are independent risk factors for anal disease, but the mechanisms by which immunosuppression contributes to anal disease are unclear.

There are still relatively few data on the natural history of ASIL in HIV-positive and HIV-negative men. Early studies of the natural history of anal disease in men with group IV disease suggested that anal disease in this population may progress rapidly (33). Thirty-seven homosexual men with group IV HIV disease were followed for an average of 17 months. During the study, 14 subjects (38%) developed anal cytological abnormalities. The number of subjects with any grade of ASIL rose from 3 (8%) to 12 (32%), with HSIL increasing from none to 6 (16%) subjects. In another study in Seattle, HSIL developed in 24 of 158 (15%) HIV-positive and 8 of (5%) 147 HIV-negative men entering the study with no anal disease, who were followed for an average of 19 months (34). The primary risk factors for HSIL in that study were HIV-induced immunosuppression, HPV type (higher risk associated with oncogenic HPV types), and level of detection of HPV. In a separate study of 259 HIV-positive and 217 HIV-negative homosexual men in San Francisco, the projected 4-year incidence of HSIL among all HIV-positive men was 49% (95% CI, 41–56), whereas that of HIV-negative men was 17% (95% CI, 12–23) (JM Palefsky, unpublished data).

In the foregoing studies, atypical squamous cells of undetermined significance (ASCUS) and low-grade squamous cell lesions (LSIL) were more common than HSIL. Based on the analogy with cervix, these lesions likely pose little or no risk for direct progression to invasive anal cancer. However, in a recent study, the 2-year progression rate of LSIL to HSIL was 62% among 169 HIV-positive and 36% among HIV-negative men (JM Palefsky, unpublished data). LSIL is, therefore, clinically important for the high rate at which it may progress to HSIL. ASCUS may be important for the same reason, particularly in HIV-positive men, because 33% of HIV-positive men with ASCUS at baseline progressed to HSIL within 2 years. Among HIV-negative men, 8% of those with ASCUS at baseline progressed to HSIL within 2 years of follow-up.

Anal cytological abnormalities are also more common among HIV-positive women than high-risk HIV-negative women (9,32). Among the HIV-positive women, anal cytological abnormalities were at least as common as cervical abnormalities, although the severity of anal disease was less marked than that of cervical disease. Of HIV-positive women, 14% had abnormal anal cytology and, consistent with data obtained in studies of men, anal cytological changes were associated with HIV infection and lower CD4 cell counts (9). The natural history of anal abnormalities and its relation to the natural history of cervical lesions in HIV-positive women are not yet known.

V. SCREENING FOR ASIL IN HIV-POSITIVE MEN AND WOMEN

Progression from anal HSIL to invasive anal cancer has never been documented, primarily because there are no reported studies of the natural history of HSIL. Moreover, in the current studies of ASIL, for ethical reasons, subjects identified with HSIL are referred for treatment. However, the strong similarities between anal and cervical cancer and the similarity between ASIL and CSIL suggest that many, if not most, cases of anal cancer arise from anal HSIL. If this assumption is true, then a screening program for ASIL, and HSIL in particular, may be useful to prevent development of anal cancer, similar to the program currently in place to prevent development of cervical cancer. The critical elements of any screening program for anal disease must include (1) identification of populations most likely to benefit from screening; (2) an acceptable screening test; and (3) a treatment program for the lesions identified by the screening test that lowers the incidence of anal cancer in the target groups.

Current data permit the identification of groups most likely to benefit from screening, and data are also emerging on the performance characteristics of screening tests that may be used. There is currently little information on the efficacy of therapy for prevention of anal cancer, and demonstration of the efficacy of a screening program for anal disease may have to await performance of large-scale treatment trials for ASIL.

Several different populations may be considered to be at high risk of anal cancer and would be appropriate target groups for screening. One high-risk group would be all homosexual HIV-positive men. In this group, those at highest risk of anal cancer would likely be men with HSIL and the likelihood of survival for several more years. HSIL has been documented in men at all levels of CD4 cell counts. Among men receiving some of the newer combinations of therapy for HIV, including protease inhibitors, even those with low CD4 cell levels may survive for several years. Therefore, HIV-positive men with good functional status should be considered for screening, regardless of CD4 count. Conversely, men with HSIL and a poor prognosis would be unlikely to benefit from screening and treatment of HSIL, and should not be included in a screening program. As measurement of HIV plasma RNA levels may provide a better clinical indicator of survival than CD4 cell levels (35), they may also be useful in estimating the expected benefit from participating in a screening program.

A second high-risk group that should be considered for screening is homosexual HIV-negative men. Identification of HSIL would be of concern in this group because their normal life expectancy may provide them with sufficient time for the lesion to progress to invasive cancer. More information is needed to design an effective screening program in this group, but because anal cancers typically occur in this group after the age of 50, it may be reasonable to restrict screening to men in their late 40s or older. Since infection with HPV is an important risk factor for anal lesions in this group, detection of anal HPV DNA may also serve to identify HIV-negative men at high risk of ASIL. The exact role of routine HPV DNA testing in the anal canal in the management algorithm of anal disease has not yet been established.

As described previously, anal cancer was historically more common among women than among men (22). There are currently no data on the incidence of anal cancer in HIV-positive women, but a strong association between anal and cervical HSIL and cancer has been shown (36,37). These data suggest that HIV-positive women with CSIL may be at particularly high risk of ASIL. Further studies of HIV-positive and HIV-negative women are needed to make definitive recommendations for screening. However, all HIV-positive and HIV-negative women who have CSIL or lesions on the vulva or vagina may also be at risk of anal disease. Because previous studies have shown that ASIL may be common among HIV-positive women, it is also possible that HIV-positive women with good functional status may benefit from anal screening, whether or not they have cervicovaginal or vulvar disease. Therefore, all HIV-positive women with good functional status and HIV-negative women with evidence of cervical or vulvo-vaginal lesions may be good candidates for anal screening.

On the basis of the CSIL screening model, high-risk men and women would be screened with anal cytology, performed as previously described (38). To perform anal cytology, a Dacron swab is moistened in saline or tap water and inserted to the distal rectum, at least 5 cm (2 in.) inside the anal opening. The swab is rotated as it is withdrawn, and mild pressure is exerted on the walls of the anal canal. After withdrawal, the material collected on the swab is immediately smeared onto a glass slide, which should be placed as quickly as possible in an alcohol bottle. The entire time from withdrawal of the swab to fixation should not exceed 10 s, because anal swabs are highly prone to artifacts caused by air-drying. Although hair spray may be used instead of an alcohol bottle, in our experience, the cells are not as well preserved and are more prone to the effects of air-drying. Smears are then stained using routine Papanicolaou staining methods. Because of the difficulty in obtaining adequate smears in some clinical settings, we recently compared the foregoing method to the ThinPrep method, a newer technique used to collect cells for cervical cytological examination (39). Our studies showed that the two techniques were equivalent in sensitivity for the detection of anal lesions, and this method may be preferable for use by clinicians with limited experience performing anal cytological assessment or limited access to alcohol bottles for cytological preservation.

Earlier studies of a small number of subjects have shown a wide range of sensitivity of anal cytological examination for the detection of anal lesions (33,40). To assess anal cytological examination as a screening tool for anal lesions in a larger population, we recently performed a comparison on assessment by anal cytology with anoscopy and histopathology of anal biopsies (41). A total of 2958 anal examinations were performed on 407 HIV-positive and 251 HIV-negative homosexual or bisexual men participating in a prospective study of ASIL. When defining abnormal cytology as including both ASCUS and ASIL, the sensitivity of anal cytological evaluation for detection of biopsy-proved ASIL was 69% (95% CI, 60–78) in HIV-positive and 47% (95% CI, 26–68) in HIV-negative men at their first visit, and 81 and 50%, respectively, for all subsequent visits combined.

In the cervix, adequacy of the cytological smear is partly judged by the presence or absence of endocervical columnar cells. For anal cytology, the presence of rectal columnar cells would indicate that the swab reached past the anorectal transformation zone (TZ), where many of the lesions arise, and that the TZ has been sampled. In our study, the absence of columnar cells did not affect the sensitivity, specificity, or predictive value of anal cytological evaluation.

These data showed that anal cytology may be a useful screening tool to detect ASIL, particularly in HIV-positive men. The lower sensitivity of anal cytology in HIV-negative men likely reflects the smaller size of the anal lesions compared with those of the HIV-positive men. Because the sensitivity of any one cytological test was limited among both HIV-positive and HIV-negative men, as with cervical cytology, at least three consecutive normal cytological smears at several-month intervals would be needed to minimize the likelihood of a false-negative result.

The grade of disease on anal cytological testing did not always correspond to that of histological appearance and, as with cervical cytology, anal cytology should be used in conjunction with histopathological confirmation. Therefore, if an abnormality is detected on anal cytology, it should be followed by anoscopy and biopsy of the lesion. To perform anoscopy, an anoscope is inserted to allow placement of a Q-Tip wrapped with a gauze pad that has been soaked in 3% acetic acid. The anoscope is removed and the gauze is left in place in contact with the anal mucosa for 1 min. After removal of the gauze-wrapped Q-tip, the anoscope is reinserted and the anal canal is examined under colposcopic magnification.

The goal of performing anoscopy is to identify and biopsy lesions with the highest grade of abnormality. In the cervix, there is a well-defined set of colposcopic criteria that identify lesions likely to be LSIL or HSIL. To determine if the colposcopic characteristics of anal and cervical disease are similar, we performed a study on the colposcopic characteristics of 385 anal lesions from 123 HIV-positive and 29 HIV-negative homosexual men and correlated the results with those of histopathology. Ninety-one percent of lesions that were acetowhite, raised, and smooth, with warty characteristics showed LSIL on histopathological evaluation, whereas 65% of lesions that were acetowhite and flat with vascular changes showed HSIL. The positive predictive value (PPV) for anal HSIL in lesions with characteristics typical of cervical LSIL was 7.7% (95% CI, 1.8–14), whereas the PPV for anal HSIL in lesions with characteristics typical of cervical HSIL was 49% (95% CI, 40–58). We concluded that the colposcopic appearance of different grades of anal SIL was similar to those described for the cervix and that incorporation of cervical colposcopic criteria into assessment of anal lesions could aid in distinguishing LSIL from HSIL for diagnosis and treatment. Examples of anal lesions demonstrating different colposcopic characteristics are shown in Fig. 1.

The complication rate of anal biopsy when properly performed is very low and consists of postbiopsy bleeding and discomfort, and rarely, anal fissures and fistulas. Contraindications to anal biopsy include thrombocytopenia (less than 75,000 platelets per cubic millimeter), neutropenia (less than 500 polymorphonuclear cells per cubic millimeter), concurrent bacterial infection of the anal canal, or concurrent herpes simplex virus infection. Unless performed in a setting where hemostasis is readily achieved, recent intake of acetylsalicylic acid is a relative contraindication. In most situations, postbiopsy bleeding can be controlled with pressure from a swab or with application of Monsell's solution.

Screening for anal disease should also include inspection of the perianal region because both HSIL and invasive anal cancer may originate in the keratinized epithelium external to the anal verge. Bowen's disease of the perianal region is a common manifestation of anal HSIL and presents as pigmented papules or plaques. Condyloma acuminatum is another common manifestation of HPV infection in the perianal region, and although it usually contains low-grade changes, HSIL may also be focally present, particularly in HIV-positive individuals. Therefore, these lesions should routinely have biopsies taken to exclude HSIL.

A summary of an algorithm of screening and diagnosis of ASIL is presented in Fig. 2. Patients with ASCUS, LSIL, or HSIL on cytological examination should undergo anoscopy with biopsy of visible lesions. Patients with normal cytological results should be retested at least three times. HIV-positive men and women with

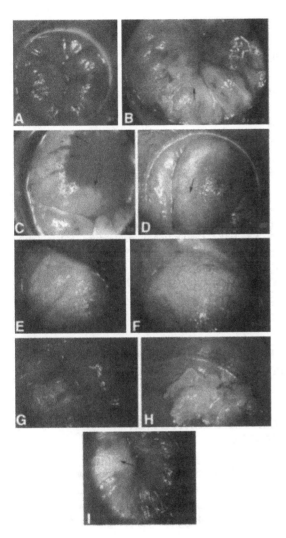

Figure 1 (A, B) Anal canal pre- and postapplication of 3% acetic acid; (C) the transition zone after application of acetic acid: Columnar epithelium, corrugated with fine punctation is noted by thin arrow. A thin border of AWE and gland neck openings representing metaplasia separates the columnar from the squamous epithelium and is noted by the thick arrow. (D) AWE ringed-gland openings are the most prominent finding in this flat, indistinct HSIL AWE lesion. (E) A flat, distinct HSIL lesion with coarse punctation; (F) coarse mosaic pattern and coarse punctation in a HSIL AWE lesion, with a shallow ulceration; (G) LGSIL (condyloma acuminata) with papillae and warty vessels; (H) This raised wart-like lesion was diagnosed as HSIL by histology; (I) A LSIL (flat condyloma) adjacent to friable scar tissue from previous surgery.

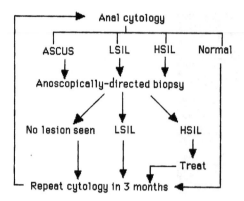

Figure 2 Screening algorithm for anal squamous intraepithelial lesions among high-risk HIV-positive men and women. See text for definition of risk groups. Patients with normal cytology can be screened at 3-month intervals or longer. LSIL should be considered for treatment if symptomatic. ASCUS, atypical squamous cells of undetermined significance; LSIL, low-grade squamous intraepithelial lesions; HSIL, high-grade squamous intraepithelial lesions.

normal cytological results could be screened annually thereafter, whereas HIV-negative men and women with such results may be screened at longer intervals.

VI. TREATMENT OF ASIL IN HIV-POSITIVE MEN AND HIV-POSITIVE WOMEN

Given the foregoing considerations, the decision to treat or follow the patient without treatment will depend on several factors, including the grade of disease and prognosis for long-term survival. The presence of symptoms may also dictate treatment, as some patients report severe itching and bleeding with ASIL. Cosmetic considerations may also apply.

Of the factors just described, the grade of the lesion is probably the most important. From the cervical model, HSIL should be treated to prevent development of anal cancer. LSIL need not be treated for this indication, but must be followed carefully because of its propensity to progress to HSIL. Likewise, patients with ASCUS should be followed carefully for progression. The intervals at which patients should be followed with cytology and anoscopy examinations have not yet been established. Among HIV-negative men and women with normal cytological results, an interval of several years might suffice, but among HIV-positive men and women, screening for those with normal cytology every year and, as shown in Fig. 2, screening those with LSIL and ASCUS every 3–6 months may be appropriate.

There currently are no data on the efficacy of different treatment regimens for ASIL, nor are there regimens directed specifically against HPV gene products. Therefore, current approaches rely on nonspecific removal of lesional tissue. These methods do not treat the HPV infection per se, and this may account for the high recurrence rate of disease following therapy. Among the therapeutic options currently available for internal anal disease are electrocautery or cold scalpel excision, liquid nitrogen, and application of local therapies, such as 80% trichloroacetic (TCA) or bichloroacetic acid. Liquid nitrogen and TCA are best used for small, focal lesions, whereas surgical excision or electrocautery are the current treatments of choice for larger lesions. As much anal tissue as possible should be sent for histopathological assessment both to exclude invasive disease and to establish the margins of the lesion.

Given the multifocal nature of anal lesions, a systemic approach to treatment would be ideal. Systemic interferon is active against HPV-related lesions, but is not practical because of the severe side effects noted at the usual doses administered. Oral therapy with retinoids represents another therapeutic option, but has not been studied in formal clinical trials. Isotretinoin can be given at doses of up to 1 mg/kg per day, but may be associated with side effects, such as skin peeling and biochemical abnormalities, including hypertriglyceridemia. Topical therapies with newer drugs such as HPMPC and imiquimod would represent another therapeutic option for internal lesions, but these drugs are not currently available in suppository form.

Another form of systemic therapy that must be considered are treatment regimens directed against HIV. If HIV-related immunosuppression is playing a role in the pathogenesis of HSIL, then therapies directed toward reducing HIV replication, such as the newer combinations of drugs for HIV might be expected to influence the natural history of ASIL. To date, regression of preexisting HSIL lesions among men receiving protease inhibitor therapy for at least 3 months has not been seen (JM Palefsky, unpublished data), a finding consistent with low regression rates of HSIL among HIV-negative men. The effect of these therapies on the natural history of low-grade lesions or on progression of HSIL to cancer is unknown. Paradoxically the longer lifespan afforded by these drugs may increase the risk of development of cancer if they do not substantially reduce the incidence of HSIL.

Treatment of external lesions may differ from internal lesions because topical therapy may be used. TCA and podophyllin or podophyllotoxin may be applied topically to these lesions. 5-Fluorouracil cream may also be applied to the lesion, but is associated with burning and ulcerations. HPMPC and imiquimod are new drugs currently under trial for treatment of external warts and might represent therapeutic options in the future for HIV-positive patients. The success rate of these treatments for LSIL compared with HSIL is unknown.

Treatment complications following therapy have not yet been systematically studied. Complications of therapy of internal disease may include anal strictures, which are most likely to occur following excision of large, circumferential internal anal lesions. Therefore, the extent of the lesions and their topographical location should be considered when attempting to minimize the risk of complications, and a multistage procedure may be necessary. Abscesses, fissures, or fistulas may also occur as rare complications of surgery or nonsurgical treatment. Temporary local discomfort is common, as is postsurgical bleeding. Postsurgical pain is often due to anal sphincter spasm and may respond to muscle relaxants, such as benzodiazepines, and local measures, such as sitz baths.

There are also few data on disease recurrence following treatment with these modalities. Consequently, it would be prudent to continue to follow the patient closely after treatment. It is currently our practice to follow patients every 3 months after treatment with anal cytology and by anoscopy if the cytology is abnormal.

VII. SUMMARY

When compared with high-risk HIV-negative men and women, HIV-positive men and women have higher rates of anogenital HPV infection, higher number of HPV types in anogenital samples, and higher levels of HPV replication, as indicated by higher levels of viral DNA. Consistent with these findings are higher rates of anogenital disease, higher rates of multifocal disease, and more rapid disease progression. Among HIV-positive women being treated for CSIL, higher failure rates of standard therapy have been shown, as have higher recurrence rates once the lesions are treated. These observations suggest that HIV-positive men and women with anal HSIL may have a high risk of progression to invasive cancer if not screened and treated aggressively. ASIL has only recently been recognized as a clinical problem and much remains to be learned about its natural history. Optimal regimens for screening and treatment for anal disease have not yet been established, and further research is needed to improve therapeutic regimens, including the development of therapies directed specifically against HPV gene products. With increasing survival owing to improved medical therapy for HIV, HIV-related complications may shift toward morbidity and mortality from illnesses with a long natural history, such as malignancies. Given the high rates of ASIL among HIV-positive men and women, anal cancer must be considered among those malignancies poised to increase in the era of improved therapy for HIV. Unlike many of the other cancers that may occur, anal cancer may be preventable and studies are now needed on the natural history of anal HPV infection and ASIL among men and women being treated with newer drug combinations for HIV. Research on the role of the immune response to HPV in the pathogenesis of ASIL is needed, as is clinical research on therapeutic vaccines directed against HPV. Research is also needed to delineate the role, if any, of ASIL in HIV transmission.

REFERENCES

1. A Schneider, L Koutsky, eds. Natural History and Epidemiologic Features of Genital HPV Infection. Lyon: IARC, 1992. (Munoz N, Bosch FX, Shah KV, Meheus A, ed. IARC Scientific Publications; vol 119).
2. DS MacDougall, Ritonavir: first to prolong survival. J Int Assoc Physicians AIDS Care 2:38–44, 1996.
3. M Laga, M Alary, N Nzila, AT Manoka, M Tuliza, F Behets, J Goeman, M St Louis, P Piot. Condom promotion, sexually transmitted diseases treatment, and declining incidence of HIV-1 infection in female Zairian sex workers. Lancet 344:246–248, 1994.
4. M Laga, A Manoka, M Kivuvu, et al. Non-ulcerative sexually transmitted diseases as risk factors for HIV-1 transmission in women: results from a cohort study. AIDS 7:95–102, 1993.
5. KK Smith-McCune, N Weidner. Demonstration and characterization of the angiogenic properties of cervical dysplasia. Cancer Res 54:800–804, 1994.
6. AM Beckmann, JR Daling, KJ Sherman, C Maden, BA Miller, RJ Coates, NB Kiviat, D Myerson, NS Weiss, TG Hislop. Human papillomavirus infection and anal cancer. Int J Cancer 43:1042–1049, 1989.
7. JM Palefsky, J Gonzales, RM Greenblatt, DK Ahn, H Hollander. Anal intraepithelial neoplasia and anal papillomavirus infection among homosexual males with group IV HIV disease. JAMA 263:2911–2916, 1990.
8. SR Zaki, R Judd, LM Coffield, P Greer, F Rolston, BL Evatt. Human papillomavirus infection and anal carcinoma. Retrospective analysis by in situ hybridization and the polymerase chain reaction. Am J Pathol 140:1345–1355, 1992.
9. AB Williams, TM Darragh, K Vranizan, C Ochia, AR Moss, JM Palefsky. Anal and cervical human papillomavirus infection and risk of anal and cervical epithelial abnormalities in human immunodeficiency virus-infected women. Obstet Gynecol 83:205–211, 1994.
10. E Hughes, AM Cuthbertson, MK Killingback, eds. Colorectal Surgery. New York: Churchill-Livingstone, 1983.
11. EA Holly, AS Whittemore, DA Aston, DK Ahn, BJ Nickoloff, JJ Kristiansen. Anal cancer incidence: genital warts, anal fissure or fistula, hemorrhoids, and smoking. J Natl Cancer Inst 81:1726–1731, 1989.
12. JR Daling, NS Weiss, TG Hislop, C Maden, RJ Coates, KJ Sherman, RL Ashley, M Beagrie, JA Ryan, L Corey. Sexual practices, sexually transmitted diseases, and the incidence of anal cancer. N Engl J Med 317:973–977, 1987.

13. RK Peters, TM Mack, L Bernstein. Parallels in the epidemiology of selected anogenital carcinomas. J Natl Cancer Inst 72:609–615, 1984.
14. RK Peters, TM Mack. Patterns of anal carcinoma by gender and marital status in Los Angeles County. Br J Cancer 48:629–636, 1983.
15. DF Austin. Etiological clues from descriptive epidemiology: squamous carcinoma of the rectum or anus. Natl Cancer Inst Monogr 62:89–90, 1982.
16. JR Daling, NS Weiss, LL Klopfenstein, LE Cochran, WH Chow, R Daifuku. Correlates of homosexual behavior and the incidence of anal cancer. JAMA 247:1988–1990, 1982.
17. JR Qualters, NC Lee, RA Smith, RE Aubert. Breast and cervical cancer surveillance, United States, 1973–1987. MMWR Morb Mortal Wkly Rep 41:1–15, 1992.
18. CS Rabkin, F Yellin. Cancer incidence in a population with a high prevalence of infection with human immunodeficiency virus type 1. J Natl Cancer Inst 86:1711–1716, 1994.
19. M Melbye, TR Cote, L Kessler, M Gail, RJ Biggar. High incidence of anal cancer among AIDS patients. The AIDS/Cancer Working Group. Lancet 343:636–639, 1994.
20. J Young Jr, CL Percy, AJ Asire, JW Berg, MM Cusano, LA Gloeckler, JW Horm, W Lourie Jr, ES Pollack, EM Shambaugh. Cancer incidence and mortality in the United States, 1973–77. Natl Cancer Inst Monogr 57:1–187, 1981.
21. M Frisch, M Melbye, H Moller. Trends in incidence of anal cancer in Denmark. Br Med J 306:419–422, 1993.
22. F Holmes, D Borek, M Owen-Kummer, R Hassanein, J Fishback, A Behbehani, A Baker, G Holmes. Anal cancer in women. Gastroenterology 95:107–111, 1988.
23. DJ Bolling. Prevalence, goals, and complications of heterosexual intercourse in a gynecologic population. J Reprod Med 19:120–124, 1977.
24. N Kiviat, A Rompalo, R Bowden, D Galloway, KK Holmes, L Corey, PL Roberts, WE Stamm. Anal human papillomavirus infection among human immunodeficiency virus-seropositive and -seronegative men. J Infect Dis 162:358–361, 1990.
25. CW Critchlow, KK Holmes, R Wood, L Krueger, C Dunphy, DA Vernon, JR Daling, NB Kiviat. Association of human immunodeficiency virus and anal human papillomavirus infection among homosexual men. Arch Intern Med 152:1673–1676, 1992.
26. JM Palefsky, S Shiboski, A Moss. Risk factors for anal human papillomavirus infection and anal cytologic abnormalities in HIV-positive and HIV-negative homosexual men. J Acquir Immune Defic Syndr 7:599–606, 1994.
27. PL Breese, FN Judson, KA Penley, J Douglas, Jr. Anal human papillomavirus infection among homosexual and bisexual men: prevalence of type-specific infection and association with human immunodeficiency virus. Sex Transm Dis 22:7–14, 1995.
28. J Palefsky, E Holly, M Ralston, S Arthur, C Hogeboom, T Darragh. Anal cytologic abnormalities and anal HPV infection in men with Centers for Disease Control Group IV HIV disease. Genitourin Med 73:174–180, 1997.
29. D Caussy, JJ Goedert, J Palefsky, J Gonzales, CS Rabkin, RA DiGioia, WC Sanchez, RJ Grossman, G Colclough, SZ Wiktor. Interaction of human immunodeficiency and papilloma viruses: association with anal epithelial abnormality in homosexual men. Int J Cancer 46:214–219, 1990.
30. M Melbye, J Palefsky, J Gonzales, LP Ryder, H Nielsen, O Bergmann, J Pindborg,

RJ Biggar. Immune status as a determinant of human papillomavirus detection and its association with anal epithelial abnormalities. Int J Cancer 46:203–206, 1990.

31. N Kiviat, C Critchlow, K Holmes, J Kuypers, J Sayer, C Dunphy, C Surawicz, P Kirby, R Wood, J Daling. Association of anal dysplasia and human papillomavirus with immunosuppression and HIV infection among homosexual men. AIDS 7:43–49, 1993.

32. M Melbye, E Smith, J Wohlfahrt Nielson, A Østerlind, M Orholm, OJ Bergmann, L Mathiesen, T Darragh, J Palefsky. Anal and cervical abnormality in women: prediction by NPV tests. Int J Cancer 68:559–564, 1996.

33. JM Palefsky, EA Holly, J Gonzales, K Lamborn, H Hollander. Natural history of anal cytologic abnormalities and papillomavirus infection among homosexual men with group IV HIV disease. J Acquir Immune Defic Syndr 5:1258–1265, 1992.

34. CW Critchlow, CM Surawicz, KK Holmes, et al. Prospective study of high grade anal squamous intraepithelial neoplasia in a cohort of homosexual men: influence of HIV infection, immunosuppression and human papillomavirus infection. AIDS 9:1255–1262, 1995.

35. JW Mellors, LA Kingsley, C Rinaldo Jr. JA Todd, BS Hoo, RP Kokka, P Gupta. Quantitation of HIV-1 RNA in plasma predicts outcome after seroconversion. Ann Intern Med 122:573–579, 1995.

36. JH Scholefield, WG Hickson, JH Smith, K Rogers, F Sharp. Anal intraepithelial neoplasia: part of a multifocal disease process. Lancet 340:1271–1273, 1992.

37. M Melbye, P Sprogel. Aetiological parallel between anal cancer and cervical cancer. Lancet 338:657–659, 1991.

38. J Palefsky. Anal cancer in HIV-positive individuals: an emerging problem. AIDS 8:283–295, 1994.

39. T Darragh, EA Holly, CJ Hogeboom, JM Palefsky. Comparison of conventional cytologic smears and ThinPrep preparations of the anal canal. Acta Cytol 41:1167–1170, 1997.

40. C Sonnex, JH Scholefield, G Kocjan, G Kelly, C Whatrup, A Mindel, JM Northover. Anal human papillomavirus infection: a comparative study of cytology, colposcopy and DNA hybridisation as methods of detection. Genitourin Med 67:21–25, 1991.

41. JM Palefsky, EA Holly, CJ Hogeboom, N Jay, M Berry, TM Darragh. Anal cytology as a screening tool for anal squamous intraepithelial lesions. J Acquir Immune Defic Syndr 14:415–422, 1997.

7

The Management of Cervical Neoplasia in HIV-Infected Women

Mitchell Maiman
Staten Island University Hospital,
Staten Island, New York

I. INTRODUCTION

Human immunodeficiency virus (HIV) infection continues to be a national and international health problem of epidemic proportions. Despite that new AIDS cases increased by less than 5% for the fifth year in a row, a number well below the rate of increase in the epidemic's first decade, the incidence of acquired immunodeficiency syndrome (AIDS) cases among women continues to increase, particularly in minority women. Approximately 19% of new adult and adolescent cases of AIDS in the United States last year were in women, and women represent the subgroup with the greatest rate of increase compared with any other defined population in North America. As with cervical neoplasia, HIV infection is largely a disease of women in their reproductive years, with the incidence of both diseases significantly higher in women of color. Even with widespread screening efforts, an estimated 15,000 new cases of invasive cervical carcinoma are diagnosed each year in the United States. This number represents only a fraction of the women treated for preinvasive cervical neoplasia and evaluated for abnormal cytology. Cervical intraepithelial neoplasia (CIN) has long represented the model of transition from a precursor lesion to invasive disease.

The coexistence of cervical neoplasia in women infected with HIV represents one of the most serious challenges in the oncological care of immunosuppressed patients. Whereas the development of most illnesses and malignancies in HIV-infected patients can largely be attributed to immunodeficiency, the relation between cervical neoplasia and HIV infection is quite unique. Both cervical carcinoma and HIV infection are, in part, sexually transmitted diseases, with onco-genic types of human papillomavirus (HPV) infection the implicated viral carcin-ogen associated with cervical cancer. Therefore, an association between cervical cancer and HIV can be anticipated, not only on the basis of immunosuppression, but also because of shared common sexual behavioral risk factors. Thus, while immunosuppressed women, such as renal transplant patients receiving highly im-munosuppressive drugs, are at high risk for lower genital tract neoplasia, immu-nodeficient HIV-infected women are perhaps the highest-risk subgroup that we know. Although these factors likely play the major role in the pathogenesis of cervical neoplasia in HIV-infected women, direct interactions between HIV and HPV at the molecular level, the effects of HIV on the local mucosal immune response, enhancement of HPV regulatory expression by the HIV-1 Tat protein, and HIV-induced perturbations of paracrine or autocrine factors that influence HPV gene expression must also be considered.

II. IMMUNOSUPPRESSION AND HPV

Immunodeficiency, whether congenital, iatrogenic, or acquired, predisposes to the development of neoplasia. This phenomenon has been demonstrated in indi-viduals with rare congenital immunodeficiency disorders, organ transplant pa-tients receiving immunosuppressive drugs, and patients receiving cytotoxic che-motherapy. The AIDS epidemic has enabled us to study the most glaring example of acquired immunodeficiency. Neoplasia in all such patients represents an accel-erated version of the long-term course of such lesions in immunocompetent hosts. Immunosuppressed individuals demonstrate a heightened susceptibility to HPV infection, which increases as the immune system becomes more compromised and the duration of immune dysfunction is prolonged. There is abundant evidence that HPV is a necessary, but not sufficient, cofactor related to malignant and premalignant neoplasia of the cervix, and certain HPV subtypes are more onco-genic than others in their association with invasive cervical cancer and progres-sive aneuploid dysplasia.

Although reported rates of cervical neoplasia in renal transplant patients range from 5 to 40%, with the risk of anogenital neoplasia in such patients being 9–14 times that of matched control subjects (1), HIV-positive patients represent the subgroup of immunosuppressed women at greatest risk, probably because the sexual behavioral risk factors for developing HIV and HPV are similar. Petry et al. (2), in a study of cellular immunodeficiency of HPV-associated cervical lesions, compared HIV-seropositive women and female allograft recipients. The HIV-infected patients were three times more likely to have HPV–DNA-positive swabs than the transplantation group, as well as higher rates of oncogenic HPV types and CIN lesions. Without HPV infection, even severely immunosuppressed women may remain free of lower genital cancer; however, HPV infections are more common among HIV-seropositive women at all levels of immunosuppression.

The HIV-infected women have as much as an 18-fold risk for the development of genital condylomata (3), which are related to the "benign" subtypes of HPV, and cervical HPV infection is especially prevalent in the HIV-positive female population, with an altered ratio of clinically expressed to latent lesions, when compared to HIV-negative women. HIV-infected women have more consistent cytological and histological evidence of HPV infection than do matched controls (4), and the risk of HPV-associated cervicovaginal infection is at least 1.4–7.8 times that in HIV-noninfected women in a series of studies from Africa and the Netherlands (5–7). HPV infection is common in the lower genital tract of HIV-seropositive women and may further facilitate HIV transmission through disruption of mucosal integrity or altered local immune surveillance.

Higher rates of more oncogenic HPV subtype infection, multiple type HPV infection, and unspecified type HPV infection have been reported by numerous investigators, and may help explain the more aggressive cervical pathology that develops in HIV-infected women. Sun et al. found infections with HPV type-16, 18, and more than one type to be more common in the HIV-seropositive patients (8), whereas Maiman et al. (9) found the only independent risk factor for CIN was an oncogenic HPV type. Results from an African study suggested that types not detected by the usual probes are common in HIV-infected women (6), whereas other studies of dysplastic cervical tissue in such patients have described infections with combinations of all HPV subtypes. Johnson et al., in a study of patients with CIN and CD4 cell counts of fewer than 200/mm^3, recovered HPV-18, the most oncogenic of subtypes, in 50% of specimens (10), whereas Vernon et al. (11) found a high prevalence of HPV types 31, 33, and 35. The altered nature of HPV infection in such individuals may be viewed as opportunistic complication of HIV infection.

Although systemic immunosuppression plays the major role on the pathogenesis of HPV-associated neoplasia in the HIV-infected women, the effects of HIV on mucosal immune response and direct interactions between HIV and HPV at the molecular level must be considered. Local cervical immunity, as evaluated by Langerhans cell counts, is impaired in HIV-seropositive women, with the severity of impairment correlating with the stage of HIV disease (12). HIV may have direct effect on cells participating in the local cervical immune response. In addition, soluble HIV proteins, such as Tat, which can activate HPV protein expression in vitro, may diffuse from the stroma to the epithelium. Vernon et al. (13) described how the HIV-1 Tat protein enhances E2-dependent HPV-16 transcription, and Tornesello et al. (14) showed that Tat protein alone can increase the enhancer activity of regulatory regions of HPV-transforming genes. The relation between HIV and HPV is obviously quite complex and awaits further clinical, immunological, and molecular biological investigation.

III. SCREENING ISSUES

Because a well-defined precursor lesion for cervical cancer can be detected by screening, organized screening programs for cervical neoplasia can be expected to reduce both the incidence and the mortality rates. As the prevalence of disease is far greater in HIV-positive patients than the general population, optimal screening strategies take on an increased importance. HIV-positive women have as much as a tenfold increased rate of abnormal cytology, including a wide range of cellular and inflammatory changes, such as hyperkeratosis, parakeratosis, infection with trichomonas and herpes, inflammatory atypia, HPV-related changes, and varying degrees of cervical neoplasia (15). Higher rates of abnormalities have also been demonstrated after seroconversion than before seroconversion (14). Studies from several centers have demonstrated that women who are immunodeficient from HIV infection have cytological abnormality rates (including inflammatory Papanicolaou [Pap] smears) of between 30 and 60% (16–18) and Pap smears consistent with cervical dysplasia from 15 to 40% (19). Most studies also consistently demonstrate that the prevalence of such abnormalities increases as immunodeficiency becomes more severe.

Screening strategies in HIV-positive women must take into account the high prevalence of cervical dysplasia in this subgroup as well as the limitations of cytological screening, the relatively high noncompliance rate, and the possibility of accelerated progression of disease. These factors make initial accurate diagnosis critical. Although the Centers for Disease Control and Prevention (CDC) continues to recommend Pap smears as the sole screening method, numerous authors have advocated the need for baseline colposcopy in HIV-infected women because of the inaccuracy of cytology in consistently predicting histology, low negative predictive values of the Pap smear, decreased sensitivity, and discordances between cytological smear and biopsy results (20–24). Other authors have found HIV-infected women had significantly more smears of limited adequacy owing to obscuring blood or inflammation, and higher rates of concomitant vaginal infections leading to "underread" smears (25). Maiman et al. (9), in a unique study of 248 HIV-infected women, all of whom had had cytology, colposcopy, and biopsy, found that 38% of all CIN would have been missed if routine colposcopy and biopsy were not performed. Interestingly, similar high false-negative rates of cytological tests have been reported in immunosuppressed women after renal transplantation (26).

The limitations of cytological screening become more glaring as the prevalence of cervical dysplasia increases in a given population. Although more frequent cytological screening (every 6 months) is to be advocated, a reasonable approach would involve baseline colposcopy or cervicography in HIV-positive women once the diagnosis is made (Fig. 1). Patients with normal colposcopy could then undergo more aggressive cytological screening than the normal population, whereas those diagnosed and treated for CIN undergo colposcopy with liberal biopsy every 4–6 months for 2 years and semiannual Pap smears thereafter. Alternatively, screening strategies may be based on baseline immune status, with more aggressive techniques reserved for patients with CD4 cell counts of fewer than 500/mm^3. All strategies must take into account availability of colposcopic resources and individualized knowledge of risk in given patient populations.

Recent studies have begun to delineate the role of HPV DNA testing in the clinical management of patients, particularly for primary screening and secondary screening of the minimally abnormal Pap smear. Molecular techniques, including

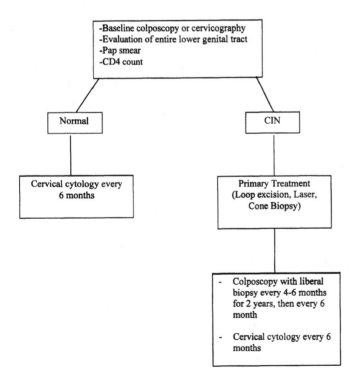

Figure 1 Screening for CIN in HIV-positive women.

consensus primer polymerase chain reaction (PCR) and hybrid capture, have become less expensive and more reliable and can readily distinguish between low-risk (HPV-6 and 11), intermediate-risk (HPV-31, 33, 35, 51, and 52), and high–oncogenic-risk (HPV-16, 18, 45, and 56) HPV subtypes. Accurate, precise, and cost-effective viral tests for oncogenic HPV may have a significant role in future screening programs, and may be particularly useful in the clinical care of HIV-positive women.

In contrast with the inherent lack of sensitivity of normal cervical cytology, abnormal cytology is extremely accurate in predicting CIN on histology and Pap smears, indicating CIN must be taken very seriously (27). Specificities of 84% or greater have been reported, with even higher predictive values (24). Therefore, virtually all such patients will indeed have cervical pathology, justifying immediate treatment during initial colposcopic evaluation of a significantly abnormal Pap smear. This ''see-and-treat'' approach using excisional methods, such as loop electrosurgical excision procedure, may be particularly appropriate for the HIV-infected woman.

In addition to screening for cervical neoplasia, the early identification of asymptomatic HIV-infected women by virtue of their cervical disease is an important screening issue. HIV counseling and testing in such women provides a unique opportunity for early medical intervention for HIV disease, as well as the chance to limit both heterosexual and vertical transmission. The risk of HIV infection in women with abnormal Pap smears will vary with the prevalence of HIV infection in a given population. Overall HIV seropositivity rates of 11–13% have been reported in colposcopy clinics in Brooklyn (28) and Queens (29), New York with the highest risk being among women aged 30–39. Screening programs in such high-risk clinics have yielded HIV-positivity rates of between 6 and 7%. Although HIV counseling and testing should be advocated for all sexually active women, more cost-effective screening programs in lower-risk areas are reasonable, to include women with recurrent, multifocal, or high-grade dysplasia.

The prevalence of HIV infection in women with invasive cervical carcinoma may be even higher than in those with preinvasive disease. Maiman et al. reported a 19% seropositivity rate in women younger than the age of 50 in a high-risk population in Brooklyn (30). Most importantly, most of these women were asymptomatic for HIV disease and died of cervical cancer, not AIDS; therefore, only HIV-screening programs would have detected their positive serostatus. We currently recommend HIV counseling and testing in all younger (less than age 50) patients with cervical cancer, as test results may have a significant influence on oncological therapeutic strategies. The Gynecologic Oncology Group (GOG) is currently conducting a nationwide screening study involving HIV testing and follow-up of newly diagnosed patients with invasive cervical carcinoma.

IV. PREINVASIVE CERVICAL NEOPLASIA

A. Characteristics of Disease

The HIV-seropositive women represent perhaps the highest risk group encountered for the development of cervical intraepithelial neoplasia (CIN). In the most recent classification system of HIV-related diseases, the CDC has identified moderate to severe cervical dysplasia and carcinoma in situ as category B conditions. Independent studies have estimated the prevalence of CIN in this subgroup to be between 20 and 50% (16,18,20,24). Maiman et al., in a study of HIV-positive women without AIDS-defining illness, found the prevalence of CIN on histology to be 32% in a cohort of 248 patients (9). Cervical dysplasia of HIV-positive women may be of higher grade than in seronegative women, with more extensive involvement of the lower genital tract with HPV-associated lesions (4). Extensive cervical involvement, endocervical involvement, and multisite (vagina, vulva, and perianal) disease are more common. Natural history studies examining the biological behavior of cervical HPV and CIN strongly suggest that disease is more aggressive in HIV-positive patients. Conti et al. (31) found fourfold higher progressions and threefold lower regression rates of untreated HPV-related cervical lesions in infected women compared with HIV-negative controls, and Petry (2) found only a 27% regression rate of CIN I lesions in immunosuppressed HIV-positive and transplant patients compared with 62% in immunocompetent controls.

Numerous studies have demonstrated the relation between HIV-associated immunosuppression and the development of CIN, and the presence and severity of cervical neoplasia are correlated with both quantitative and qualitative T-cell function (20,32). In one study, HIV-positive patients with CIN had absolute CD4 cell counts and T4/T8 ratios roughly half those of HIV-positive patients without CIN (Fig. 2), and patients with AIDS-defining illness are more likely to have cervical disease than are asymptomatic HIV-positive patients. Wright et al. (33) concluded that a CD4 lymphocyte count of $200/m^3$ was independently associated with CIN. The concept of worsening immunodeficiency increasing the risk of cervical pathology may be used to individualize screening and surveillance strategies in HIV-positive women.

B. Management

The treatment of preinvasive cervical disease in HIV-infected women is among the most challenging and frustrating tasks faced by the practicing gynecologist. In general, standard therapeutic strategies for immunocompetent women apply, but the increased risk for treatment failures and chronic nature of disease in such women is well documented.

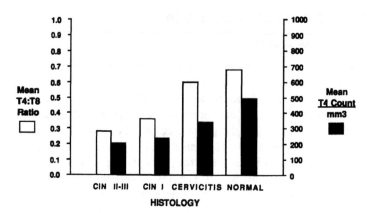

Figure 2 Absolute T4 count and T4/T8 ratio by cervical histology in HIV-positive patients. (From Ref. 20.)

Excisional methods, which include loop electrosurgical excision procedure (LEEP), laser cone and cold knife cone biopsy, are preferred over ablative methods, such as cryotherapy and laser vaporization. Excisional methods have the advantage of confirmation of histology and documentation of negative margins, which is of particular importance in HIV-positive women in whom disease may be more extensive. DelPriore et al. (34) reported that colposcopically directed biopsies may be poor predictors of histology on excisional cone specimens in HIV-seropositive women, as 47% with CIN II–III on cone biopsy had only CIN I or HPV on punch biopsy, as compared with only 9% in HIV-seronegative patients. Additionally, with advances in the technology in electrosurgical generators and the development of large wire loops with insulated bases, LEEP has allowed excision of the cervical transformation zone and distal canal with a single-pass of the loop, with the patient under local anesthesia in an outpatient setting. Therefore, in most centers LEEP excision has become the preferred treatment, although laser ablation is still quite adequate if the CIN lesion lies within the range of satisfactory colposcopic assessment. Although the use of cryotherapy in HIV-positive women may seem particularly attractive because of the absence of bleeding and reduced theoretical risk of iatrogenic transmission of HIV, studies have indicated that the use of this modality in HIV-infected women may offer a specific treatment disadvantage. In one study (35), 48% of HIV-infected women with low-grade CIN receiving cryotherapy developed recurrence, compared with 1% of seronegative women.

Diagnostic procedures, such as coldknife cone conization, diagnostic LEEP, or laser cone must be performed for the usual indications, including

1. The transformation has not been fully visualized colposcopically.
2. The endocervical curettage (ECC) is positive.
3. There is a two-step or more discordance between cytology and histology.
4. There is suspicion of microinvasion.

Diagnostic procedures may then be considered therapeutic if histological results are favorable. An algorithm for the management of CIN in HIV-positive patients is presented in Fig. 3. Recurrence rates for CIN in HIV-positive women with standard therapies have been reported to be as high as 40% at 1 year and 60% with longer follow-up (35,36). Maiman et al. (35) and Petry et al. (2) reported recurrence rates of 39 and 40%, respectively, compared with 9 and 10% on seronegative controls. Fruchter et al. (37), at 36 months, reported a 62% failure rate (Fig. 4), compared with 18% in controls, with an 87% failure rate in patients with CD4 cell counts of fewer than 200/mm³. In addition, progression to higher-grade dysplasia was more common in HIV-positive patients, as well as multiple episodes of recurrent disease requiring many repeated procedures. The frequency of recurrence is closely related to immune function. Patients with CD4 cell counts of fewer than 500/mm³ are at extremely high risk for recurrence (>60%), whereas

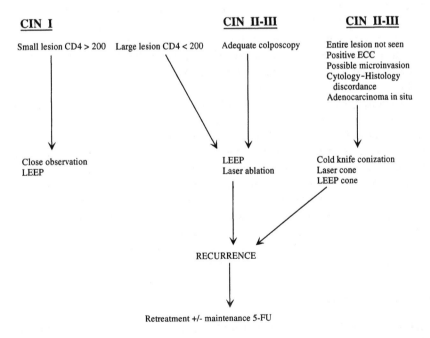

Figure 3 Treatment options for CIN in HIV-positive women.

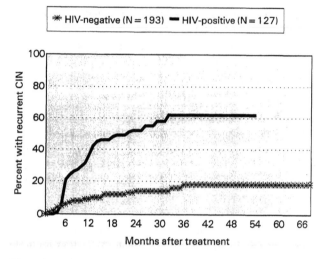

Figure 4 Recurrence of cervical intraepithelial neoplasia after treatment by HIV status in 127 HIV-infected and 193 HIV-negative women. (From Ref. 37.)

women with counts of more than 500/mm³ may be expected to recur at about twice the rate (18%) of seronegative women (Fig. 5). Therefore, diagnostic and therapeutic strategies may be stratified based on the degree of immunosuppression. Unfortunately, complications after treatment for CIN in HIV-positive women may be increased, as one study demonstrated higher rates of excessive bleeding and cervicovaginal infections (38).

    Although poor treatment results of standard ablative and excisional therapies in HIV-infected women with CIN certainly warrant unique therapeutic strategies, one must recognize that close and meticulous posttherapy surveillance and repetitive aggressive retreatment for persistent and recurrent disease have been successful in preventing progressive neoplasia and invasive cervical carcinoma and, therefore, should not be abandoned. Hysterectomy, which is rarely used today in the management of CIN in immunocompetent patients, may be considered in individual cases in HIV-seropositive women, and be particularly reserved for the multiparous patient with relatively good immune function who has undergone multiple therapeutic procedures for recurrent high dysplasia, and in whom repeated evaluation is exceedingly difficult.

C. Clinical Trials

In response to the high rates of treatment failures for preinvasive cervical disease in HIV-positive women, the AIDS Clinical Trials Group (ACTG) is investigating

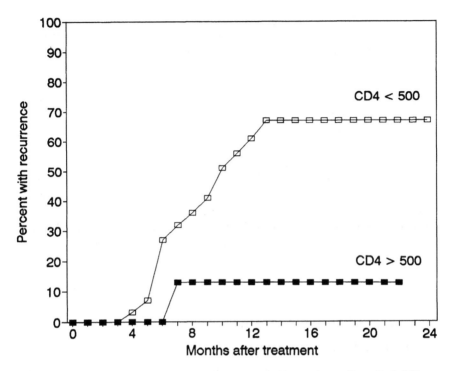

Figure 5   Recurrence by CD4 cell count in HIV-positive patients. (From Ref. 35.)

novel therapeutic approaches. For patients with high-grade dysplasia (CIN II–III), ACTG 200 examined the role of topical vaginal 5-fluorouracil (5-FU) cream maintenance therapy as prophylaxis against recurrent CIN. In this study, patients were randomized to receive standard ablative or excisional therapy alone versus standard therapy plus 2 g of vaginal FU every 2 weeks, for 6 months. 5-FU has previously been used with considerable success in the care of immunocompromised women with lower genital tract neoplasia, especially after conventional therapy has resulted in repetitive recurrence. Krebs (39) found that prophylactic maintenance therapy with vaginal 5-FU was effective in the treatment of HPV-associated lesions of the vulva and vagina, especially in immunosuppressed women with multiple organ involvement. Effective local adjunctive therapy with topical chemotherapeutic agents is particularly attractive in HIV-positive patients in light of their favorable therapeutic index, and results of such randomized, controlled studies are extremely important.

ACTG 293 is a study involving the treatment of HIV-positive patients with CIN I. Although the standard of care today in immunocompetent women with

CIN I (mild dysplasia) is close follow-up only, without surgical therapy, it is unknown whether this conservative strategy is safe in seropositive patients in light of reports of more aggressive and progressive disease. In this trial, patients are randomized between observation-only without any surgical therapy, versus oral isotretenoin 0.5 mg/kg per day for 6 months, with close attention to follow-up for regression, persistence, or progression. The results of this trial are likely to have implications for women with CIN in general.

Optimization of immune function and lowering of viral load with proven and newer anti-HIV drugs is also desirable, and many patients today are placed on multiple drug regimens. It is unknown whether any of such interventions has any effect on cervical disease, and the presence of multiple confounding variables will make this issue exceedingly difficult to study. At present, the principles of aggressive initial evaluation, more frequent cytological screening, and meticulous posttherapy surveillance, with liberal repeat colposcopy and retreatment for recurrent dysplasia, in managing preinvasive disease in HIV-infected women seem prudent as we investigate novel treatment strategies in clinical trials.

V. INVASIVE CERVICAL CARCINOMA

A. Characteristics of Disease

On January 1, 1993, the CDC expanded the surveillance case definition of AIDS to include HIV-positive women with invasive cervical cancer. As an AIDS-defining illness, it is required that physicians and hospitals report cases of cervical cancer in HIV-infected women to their local health departments. These changes have served to educate the health care community concerning this relation and to stimulate more aggressive testing programs. In the first year of the expanded definition, approximately 1.3% of women with AIDS-defining illnesses 13 years of age or older had cervical cancer (40). However, HIV testing in women with cervical cancer was far from routine, and documentation of AIDS cases varied considerably based on the reporting practices of physicians and hospitals. In addition, cancer registry reports, which may be expected to be highly accurate in surveilling cases of cervical cancer, are relatively ineffective in AIDS case surveillance, and hospital discharge summaries, which document multiple diagnoses very well are infrequently used. Other factors may also contribute to the underdiagnosis of cervical cancer in HIV-infected women, including lack of HIV testing in older women, poor access to health care, and the coexistence of more acute and life-threatening AIDS-defining opportunistic infections that inhibit both the diagnosis and the reporting of cervical cancer. In an urban population at high risk for both diseases in Brooklyn, New York where a routine HIV-testing program was instituted in all cervical cancer patients 50 years of age or younger (41), cervical cancer was the sixth most common AIDS-defining illness in women, representing 4% of the subjects, as well as the most common AIDS-related malignancy in women (55%), followed by lymphoma (29%), and Kaposi's sarcoma (16%).

B. Clinical Issues in Invasive Cervical Carcinoma

The signs and symptoms of cervical cancer may take on typical or atypical presentations in HIV-infected women. Ideally, the disease should be diagnosed by classic screening methods of cytology, colposcopy, and biopsy if disease is to be detected in the preinvasive or early invasive phase. When patients present with symptoms, more-advanced disease is often found, and vaginal bleeding or postcoital bleeding is most commonly reported. Malodorous vaginal discharge is also quite common, as is pelvic pain, back pain, or lower abdominal pain. Leg pain, edema, weight loss, or obstructive uropathy is indicative of more advanced disease. In HIV-positive patients, metastatic disease may occur in both common and uncommon sites (4), and unusual extracervical metastases have been described in the psoas muscles, periclitoral area, and spinal cord, as well as malignant ascites (42,43). Diagnosis can be even more difficult, because the classic signs of systemic cancer may mimic the subtle manifestations of HIV disease. Low-grade fevers, unexplained weight loss, gastrointestinal disturbances, and fatigue may occur in both disease processes. Lymphadenopathy, either clinically detected in the left supraclavicular (scalene) nodes or inguinal nodes, or retroperitoneal (pelvic or paraaortic) nodes, discovered at the time of surgery, or on radiologic imaging, must not be assumed to be metastatic cancer; HIV-infected patients will often have very large, suspicious nodes that may be secondary to follicular hyperplasia, not to a tumor. This pathological diagnosis, which includes mononuclear cell proliferation, polykaryocytes, epithelioid histiocytes, and mantle-zone loss, although not pathognomonic for HIV, is highly suggestive.

In addition, coexistent pelvic infection may present diagnostic and therapeutic dilemmas. HIV-infected women have high rates of concomitant pelvic inflammatory disease, which is more often refractory to antibiotic therapy. Pelvic abscesses may mimic metastatic cervical cancer, and pelvic infection may contribute to the development and spread of disease and increase the failure rate and morbidity of therapeutic interventions.

Cervical cancer is the only gynecological malignancy that is clinically staged, which is assigned by the current staging system of the International Federation of Gynecology and Obstetrics (FIGO; Table 1). Once a clinical stage is assigned and treatment has been initiated, the stage must not be changed because of subsequent findings by either extended clinical or surgical staging. Bimanual rectovaginal pelvic examination, performed under anesthesia if necessary, is the most important part of clinical staging, and only certain additional studies for

Table 1   Staging for Carcinoma of the Cervix Uteri

Stage I

The carcinoma is strictly confined to the cervix.

    Stage IA

    Invasive cancer is identified only microscopically. All gross lesions even with superficial invasion are stage IB cancers. Invasion is limited to measured stromal invasion, with maximum depth of 5.0 mm and no wider than 7.0 mm.

        Stage IA-1

        Measured invasion of stroma no greater than 3.0 mm in depth and no wider than 7.0 mm.

        Stage IA-2

        Measured invasion of stroma greater than 3.0 mm, but no greater than 5.0 mm, and no wider than 7.0 mm.

    Stage IB

    Clinical lesions confined to the cervix or preclinical lesions greater than IA.

        Stage IB1

        Clinical lesions no greater than 4.0 cm in size.

        Stage IB2

        Clinical lesions greater than 4.0 cm in size.

Stage II

The carcinoma extends beyond the cervix, but has not extended to the pelvic wall. The carcinoma involves the vaginal, but does not extend as far as the lower third.

    Stage IIA

    No obvious parametrial involvement.

    Stage IIB

    Obvious parametrial involvement.

Stage III

The carcinoma has extended to the pelvic wall. On rectal examination, there is no cancer-free space between the tumor and the pelvic wall. The tumor involves the lower third of the vagina. All cases with a hydronephrosis or nonfunctioning kidney are included unless they are known to be due to other causes.

    Stage IIIA

    No extension to the pelvic wall.

    Stage IIIB

    Extension to the pelvic wall or hydronephrosis or nonfunctioning kidney.

Stage IV

The carcinoma has extended beyond the true pelvis or has clinically involved the mucosa of the bladder or rectum.

    Stage IVA

    Spread of the growth to adjacent organs.

    Stage IVB

    Spread to distant organs.

extracervical disease are allowed by FIGO, including intravenous pyelogram, barium enema, chest and skeletal x-ray films, cystoscopy, and sigmoidoscopy. However, other more practical and useful studies are often employed that provide more specific information, including computed tomography (CT), magnetic resonance imaging (MRI), and laparoscopic lymph node biopsies or extraperitoneal lymph node biopsies by laparotomy. The recommended diagnostic workup for HIV-infected patients with cervical cancer is presented in Table 2. Tumor markers, specifically squamous cell carcinoma antigen or CA-125 for the respective cell types of squamous or adenocarcinoma, are useful parameters with which to follow patients during and after treatment.

Cancer of the cervix most often spreads by direct invasion into the cervical stroma and laterally into the parametrial tissues, as well as to the vagina and corpus uteri. Lymphatic metastases are also quite common, and are involved in a progressive fashion, beginning with the pelvic (obturator, external, and internal iliac) nodes, and then involving the para-aortic, inguinal, and scalene nodes. The incidence of positive pelvic and para-aortic nodes ranges from 15 and 5%, respectively, for stage IB to 45 and 30% for stage III patients. However, HIV-positive patients may have higher-grade tumors and higher rates of lymph node involvement than expected by stage alone. Cervical cancer may also spread by blood-borne metastases or intraperitoneal implantation, or present or recur with painful bony metastases.

Table 2 Workup for Cervical Cancer in HIV-Infected Patients

All stages
Cervical biopsy
Biannual rectovaginal examination
Chest radiography
CD4 cell count (mm³)
SCC antigen
Stages IB1-IV
CT scan—abdomen and pelvis; or
MRI
Sigmoidoscopy
Cystoscopy
Optional studies
Bone scan
Lymphangiography
Surgical evaluation of lymph nodes

C. Characteristics of Disease

Although much of the data thus far has been limited to case reports and single-institution studies, it seems apparent that in some HIV-infected women the disease characteristics may take a more aggressive clinical course (30,44). This parallels the examples observed in other AIDS-related malignancies. HIV-positive women present with more advanced disease than do HIV-negative women with cervical cancer. In the largest study to date at the Health Science Center at Brooklyn, comparing 16 seropositive to 68 seronegative women, significantly more advanced disease was found in those who were HIV-positive (30). Half the seropositive patients presented with stage III or IV disease, compared with 19% in seronegative controls, and only 1 infected patient remained with early disease after careful surgical–pathological staging. Almost 70% of HIV-infected women had stage III or higher surgical–pathological stage, compared with 28% of seronegative controls. HIV-infected women with cervical cancer may be quite young, such as the case of a 16-year-old who presented with stage IIIB disease and died at age 17 (4).

Most HIV-positive patients can be expected to have squamous cell carcinomas, as was found in the foregoing study in which 15 of 16 patients had squamous cancers, with the remaining patient having an adenosquamous tumor (30). Most importantly, most patients die of cervical cancer before they succumb to AIDS and are usually asymptomatic for HIV infection. Therefore, only HIV-testing programs of such patients will enable the physician to make the diagnosis and realize the full effect of the interaction of these two disease processes. The HIV-positive women with cervical cancer have higher recurrence and death rates, with shorter intervals to recurrence and death than do HIV-negative control subjects (Fig. 6; 30). Mean intervals to recurrence are extremely short, and many patients retain persistent disease after primary treatment. Median time to death was 10 months in seropositive women, compared with 23 months in seronegative patients. Several other case reports have described examples of rapidly progressive cervical cancer in such women. As with preinvasive disease, the relation between immune function and disease status is apparent. The mean absolute CD4 cell count and CD4/CD8 ratio in such patients was $360/mm^3$ and 0.57, compared with $830/mm^3$ and 1.71, respectively, in uninfected women. One can infer from these values that the typical HIV-infected woman with cervical cancer would not meet the immunological definition for AIDS solely by CD4 count ($\leq 200/mm^3$), emphasizing the importance of the recent inclusion of seropositive women with cervical cancer as AIDS patients. Although stage of cancer may not predict CD4 cell levels, immune status does influence subsequent outcome. Patients with counts of more than $500/mm^3$ have had more favorable disease courses; therefore, management decisions in HIV-infected women with cervical cancer should carefully consider pretreatment immune function, as positive serostatus alone may

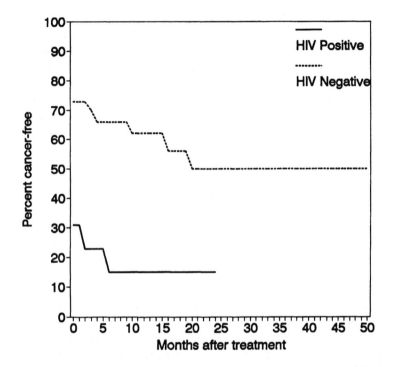

Figure 6   Progression-free interval by HIV status in treated patients with advanced stage cervical carcinoma. (From Ref. 35.)

not necessarily and uniformly confer a dismal outcome. HIV-related immunodeficiency may contribute heavily to the natural history of cervical carcinoma, and HIV-positive patients need not demonstrate other signs of immunosuppression, such as opportunistic infections, for their neoplasia to be adversely affected by HIV.

In addition to host factors specific to HIV-infected patients, classic tumor variables as prognostic factors in cervical cancer are extremely important in predicting recurrence risk and outcome. The most important of these factors in clinical (FIGO) stage, as well as tumor volume, depth of cervical invasion, presence of microscopic lymphvascular space invasion, parametrial invasion, and tumor differentiation. The presence of lymph node metastases represents the dominant prognostic factor affecting survival after radical hysterectomy. The use of quantitative flow cytometric methods, such as DNA ploidy and S-phase fraction, to characterize biological potential of individual cancer cells has not yet been proved to be of prognostic benefit in cervical cancer, as it has in a number of other solid tumors.

The characteristics of HIV disease in cervical cancer may be different in cervical cancer patients when compared with HIV-positive patients with other AIDS-related malignancies. Women with invasive cervical cancer are less immunosuppressed than women with other AIDS opportunistic illnesses, and may be expected to have CD4 cell counts about twice as high as those with Kaposi's sarcoma and non-Hodgkins lymphoma ($312-153/mm^3$; 41). In most women with cervical cancer, HIV infection was diagnosed at the time of cancer presentation, whereas in women with other malignancies, HIV diagnosis preceded cancer diagnosis by a mean on 2.7 years. Although the interval from cancer diagnosis to death may be similar in all AIDS-related malignancies, cancer was the cause of death more often with cervical cancer patients (95%), compared with those with other cancers (60%). Although patients with cervical cancer as their AIDS-defining illness may be slightly younger than those women without cervical cancer, the distribution of mode of HIV transmission (heterosexual versus injection drug abuse) and race (black versus Hispanic versus white) was remarkably similar (9).

D. Management

The management of HIV-positive patients with cervical cancer is among the most challenging tasks faced by the oncological team. In general, the same principles that guide the oncological management of cervical cancer in immunocompetent patients should be applied (Table 3). However, extremely close monitoring for both therapeutic efficacy and unusual toxicity must be instituted.

Numerous definitions of "microinvasive" cervical cancer have been used over the past two decades, and no consensus has yet been reached. The purpose

Table 3 Treatment Recommendations for Cervical Carcinoma in HIV-Infected Women

Stage	Recommended treatment
Stage Ia1	Cold knife therapeutic cone biopsy if fertility desired; otherwise, simple hysterectomy
Stages IA2 and IB1	Radical hysterectomy, with pelvic lymphadenectomy Alternatively, radiation therapy in poor surgical candidates
Stages IB2 and IIA	Radiation therapy +/− simple hysterectomy; or radical hysterectomy with pelvic lymphadenectomy; or neoadjuvant chemotherapy + radical surgery
Stage IIB–IVA	Radiation therapy +/− chemosensitization
Stage IVB	Chemotherapy +/− radiation therapy
Recurrent disease	Pelvic exenteration (central disease), otherwise palliative chemotherapy

of defining microinvasion is to identify a group of patients who are not at risk for lymph node metastases or recurrence and who, therefore, might be treated with less than radical therapy. This is particularly important in HIV-positive patients who may be quite young and very interested in childbearing. Treatment plans must be based on microscopic depth of invasion of the lesion on cone biopsy, width and breadth of the invasive area, and the presence or absence of lymphatic vascular space invasion. Patients with less than 3 mm of invasion below the basement membrane without lymphovascular invasion are candidates for simple, rather than radical, hysterectomy and even therapeutic cold knife conization if future childbearing is desired. Lymph node biopsies are probably not necessary in this group. Patients with more than 3 mm of invasion need more radical surgery, with pelvic lymphadenectomy. Because there are very little data on the safety of more conservative management of microinvasive carcinoma in HIV-positive patients specifically, close monitoring is essential.

Radical hysterectomy and pelvic lymphadenectomy should be performed in most cases of stage IA2 and IB1, and in some cases of stage IB2 and IIA cervical cancer where cervical size is not too enlarged and vaginal involvement is minimal. Radical oncological surgery in HIV-positive women can be performed for the usual indications, and surgical decisions should be based on oncological issues, not HIV status. As has been demonstrated in other types of operations in the HIV-positive patients, women with relatively good immune function tolerate surgery well, with no significant excess morbidity. Prophylactic antibiotics should be routinely used, and standard surgical precautions should be taken to prevent surgical transmission. The transmission rate of HIV from patient to health care worker is extremely low—about 1:320.

Although radiation therapy can be used in all stages of cervical cancer and has identical cure rates when compared with radical surgery in stage IB, the issues of ovarian conservation and better vaginal sexual function make radical hysterectomy the preferred modality in younger patients. Ovarian transposition should be considered at the time of surgery if postoperative pelvic radiation is a strong possibility. One may expect a urological fistula rate of 1–2% and a chronic bladder atony rate of 3% after radical hysterectomy, compared with an intestinal and urinary stricture and fistula rate of 3–5% and rate of chronic radiation fibrosis of the bowel or bladder of 6–8% with pelvic radiation therapy. Another advantage of surgery over radiation is the availability of surgical–pathological data such as lymph node status, for which postoperative therapy can then be designed.

As most HIV-infected patients with cervical cancer present with more-advanced disease, radiation therapy is usually the cornerstone of treatment and is the basis for therapy in stages II–IV. Pelvic radiation therapy begins with external beam therapy, designed to shrink the primary tumor and create better geometry for the brachytherapy insertions to follow. Pelvic fields are usually

15 × 15 cm, extending to a 2-cm margin lateral to the bony pelvis and inferiorly to the border of the obturator foramen. The superior margin can be extended to 18 cm to cover the common iliac nodes, or even higher if para-aortic lymph node metastases are evident. The usual dosages of pelvic radiotherapy delivered include 7000–8000 cGy to point A and 6000 cGy to point B. Some HIV-positive patients may respond poorly to radiation therapy alone, and regimens that incorporate radiation sensitizers that are being utilized more frequently in general should be strongly considered. The two most common sensitizing regimens include cisplatin (50 mg/m^2 week 1 and week 6) combined with 5-fluorouracil (1000 mg/m^2, continuous infusion for 4 days, weeks 1 and 6) or p.o. hydroxyurea (3 g/m^2, twice per week for 5 weeks). One must also keep in mind that pelvic radiation is associated with transient lymphopenia and depressed T-cell function, which may lead to further immunological compromise in the HIV-positive patient, and anecdotal reports of poor tolerance and increased morbidity from pelvic radiation therapy have been reported, although adequate studies have not yet been performed to evaluate this issue.

Chemotherapy should be used in cases of systemic disease (pulmonary or liver metastases) or recurrent disease after radiation failures in those patients not eligible for pelvic exenteration. However, recurrent cervical cancer in this setting is not considered curable with chemotherapy, and treatment is palliative. Regimens that incorporate drugs that are both active in cervical carcinoma and are relatively bone marrow-sparing should be used, with close monitoring of all hematological indices. Cisplatin (50–75 mg/m^2) is the drug of choice, and may be combined with bleomycin (20 U/m^2, maximum 30 U) and vincristine (1 mg/m^2). Recently, neoadjuvant chemotherapy has been employed in patients with stage IB2 or stage II cervical cancer with similar agents, followed by radical hysterectomy, with good results; however, the efficacy of this approach in HIV-positive patients is unknown.

Other novel therapeutic approaches, such as the use of interferons, retinoids, bone marrow support, or vaccine therapy, may represent future investigative treatment options. The Gynecology Oncology Group is presently evaluating the role of interferon alpha and isotretinoin, with or without antiretroviral therapy, in the neoadjuvant or advanced or recurrent setting in the treatment of HIV-infected women with cervical cancer. Innovative treatment regimens and research protocols such as these are needed to combat the interaction of these two potentially life-threatening disease processes.

Lastly, the treatment of HIV and its sequelae with anti-HIV-1 agents and prophylactic regimens is exceedingly complex and always changing. Combination therapy with nucleoside analogues and protease inhibitors is now standard and is initiated earlier in the course of HIV disease. Careful attention to overlapping side effects of these regimens when co-utilized with oncological therapy for cervical cancer, as well as potential synergistic antineoplastic effects will be an important area of future investigation.

VI. LOWER GENITAL TRACT NEOPLASIA

The female lower genital field is particularly susceptible to malignant change, possibly because its squamous epithelial tissues have a common embryonic origin and may share a common susceptibility to certain carcinogens. It is probable that, as in other immunodeficient subgroups, the immunodeficiency resulting from HIV infection allows an oncogenic virus to flourish, and inhibits the body's natural immunological defense mechanisms that suppress the development of neoplasia. The concept of the "lower genital tract field" in the female as an organ system including the cervix, vagina, vulva, perianal, and anal regions sharing a carcinogenic risk was first developed in the 1950s. Green et al. (45) noted multiple cancers in 13% of vulvar cancer patients, and Day (46) considered the possibility of a widely spread predisposition of the cervical, vaginal, and vulvar epithelium to squamous carcinoma. Numerous authors have since demonstrated the tendency of such patients to develop multicentric cancers in a "previously sensitized" lower genital field. The cervix is most often the initial site of neoplasia, and is part of the syndrome in almost all cases. It is probable that the cervix is the most common site of neoplasia because the more active metabolism of the metaplastic epithelium in the transformation zone makes the cervical epithelium more likely to incorporate viral or other carcinogenic material. Early carcinogenic initiation may be activated by the increased rate of squamous metaplasia in the teenage years, with cervical neoplasia manifested at a younger age than the neoplasia at other sites. Ostergard and Morton (47) reviewed patients with multiple lower genital primary carcinomas and found the initial neoplasm was cervical in 91%, whereas only 2% of patients had vulvar and vaginal neoplasia without cervical neoplasia. Silman et al. (48) summarized subsequent reports concerning the anogenital neoplastic syndrome, and found that 33% of patients with vaginal neoplasia and 73% of patients with vulvar neoplasia had involvement of other genital sites.

Although the vagina is the least frequent location for lower genital tract neoplasia, it is unusual in a nonhysterectomized patient for the vaginal epithelium to undergo neoplastic transformation without concomitant cervical involvement. Most lesions regress after initial treatment, but lesions may progress to invasion and careful monitoring is required. Vulvar neoplasia is the second most common anogenital site, particularly in immunosuppressed patients of all types. Penn (1), from data collected by the Cincinnati Transplant Registry, found a 100-fold increase in the incidence of carcinoma of the vulva and anus in transplant recipients, compared with the general population. Such neoplasms occurred later posttransplantation (mean 88 months), compared with an average of 56 months for all other posttransplant malignancies. Interestingly, female graft recipients are much more susceptible to external genital and anal cancers than the male. Neoplasia of the vulva has most recently been described in women infected with HIV. Korn et al. (49) found 29% of patients with vulvar intraepithelial neoplasia (VIN) reviewed over a 4-year period were infected with HIV, and relative risk of recurrence of persistence of VIN in HIV-infected women was 3.3. Cases of invasive squamous cell carcinoma of the vulva have also been described, particularly in patients diagnosed and adequately treated for preinvasive disease (50). Lastly, anal involvement by the neoplastic process may go unrecognized in women because of inadequate evaluation. Williams et al. (51) found 14% of 114 HIV-infected women had anal epithelial abnormalities in general, and 44% of those with abnormal cervical cytology also had abnormal anal cytology.

REFERENCES

1. I Penn. Cancers of the anogenital region in renal transplant recipients. Cancer 58: 611, 1986.
2. KU Petry, D Scheffel, U Bode. Cellular immunodeficiency enhances the progression of human papillomavirus-associated cervical lesions. Int J Cancer 57:836–840, 1994.
3. R Matorras, JM Ariceta, A Rementeria, J Corral, G Gutierrez de Teran, J. Diez, F Montoya, FJ Rodriguez-Escudero. Human immunodeficiency virus-induced immunosuppression: a risk factor for human papillomavirus infection. Am J Obstet Gynecol 164:42–44, 1991.
4. M Maiman, RG Fruchter, E Serur, JC Remy, G Feuer, JG Boyce. Human immunodeficiency virus and cervical neoplasia. Gynecol Oncol 38:377–382, 1990.
5. J TerMeulen, HC Eberhardt, J Luande, HN Mgaya, J Chang-Claude, H Mtiro, M Mhina, P Kashaua, S Ocker, YG Meinhardt, L Gissmann, M Pawlita. Human papillomavirus (HPV) infection, HIV infection and cervical cancer in Tanzania, East Africa. Int J Cancer 51:515–521, 1992.
6. M Laga, JP Icenogle, R Marsella, AT Manoka, N Nzila, RW Ryder. Genital papillomavirus infection and cervical dysplasia—opportunistic complications of HIV infection. Int J Cancer 50:45–48, 1992.
7. GJ Van Doornum, JA Van den Hoek, EJ Van Ameijden. Cervical HPV infection among HIV-infected prostitutes addicted to hard drugs. J Med Virol 41:185–190, 1993.
8. XW Sun, TV Ellerbrock, O Lungu, MA Chiasson, TJ Bush, TC Wright. Human papillomavirus infection in human immunodeficiency virus-seropositive women. Obstet Gynecol 85:680–686, 1995.
9. M Maiman, RG Fruchter, A Sedlis, J Feldman, P Chen, RD Burk, H Minkoff. Prevalence, risk factors and accuracy of cytologic screening for cervical intraepithelial

neoplasia in women with the human immunodeficiency virus. Gynecol Oncol 68: 233–239, 1998.

10. J Johnson, A Burnett, G Willet, MA Young, J Doniger. High frequency of latent and clinical human papillomavirus cervical infections in immunocompromised human immunodeficiency virus-infected women. Obstet Gynecol 79:321–327, 1992.

11. SD Vernon, WC Reeves, KA Clancy, M Laga, M St Louis, HE Gary Jr, RW Ryder, AT Manoka, JP Icenogle. A longitudinal study of human papillomavirus DNA detection in human immunodeficiency virus. J Infect Dis 169:1108–1112, 1994.

12. A Spinillo, P Tenti, R Zappatore, F De Seta, E Silini, S Guaschino. Langerhans cell counts and cervical intraepithelial neoplasia in women with human immunodeficiency virus infection. Gynecol Oncol 48:210–213, 1993.

13. SD Vernon, CE Hart, WC Reeves, JP Icenogle. The HIV-1 Tat protein enhances E2-dependent human papillomavirus 16 transcription. Virus Res 27:133–145, 1993.

14. ML Tornesello, FM Buonaguro, E Beth-Giraldo, G Giraldo. Human immunodeficiency virus *tp 1 tat* gene enhances human papillomavirus early gene expression. Intervirology 36:57–64, 1993.

15. D Provencher, S Valme, HE Averette, P Ganjei, D Donato, M Penalver, BU Sevin. HIV status and positive Papanicolaou screening: identification of a high risk population. Gynecol Oncol 31:184–190, 1988.

16. LK Schrager, GH Friedland, D Maude. Cervical and vaginal squamous cell abnormalities in women infected with the human immunodeficiency virus. J Acquir Immune Defic Syndr 2:570–575, 1990.

17. C Marte, P Kelly, M Cohen, RG Fruchter, A Sedlis, L Gallo, V Ray, CA Webber. Papanicolaou smear abnormalities in ambulatory care sites for women infected with the human immunodeficiency virus. Am J Obstet Gynecol 166:1232–1237, 1992.

18. AR Feingold, SH Vermund, KF Kelley, LK Schreiber, G Munk, GH Friedland, RS Klein. Cervical cytological abnormalities and papillomavirus in women infected with HIV. J Acquir Immune Defic Syndr 3:896–903, 1990.

19. JR Smith, VS Kitchen, M Bothcherby, M Hepburn, C Wells, D Gor, SM Forster, JRW Harris, P Steer, P Mason. Is HIV infection associated with an increase in the prevalence of cervical neoplasia? Br J Obstet Gynaecol 100:149–153, 1993.

20. M Maiman, N Tarricone, J Viera, J Suarez, E Serur, JG Boyce. Colposcopic evaluation of human immunodeficiency virus-seropositive women. Obstet Gynecol 78:84–88, 1991.

21. PD Kell, PM Shah, SE Barton. Colposcopic screening of HIV seropositive women—help or hindrance? Int Conf AIDS 8:B96, 1992.

22. MJ Fink, RG Fruchter, M Maiman, P Kelly, A Sedlis, Weber CA, P Chen. The adequacy of cytology and colposcopy in diagnosing cervical neoplasia in HIV-seropositive women. Gynecol Oncol 55:133–137, 1994.

23. G Del Priore, J Lurain. The value of cervical cytology in HIV positive women. Gynecol Oncol 56:395–398, 1995.

24. A Korn, M Autry, P DeRemer. Sensitivity of the Papanicolaou smear in human immunodeficiency virus-infected women. Obstet Gynecol 83:401–404, 1994.

25. RG Fruchter, M Maiman, FH Silman, L Camilien, CA Webber, DS Kim. Characteristics of cervical intraepithelial neoplasia in women infected with the human immunodeficiency virus. Am J Obstet Gynecol 171:531–537, 1994.

26. MI Alloub, BBB Barr, KM McLaren, IW Smith, MH Bunney, GE Smart. Human papillomavirus infection and cervical intraepithelial neoplasia in women with renal allografts. Br Med J 298:153–156, 1989.
27. A Adachi, I Fleming, RD Burk, GY Ho, RS Klein. Women with human immunodeficiency virus infection and abnormal Papanicolaou smears: a prospective study of colposcopy and clinical outcome. Obstet Gynecol 81:372–377, 1993.
28. M Maiman, RG Fruchter, E Serur, JG Boyce. Prevalence of human immunodeficiency virus in a colposcopy clinic. JAMA 260:2214–2215, 1988.
29. M Spitzer, D Brennessel, VL Seltzer, L Silver, MS Lox. Is human papillomavirus-related disease an independent risk factor for human immunodeficiency virus infection? Gynecol Oncol 49:243–246, 1993.
30. M Maiman, RG Fruchter, L Guy, S Cuthill, P Levine, E Serur. Human immunodeficiency virus infection and invasive carcinoma. Cancer 71:402–406, 1993.
31. M Conti. Prevalence and risk of progression of genital intraepithelial neoplasia in women with human immunodeficiency virus infection. Adv Gynecol Obstet Res 3: 283–287, 1991.
32. A Schafer, W Friedmann, M Mielke, B Schwartlander, MA Koch. The increased frequency of cervical dysplasia–neoplasia in women infected with the human immunodeficiency virus is related to the degree of immunosuppression. Am J Obstet Gynecol 164:593–599, 1991.
33. TC Wright, TV Ellerbrock, MA Chiasson, N Van Devanter, XW Sun, New York Cervical Disease Study. Cervical intraepithelial neoplasia in women infected with the human immunodeficiency virus: prevalence, risk factors and validity of Papanicolaou smears. Obstet Gynecol 84:591–597, 1994.
34. G Del Priore, PR Gilmore, T Maag, DP Warshal, TH Cheon. Colposcopic biopsies versus loop electrosurgical excision procedure cone histology in human immunodeficiency virus-positive women. J Reprod Med 41:653–657, 1996.
35. M Maiman, RG Fruchter, E Serur, PL Levine, C Arrastia, A Sedlis. Recurrent cervical intraepithelial neoplasia in human immunodeficiency virus-seropositive women. Obstet Gynecol 82:170–174, 1993.
36. T Wright, J Koulos, F Schnoll, J Swanback, TV Ellerbrock, MA Chiasson, RM Richart. Cervical intraepithelial neoplasia in women infected with the human immunodeficiency virus: outcome after loop electrosurgical excision. Gynecol Oncol 55: 253–258, 1994.
37. RG Fruchter, M Maiman, A Sedlis, L Bartley, L Camilien, CD Arrastia. Multiple recurrences of cervical intraepithelial neoplasia in women with human immunodeficiency virus. Obstet Gynecol 87:338–344, 1996.
38. S Cuthill, M Maiman, RG Fruchter, I Lopatinsky, CC Cheng. Complications after treatment of cervical intraepithelial neoplasia in women infected with the human immunodeficiency virus. Reprod Med 40:823–828, 1995.
39. HB Krebs. Prophylactic topical 5-fluorouracil following treatment of human papillomavirus-associated lesions of the vulva and vagina. Obstet Gynecol 68:837, 1986.
40. MR Klevens, PL Fleming, MA Mays, R Frey. Characteristics of women with AIDS and invasive cancer. Obstet Gynecol 88:169–173, 1996.
41. M Maiman, RG Fruchter, M Clark, CD Arrastia, R Matthews, EJ Gates. Cervical cancer as an AIDS-defining illness. Obstet Gynecol 89:76–80, 1997.

42. GS Singh, JK Aikins, R Deger, S King, JJ Mikuta. Case report on metastatic cervical cancer and pelvic inflammatory disease in the AIDS patient. Gynecol Oncol 54: 372–376, 1994.

43. LB Schwartz, ML Carcangiu, L Bradham, PE Schwartz. Rapidly progressive squamous cell carcinoma of the cervix coexisting with human immunodeficiency virus infection: clinical opinion. Gynecol Oncol 41:255–258, 1991.

44. MA Relliman, DP Dooley, TW Burke, ME Berkland, RN Longfield. Rapidly progressing cervical cancer in a patient with human immunodeficiency virus infection. Gynecol Oncol 36:435–438, 1990.

45. TH Green Jr, H Ulfelder, JV Meigs. Epidermoid carcinoma of the vulva. Am J Obstet Gynecol 75:834, 1958.

46. JC Day. The second primary malignant tumor in gynecology—a review of the literature and a series presentation. Am J Obstet Gynecol 75:976, 1958.

47. DR Ostergard, DG Morton. Multifocal carcinoma of the female genitals. Am J Obstet Gynecol 99:1006, 1967.

48. FH Sillman, A Sedlis, JG Boyce. A review of lower genital intraepithelial neoplasia and the use of topical 5-fluorouracil. Obstet Gynecol Surv 40:190, 1985.

49. AP Korn, PD Abercrombie, A Foster. Vulvar intraepithelial neoplasia in women infected with human immunodeficiency virus-1. Gynecol Oncol 61:384–386, 1996.

50. TC Wright, JP Koulos, P Liu, XW Sun. Invasive vulvar carcinoma in two women infected with human immunodeficiency virus. Gynecol Oncol 60:500–503, 1996.

51. AB Williams, TM Darragh, K Vranizan, C Ochia, AR Moss, JM Palefsky. Anal and cervical human papillomavirus infection and risk of anal and cervical epithelial abnormalities in human immunodeficiency virus-infected women. Obstet Gynecol 83:205–211, 1994.

8

Cytokines, Viruses, Angiogenesis
New Therapies for Kaposi's Sarcoma

Steven A. Miles
University of California, Los Angeles, Los Angeles, California

I. CYTOKINES, VIRUSES, AND ANGIOGENESIS

Kaposi's sarcoma (KS) is by far the most common malignancy that affects patients with human immunodeficiency virus (HIV) infection (1). The risk for Kaposi's sarcoma in persons with HIV infection is approximately 13,000 times the risk for non–HIV-infected persons and can occur at any stage of HIV infection (1–4). The complex biology of this tumor has challenged many scientists over the years. Yet recent advances in molecular virology and a better understanding of cytokine regulation gives rise to hope that therapeutic breakthroughs are imminent. These studies suggest that Kaposi's sarcoma is the end result of a complicated interplay of cytokines, viruses, angiogenesis, and human genetics. Understanding these elaborate interactions will be the key to improving therapy for this cancer.

A. Multiple Cytokines Are Implicated in HIV-Associated Kaposi's Sarcoma

The development of techniques for the isolation, characterization, and long-term growth of cells derived from Kaposi's sarcoma lesions make possible the study of cytokines and other growth factors that may be involved in the development and progression of Kaposi's sarcoma (5–10). Initial studies identified cytokines in the supernatants from retrovirus-infected T cells as being important in the long-term maintenance of these cells and culture. Several groups identified various growth factors in these supernatants as either autocrine or paracrine growth factors. These factors include interleukin-6 (IL-6), interleukin-1β (IL-1), tumor necrosis factor alpha (TNF-α), basic fibroblast growth factor (bFGF), and vascular endothelial cell growth factor (VEGF; 8,11–21). Manipulation of the level of these cytokines or their function with oligonucleotides, soluble receptors, or neutralizing antibodies inhibits growth.

1. Interleukin-6

Many of the mechanisms that control proliferation of Kaposi's sarcoma-derived cells in culture are similar for different cytokines. For example, IL-6 is an autocrine growth factor for Kaposi's sarcoma (12). Several inhibitors of IL-6 expression or function, including IL-6 antisense oligonucleotides, soluble receptors, and retinoids, interfere with the growth of Kaposi's sarcoma cells in vitro (12,22–25). Monoclonal antibodies that neutralize IL-6 as well as soluble IL-6 gp130 receptor molecules inhibit the proliferation of Kaposi's sarcoma cells (26,27). To a large extent adding exogenous IL-6 reverses this inhibition. Dexamethasone, a potent glucocorticoid, synergistically enhances gp130 receptor-mediated growth of Kaposi's cells. Anti–IL-6 gp130 antibodies or the glucocorticoid antagonist mifepristone (RU 486) abolishes this synergistic effect. Dexamethasone has additive but not synergistic effect on the stimulation of KS cells by IL-1β or TNF-α, the signals of which are not mediated through IL-6 gp130 receptor subunits (26,28,29). Stimulation of KS cells with soluble IL-6 receptor α-chain, IL-6, or oncostatin-M induces rapid phosphorylation of the transcription factor STAT3 (26,30,31). Dexamethasone enhances the accumulation of phosphorylated STAT3 that has increased DNA-binding activity. In vitro studies show similar results for IL-1 and TNF-α. Soluble cytokine receptor antagonists, neutralizing antibodies, or chemicals that decrease expression of these cytokines inhibit proliferation of the KS cells.

2. Basic Fibroblast Growth Factor

Recent work has suggested a more prominent role for bFGF in control and regulation of KS growth. Basic fibroblast growth factor, one of many cytokines in the supernatants from retrovirus-infected T cells, induces the expression of integrin receptors on the surface of endothelial cells as well as KS cells (19,20). Induction of integrin receptors facilitates the attachment of HIV *tat* to the surface of endothelial cells (20,32–34). HIV *tat* is bound to cells, where it increases proliferation. HIV *tat* acts as both a cell-attachment factor and a direct mitogen (14,19,35–40). In animal models, bFGF and HIV *tat* are synergistic as mitogens (19). Phosphorothioate antisense oligonucleotides directed against bFGF mRNA inhibit both the growth of AIDS KS-derived cells and the angiogenic activity associated with these cells.

3. Vascular Endothelial Cell Factor

Vascular endothelial cell growth factor is another potent angiogenic factor for AIDS KS-derived spindle cells and a potential target for therapy (21). Supernatants from AIDS KS cells are rich in VEGF and a combination of anti-VEGF and anti-bFGF antibodies completely inhibit the endothelial cell growth-promoting activities of AIDS KS cells. VEGF is an autocrine growth factor for AIDS KS cells, and cells express high levels of both Flt-1 and KDR (41), the receptors for VEGF. VEGF antisense oligonucleotides block VEGF mRNA and protein production, inhibiting KS cell growth in a dose-dependent manner (21).

4. Alterations of Cytokines In Vivo

Biopsies of KS lesions demonstrate large amounts of IL-6 as well as IL-6 gp130 receptor subunits. The α-chain of the IL-6 receptor is generally not expressed. There is strong expression of platelet-derived growth factor (PDGF) as well as platelet-derived growth factor receptors (PDGFRs). There is little oncostatin-M in most KS lesions, despite its potent growth activity in vitro (16). Abnormalities of FGF and FGF receptor expression are also seen (42–44). Basic fibroblast growth factor is largely expressed in basal and super-basal keratinocytes as well as around endothelial cells in KS lesions. Spindle cells express Flt-1 and KDR, the receptors for VEGF, whereas there is little expression in adjacent normal skin (41). There is conflicting data on the amounts of VEGF mRNA and protein present in spindle cells in vivo. Nonetheless, the in vivo studies of cytokine receptor expression largely mirror the in vitro findings (45).

Interleukin-6 along with TNF-α are two of several interleukins that are perturbed in patients with HIV infection (46,47). Case-controlled studies demonstrate that patients with Kaposi's sarcoma have elevated levels of IL-6 relative to CD4 cell number-, age-, and sex-matched controls (48,49). Moreover, this elevation in IL-6 is seen on the visit before the development of clinical disease, suggesting that IL-6 is a precipitating cause and not a result of the development of KS. In a larger, nested case–control study, IL-6 more closely correlated with the development of opportunistic infections than with KS (47). However, there is a close interaction between opportunistic infection and the development of KS. Thus it is difficult to determine whether elevated IL-6 levels are the result of opportunistic infections or KS. There is no correlation between oncostatin-M levels and KS.

B. Viruses and Kaposi's Sarcoma: The Roles of HIV and KSHV

Although HIV does not directly cause KS, HIV infection alters the natural history of this malignancy (50,51). HIV results in profound immune suppression with loss of CD4 cells and impairment of residual CD4 cell function (52). This decreases immune surveillance and can facilitate the development of KS. Multiple cytokines, including IL-1β, TNF-α, and IL-6, are perturbed as a result of HIV infection and increase with the advancement of HIV disease (52,53). In vitro these increase the rate of growth of KS-derived cells (54). The concept that HIV infection directly perturbs the expression of multiple cytokines, which in turn, alter the rate of growth of KS, is sound.

Finally, proteins derived from HIV, specifically the HIV *tat* protein, are direct mitogens for KS-derived cells (35,37). Two groups have demonstrated that the proliferation of KS cells is increased by exposure to either recombinant HIV *tat* protein or HIV DNA vectors expressing HIV *tat* proteins (37,55). Moreover these effects appear to be specific and limited to AIDS KS-derived cells.

Tat acts extracellularly by two different mechanisms. It binds directly to the $\alpha_5\beta_1$ (fibronectin) and $\alpha_v\beta_3$ (vitronectin) integrin receptors acting as an attachment factor for progenitor cells (56). Separately, the basic domain of *tat* facilitates cellular uptake (39). *Tat* then directly transactivates the IL-6 promoter causing an increase in IL-6 expression (57). Thus, there is a cooperative interaction between *tat* (37), inflammatory cytokines (34), and bFGF (19) that leads to KS cell growth. In nude mice, the injection of *tat* with bFGF results in synergistic production of KS-like lesions (19). The complex effects of the inflammatory cytokines such as bFGF and the *tat* protein of HIV results in angiogenesis that can be partly inhibited in animal models by the tissue inhibitor of metalloproteases-2 (TIMP-2; 58). Thus, HIV infection, either directly or indirectly, can increase both the incidence of KS as well as modulate its growth during HIV-related disease.

C.   KSHV:A Novel Gammaherpesvirus Linked to KS

The identification in 1994 by Moore and colleagues of a novel human herpesvirus (HHV) as a potential etiologic agent of KS is a major turning point in our understanding of the disease's biology (59). By using representational difference analyses and polymerase chain reaction (PCR) techniques, Chang and colleagues identified sequences of a novel human herpesvirus in 27 of 29 KS lesions. In addition, 3 of 12 primary extranodal lymphomas (PEL) also contained herpesvirus-related sequences. They identified several poorly characterized lymphadenopathies, such as angioimmunoblastic lymphoproliferative disease (AILD) and Castleman's disease with KS herpesvirus sequences.

Subsequent studies now strongly suggest that KSHV is intricately involved in the pathogenesis of KS (60–66). Published studies report finding KSHV DNA sequences in nearly all KS lesions, the peripheral blood lymphocytes (67) of most patients with KS, but less frequently in the lymphocytes of HIV-infected hemophilia patients or those without KS. In addition, patients with KS develop antibodies to both latent (68) and lytic KSHV antigens (69–71) before the development of clinical disease. KSHV antibodies are readily detectable in most individuals with KSHV-related malignancies (72). A comparative trial of current KSHV serological assays demonstrated that it is possible with some assays, in particular ORF65 enzyme-linked immunosorbent assay (ELISA) and BCP-1 immunofluorecence assays, to detect KSHV infection in most patients with KS (72).

In vitro studies using either KSHV reactivation from latent cells (73) or transmission to primary dermal microvascular cells (74) demonstrate that foscarnet, ganciclovir, PMEA, and lobucavir are potent inhibitors of KSHV infection and reactivation. Acyclovir and penciclovir have no activity (74). These findings are important because they link observations about the ability of certain antivirals to inhibit KSHV with their ability to decrease the incidence of KS in HIV-infected patients (75–77).

For example, three published retrospective studies demonstrate that there may be a reduction in KS in HIV-infected patients treated with either foscarnet, or ganciclovir. Jones et al. (78) retrospectively reviewed patients with HIV infection and found that patients who received foscarnet or ganciclovir had a reduced relative risk of KS compared with individuals who did not receive these medications. Glesby et al. (75) reviewed 935 men in the Multicenter AIDS Cohort Study (MACS). Although not statistically significant, they found the relative risk for development of KS over the observation period was reduced 46% in men with CMV disease who received ganciclovir (relative risk [RR], 0.56; 95% CI, 0.22–1.44; $p = 0.23$) and 60% (RR, 0.40; 95% CI, 0.051–3.10; $p = 0.38$) in men who received foscarnet (75). A third retrospective study (79) showed a risk reduction of 61% in 3688 patients with HIV infection who had received foscarnet (RH, 0.38; 95% CI, 0.15–0.95; $p = 0.038$) and 61% (RH, 0.39; 95% CI, 0.19–0.84; $p = 0.015$) in patients who had received ganciclovir. There was no reduction in incidence in patients who received acyclovir (RH, 1.10; 95% CI, 0.88–1.38; $P = 0.40$). Thus, the in vitro activity of antiherpes medications against KSHV may mirror their clinical usefulness in preventing the development of KS (74). Given new assays to detect KSHV exposure (72), the in vitro studies suggest the exciting possibility of providing once-daily oral prophylaxis with a medication, such as lobucavir (74) to those HIV-infected patients at highest risk for developing KS. However, prospective, controlled studies will be required to determine the actual ability of these drugs to prevent KS.

The complete sequencing of KSHV (80,81) led to the identification of several genes that are homologous with human cytokines or cytokine receptors. These include IL-6 (82), macrophage inhibitory proteins (MIP) 1α and 1β (82), the IL-8 receptor, and the interferon (IFN) response factor. Viral IL-6 is functional and can substitute for human IL-6 in supporting the growth of human IL-6–dependent cell lines (80). The viral MIP-1α and β are also functional. In addition to binding and interfering with the CCR5 receptor, the viral MIP-1α is a potent inhibitor of HIV entry. In animal studies, the KSHV viral MIP-1α, and to a lesser extent the viral MIP-1β, induces angiogenesis in the chorioallantoic membrane assay (83). The angiogenesis is nearly equal to that seen with other angiogenesis factors such as VEGF. Human MIP-1α does not induce angiogenesis in this assay. The human IL-8 receptor homologue is active (84) and increases cell proliferation. Both the IL-8 receptor homologue and the viral interferon-related factor transform NIH 3T3 cells and induce angiogenic tumors in nude mice (85–87). The identification of viral homologues of several human cytokines and their potential to cause angiogenesis in animal studies leads to the possibility that there may be a direct relation between human cytokines, human viruses, and angiogenesis.

There may be a spectrum of KSHV disease, ranging from pure angiogenesis (KS) to B-cell proliferation (multiple myeloma; 88,89). There may be stops along the way where angiogenesis is mixed with B-cell proliferation to varying degrees and accompanied by immunoglobin abnormalities. These intermediate steps could include Castleman's disease and AILD. This spectrum of disease could be mirrored in the spectrum of cytokine abnormalities observed. The severity of immune deficiency, the presence of other opportunistic infections, and the acquisition of chromosomal abnormalities further influence the clinical manifestations.

Preliminary data from our laboratory suggest that there may be differential induction of human cytokines in different target cells. It appears that human IL-6 and IL-8 are induced in endothelial cells, whereas other human cytokines may be induced in other target cells. These findings are important for several reasons. For the first time, it links the virus that may cause KS with cytokines that have been implicated in the pathogenesis of the disease. Second, it demonstrates that KSHV could increase local effective IL-6 concentrations through two mechanisms: production of viral IL-6 or induction of human IL-6. Third, it provides a link between major cytokines involved in neoangiogenesis (bFGF and VEGF), cytokines involved in B-cell proliferation (IL-6) and infection with KSHV.

D. Angiogenesis: A New Model of KS Pathogenesis

Together these findings place KS in a more traditional model for the development of malignancy. In this model, infection of target mesenchymal progenitor cells with KSHV would alter cytokines and cytokine receptor expression, including the production of viral cytokines and receptors during the lytic cycle. These cytokines would stimulate the replication of surrounding cells, some of which may be infected with KSHV. These same cytokines are also perturbed in HIV infection and could increase integrin receptor expression (83) on the surface of target cells. Depending on the type of infected cell, there may be induction of human cytokines that would result in further growth of the angioblastic lesion. At this point, these proliferating cells are oligoclonal. Whether they disseminate through the bloodstream is unknown. Together with the cytokine perturbations associated with HIV (53), the production of HIV *tat* protein (19,35,39,40), and the lack of effective immune surveillance (52), the risk of KS would increase dramatically. With time, some of these oligoclonal cells would acquire secondary mutations that would result in the repression of apoptosis and clonal expansion. This clonal expansion is recognized as malignant KS (90,91).

Several lines of evidence suggest that neoangiogenesis is a major part of KS pathogenesis. First, the lesion is angioblastic and bears all the hallmarks of neoangiogenesis, including the production of collagenase type IV (gelatinase) and stromelysin metalloproteases, and the digestion of the normal extravascular basement membrane. The lesions stain with markers, such as both α_5 and α_v integrin receptor subunits and intracellular adhesion molecule (ICAM)-1 suggesting a possible role for inflammatory cytokines in spindle cell formation. The spindle cell compartment is rich in collagen, laminin, fibronectin, and tenascin, suggesting an important reactive component in the evolution of KS (92). The lack of thrombospondin expression in the spindle cells favors the contention that they could be transitional, proliferating cells of endothelial origin. c-*ets-1*, A proto-oncogene that is a transcription factor expressed in endothelial cells during tumor vascularization and other forms of angiogenesis in humans is found in KS lesions (93). c-*ets* protein activates transcription through a PEA3 motif that plays a role in the stimulation of transcription of urokinase-type plasminogen-activator (u-PA), stromelysin, and collagenase genes. These gene products have all been detected in KS lesions. TNF-α, a cytokines increased early in HIV infection and increased at times of opportunistic infections (53) increases transiently the amount of both c-*ets-1* and u-PA mRNA in confluent human umbilical vein endothelial cells. This provides a model for interaction between the immune response to HIV and opportunistic infections, induction of matrix-degrading proteases, and endothelial cell proliferation.

In vitro AIDS KS–cell-conditioned medium induces endothelial cells to form invasive clusters in addition to tubes. KS–cell-conditioned medium, when placed in the lower compartment of a Boyden chamber, stimulates the migration of human vascular endothelial cells across filters coated with either small amounts of collagen IV (chemotaxis) or a Matrigel barrier (invasion; 5). Antibodies to bFGF inhibit but do not prevent, the invasive activity induced by the AIDS KS–cell-conditioned medium (94). However, specific inhibitors of laminin and collagenase IV action block the invasiveness of the AIDS KS–cell-activated endothelial cells. Finally, TIMP-2 and a synthetic peptide from the metalloprotease MMP-2 propeptide region (peptide 74), inhibits endothelial cell invasion induced by AIDS KS cell supernatants (95). Smooth muscle cells are much less sensitive to these inhibitors. Therapy that is directed at selected angiogenesis targets, such as integrin receptor expression, metalloprotinase inhibition, cytokine propeptide proteolysis, and neutralization of bFGF, might be successful in the treatment of KS.

II. Implications for Therapeutic Intervention

To a certain extent, there are now too many therapeutic opportunities for clinical investigation to adequately evaluate them all. Based on our understanding of the pathogenesis, the most promising areas are interventions in cytokine expression, function, or response; inhibition of virus replication or enhancement of KSHV, and HIV-specific immunity; and inhibition of neoangiogenesis. For each target, there are three general sites for interfering with biological processes.

Site	Mechanism	Example
Production	Inhibit gene expression	9-*cis*-Retinoic acid
Processing	Inhibit proteolysis or glycosylation	Interleukin-1—converting enzyme inhibitors
Function	Neutralize activity of secreted or expressed product	Neutralizing antibodies or soluble (decoy) receptors

As noted in Table 1, initial trials of therapeutic agents are planned or are underway in many of these areas.

A. Interleukin-6

The area that has been best-explored is therapeutic agents that interfere with cytokine expression or function. Interleukin-4, a cytokine that inhibits IL-6 expression in circulating monocytes, was studied in a phase I–II trial (96). In patients with limited disease, IL-4 caused headaches, fever, and myalgias. Mild abnormalities of hepatic enzymes and blood counts were seen. There was no evidence of HIV stimulation. Unfortunately, there was also limited clinical activity. There were no changes in C-reactive protein levels, IL-6 levels, or those of serum albumin. These observations suggest that IL-4, at the doses studied, was ineffective in inhibiting IL-6 production.

In a trial with a neutralizing anti–IL-6 monoclonal antibody (97), transient stabilization of KS was noted. There was no significant change in HIV replication or immune parameters. In a companion trial for lymphomas, the monoclonal

Table 1 Possible Agents for Treatment of KS

Therapeutic target	Agent	Route of administration	Proposed mechanism of action	Clinical results	Stage of development
Cytokines					
Interleukin-6	Interleukin-4 (96)	Subcutaneous	Inhibition of synthesis	No activity to date	Phase I/II
	Soluble gp130	Subcutaneous	Neutralization	N/A	Preclinical
	Neutralizing IL-6 MAb (97)	Subcutaneous	Neutralization	Transient responses	Phase II
	All-*trans*-retinoic acid (23)	Oral or intravenous (liposomal)	Inhibits production	UP to ~25–30% in selected populations	Phase II
	9-*cis*-Retinoic acid (98)	Topical or oral	Inhibits production	Up to ~30% topically	Phase II/III
Interleukin-1	Soluble receptor (99)	Subcutaneous	Neutralization of IL-1, decreases IL-6	N/A	Phase I
	Interleukin-1–converting enzyme inhibitors	Oral	Inhibits production, decreases IL-6.	N /A	Preclinical
TNF-α	Soluble receptor (100)	Subcutaneous	Binds and neutralizes TNF, decreases IL-6	Well-tolerated, unknown	Phase II
	Neutralizing TNF MAb (101)	Subcutaneous	Binds and neutralizes TNF decreases IL-6	Well-tolerated, weight gain, unknown effect on KS	Phase II
	Protease inhibitors	Oral	Inhibits production	N/A	Preclinical

Table 1 Continued

Therapeutic target	Agent	Route of administration	Proposed mechanism of action	Clinical results	Stage of development
	Thalidomide (103)	Oral	Unknown	Weight gain, decreases oral ulcers, induces durable response in some cases	Phase II
	Pentoxifylline (104)	Oral	Inhibits production	Decreased mRNA, weight gain, limited effect on KS	Phase II
	Marimastat	Oral	Inhibits production, also IL-1 and IL-6	N/A	Phase II
Basic fibroblast growth factor (bFGF)	Neutralizing bFGF MAb	Subcutaneous	Binds and neutralizes bFGF decreases HIV *tat* activity	N/A	Preclinical
Antivirals					
HIV	Highly active antiretroviral therapy	Oral	Inhibits HIV, improves immune function, decreases cytokines, inhibits HIV *tat*	May be related to decreases in KS incidence by up to 50% in short term	Approved for HIV, phase III/IV
KSHV	RGD peptides	Subcutaneous	Inhibits HIV *tat*	N/A	Pre-clinical
	Ganciclovir (75)	Intravenous or Oral	Inhibits DNA polymerase decreasing KSHV replication	Retrospectively decrease KS incidence ~50% in several studies	Phase III

Foscarnet (74,105)	Intravenous, intralesional	Inhibits DNA polymerase decreasing KSHV replication	Retrospectively decrease KS incidence ~50% in several studies; causes local necrosis	Phase II/III
Bis-POM PMEA (74,105)	Oral	Inhibits KSHV production	N/A	Preclinical
Angiogenesis				
TNP-470 (106)	Oral	Decreases endothelial proliferation	Stabilization of KS lesions	Phase II
SU5412	Oral	Inhibits VEGF production	N/A	Phase Ib
Endostatin (108)	Subcutaneous	Decreases endothelial proliferation	N/A	Preclinical
Angiostatin (109)	Subcutaneous	Decreases endothelial proliferation	N/A	Preclinical
Integrins				
Vitronectin receptor MAb (45)	Subcutaneous	Binds $\alpha_v\beta_3$ receptor	N/A	Preclinical
Interferons				
alfa (110)	Subcutaneous	Inhibits new vessel formation	30–40% durable, major responses	Approved
beta (111)	Subcutaneous	Inhibits new vessel formation	Limited activity in good-prognosis patients	Approved for multiple sclerosis
gamma (112)	Subcutaneous	Inhibits new vessel formation	Increased KS growth	Approved for chronic granulomatous disease

antibody completely abrogated the acute-phase reaction as demonstrated by the normalization of C-reactive protein and fibrinogen circulating levels (p = 0.013 and p = 0.008, respectively). It increased serum albumin concentration in patients with a low albumin level (p = 0.01). It decreased B-lymphocyte hyperactivity, as reflected by decreased IgG and IgA serum levels (p = 0.008 and p < 0.001, respectively), and by a decreased production of IgG in vitro (p = 0.017). In contrast, the IgM hyperproduction was not affected by the monoclonal antibody (109). Thus, unlike IL-4, neutralizing antibodies to IL-6 modulate IL-6 activity. Unfortunately, there were too few patients treated, and the treatment duration was too short to demonstrate whether this is a viable approach.

Another approach to inhibition of IL-6 has been the use of retinoids (98). Initially based on their ability to inhibit expression of the IL-6 receptor α-chain, more recent data suggests that they work by inhibiting the expression of IL-6 directly. Clinical trials of various topical retinoids, liposomal retinoids, and more recently, oral retinoids demonstrate response rates in the 25–45% range. Abnormalities of lipids and transient elevations of liver enzymes are seen. There is still insufficient information to determine if the proposed mechanism of action—that is, inhibition of IL-6—is the mechanism responsible for the clinical responses observed. Additional clinical trials with newer retinoids that target different retinoic acid receptors are planned in an attempt to improve the observed response rates.

B. Interleukin-1

There are multiple therapeutic agents available for inhibition of IL-1. These include IL-1–converting enzyme (ICE) protease inhibitors, soluble receptors, and neutralizing antibodies. These are largely the result of previous attempts to modulate the sepsis syndrome and various rheumatological conditions. A single clinical trial of soluble IL-1 receptors in patients with KS is ongoing (99). This agent is a fusion protein of the Fc fragment of human IgG with the IL-1 receptor. The fusion protein is well tolerated and has a long half-life. Results from this phase I–II trial are pending.

C. Tumor Necrosis Factor-α

Many therapeutic agents are available to inhibit various steps in TNF production and function. These include inhibitors of production, such as pentoxifylline, thalidomide, ketotifen, and marimastat. All of these agents are oral. Pentoxifylline, a phosphodiesterase inhibitor, has been studied in three clinical trials and one KS trial (104). High-dose pentoxifylline (2400 mg/day) in patients with AIDS decreased TNF mRNA by 34% (104). Pentoxifylline did not affect HIV levels nor did it alter zidovudine pharmacokinetics. The most common toxicity was gastrointestinal. In a trial in Ugandan patients with tuberculosis, pentoxifylline decreased plasma HIV RNA and serum β_2-microglobulin and, in a subset of moderately anemic patients, improved blood hemoglobin levels. Trends were noted toward reduced TNF-α production in vitro. No effect was noted on body mass, CD4 cell count, or survival. A third trial in patients with KS demonstrated that pentoxifylline was well tolerated, but had minimal activity (104). Taken together, these studies suggest that pentoxifylline, at tolerable doses, has limited ability to inhibit TNF and is an unlikely candidate for further clinical testing in HIV infection.

Another drug with a long history of clinical trials is thalidomide (102–103,117,118). Its use in AIDS patients is based on its ability to decrease the effects of TNF. In patients with HIV and esophageal ulcers (102), thalidomide at 300 mg/day caused complete clearance of ulcers in 11 of 12 patients with endoscopic clearance in 9 of 11 patients. In a randomized, double-blind, placebo-controlled clinical trial in HIV-associated wasting syndrome (118), thalidomide at 400 mg/+ day increased weight gain and increased the Karnofsky index (p = 0.003). Mild, transient somnolence and erythematous macular skin lesions were significantly more common in the thalidomide group. Immune cells and HIV viral burden in peripheral blood mononuclear cells (PBMCs) did not change in either group. Anecdotal reports of the clinical efficacy of thalidomide in patients with KS led to clinical trials that are ongoing (103). Of the oral agents, thalidomide appears to be the most active and reasonable candidate for further clinical drug development.

Ketotifen, an in vitro inhibitor of TNF-α release from PBMCs was studied in HIV-infected patients at 4 mg/day for 84 days, followed by an additional 70-day period (105). Ketotifen decreased TNF-α release from stimulated PBMCs significantly (68 versus 155 pg/mL), but did not change TNF-α or soluble TNF receptor plasma concentrations. Subjects gained weight (+ 2.7 kg), whereas weight loss was observed after cessation of treatment (−1.6 kg). Marimastat is one of several protease inhibitors in development that decrease in vitro production of TNF-α. Clinical trials of marimastat are underway in prostate and breast cancer. Trials in KS have been proposed.

Other approaches to inhibit TNF-α include the use of soluble receptors as cytokine decoys and neutralizing antibodies. Soluble TNF receptor, similar to soluble IL-1, is a fusion protein of the Fc portion of the γ-heavy chain of immunoglobulin together with either the type I or type II receptor α-chain. Whether there is any functional difference between the two agents is unknown. Soluble TNF receptor inhibits both TNF-α and TNF-β (lymphotoxin). Trials of these agents are complicated because there are readily detectable levels of both type I and type II soluble receptors in patients at various stages of HIV infection (99,100,119). In some instances this may be associated with impaired red blood cell production. Both agents are in clinical trials in a variety of settings in HIV-infected patients (99,100,119).

Several neutralizing antibodies to TNF are available for clinical study (100). Some of these antibodies have already been studied in other HIV settings. Inhibition of TNF-α by a chimeric, humanized monoclonal antibody, cA2, was investigated in six HIV-1–infected patients with CD4 cell counts of fewer than 200/mm^3 (100). Two consecutive infusions of 10 mg/kg, 14 days apart, were well tolerated, and a prolonged serum half-life for cA2 (mean, 257 $\pm$ 70 h) was demonstrated. Serum immunoreactive TNF-α concentrations fell from a mean prestudy value of 6.4 pg/mL (range, 4.2–7.9) to 1:1 pg/mL (range, 0.5–2.2) 24 h after the first infusion and returned to baseline within 7–14 days. A similar response was seen after the second infusion. No consistent changes in CD4 cell counts or plasma HIV RNA levels were observed over 42 days.

D. Basic-Fibroblast Growth-Factor and Vascular Endothelial Cell Growth Factor

Neutralizing antibodies to VEGF are available. Anti-VEGF antibodies block neo-angiogenesis in the chick chorioallantoic membrane assay. These antibodies also block new vessel formation in mouse models of mammary tumors (45). Human breast carcinomas, similar to KS, produce large amounts of VEGF. Preliminary phase I and phase II clinical studies looking at the tolerance and efficacy of neutralizing monoclonal antibodies to VEGF are underway in patients with breast carcinoma. Various groups have also proposed VEGF antisense oligonucleotides (21), liposomal VEGF oligonucleotides, and soluble VEGF receptors. These agents are all in preclinical development.

Basic FGF is another cytokine involved in neoangiogenesis (20,32–34). This factor signals in association with integrin receptor binding and can cooperate with HIV *tat* in the proliferation of KS cells in vitro (19). In nude mouse models, neutralizing antibodies to bFGF prevents Kaposi's sarcoma-like lesion development. In vitro anti-bFGF antibodies, coupled with anti-VEGF antibodies abrogates the neoangiogenesis induced by KS-derived cells (45). Thus, it is likely that anti-bFGF antibodies or soluble receptors will have clinical activity. These agents are now in preclinical development.

E. Integrin Receptor Inhibitors

Kaposi's sarcoma cells express both α_5 and α_v integrin receptor subunits. HIV *tat* can bind to $\alpha_v\beta_3$ integrin receptors (120), resulting in cellular attachment and proliferation of KS cells. A monoclonal antibody that blocks the maturation of blood vessels exists (121). Microinjection of this antibody, LM609, disrupted the normal pattern of vascular development in experimental embryos. LM609 blocks angiogenesis in similar studies in the chick chorioallantoic membrane assay (120).

The vitronectin receptor ($\alpha_v\beta_3$ integrin receptor) also colocalizes the matrix metalloprotease-2 to the surface of invasive cells (122). Thus, in addition to acting as a binding site for HIV *tat*, the vitronectin receptor can localize the major proteolytic enzyme necessary for extracellular matrix degradation and cellular invasion. This is important because TIMP-2 inhibitors inhibit the proliferation of KS cells (121). These observations suggest that $\alpha_v\beta_3$ blockade may be important in control of Kaposi's sarcoma cells. Clinical studies of LM609 in the treatment of patients with breast carcinoma are planned (121).

F. TNP-470

TNP-470 is a fumagillin derivative that blocks endothelial cell proliferation. TNP-470 binds methionine aminopeptidase (MetAP-2) and inhibits cyclin-dependent kinase 2 (cdk2; 122). This is its presumed mechanism of antiangiogensis. TNP-470 also potently inhibits DNA synthesis of smooth-muscle cells, and this inhibition is associated with decreased levels of cdk2 mRNA and activity (123,124). In vivo, TNP-470 inhibits a wide range of metastatic murine tumor models and is effective against hormone-independent breast carcinoma cell lines (125). TNP-470 synergizes with a range of cytotoxic chemotherapy agents, including cisplation and temazolamide (126). At doses of 4.6, 9.3, 15.4, 23.2, and 43.1 mg/m^2 over a 1-h infusion, TNP-470 displayed a linear relation between its dose and both area under the curve to infinity (AUC_{inf}) and time to maximum concentration (C_{max}; 126). The C_{max} ranged between 6.6 ng/mL at the lowest dose (4.6 mg/m^2) and 597.1 ng/mL at the highest dose (43.1 mg/m^2). The agent was rapidly cleared from the circulation, with a short terminal half-life (0.88 ± 2.5 h). Peak plasma concentrations of AGM-1883, an active metabolite, ranged between 0.4 and 158.1 ng/mL. There was considerable interpatient variability in the clearance, but no evidence of saturable elimination. Kaposi's sarcoma lesions showed some stabilization of growth at the highest concentrations studied (127).

G. Angiostatin and Endostatin

Angiostatin is an endogenous angiogenesis inhibitor that specifically blocks the growth of endothelial cells (128). Angiostatin is an internal fragment of plasminogen containing the first four kringle structures. Kringles 1 and 3 harbor the antiproliferative activity of angiostatin (129). Recombinant human angiostatin inhibits experimental primary and metastatic cancers, including Lewis lung carcinoma low-metastatic phenotype metastasis.

Endostatin is a novel angiogenesis inhibitor produced by a hemangioendothelioma (108,109). It is a small protein that results from the proteolysis of the carboxy-terminal fragment of collagen XVIII. Endostatin specifically inhibits endothelial cell proliferation and is a potent inhibitor of angiogenesis and tumor cell growth. In animals with primary tumors and metastatic lesions, the primary tumors regressed to dormant microscopic lesions and metastatic lesions involuted. Immunohistochemistry demonstrates blocked angiogenesis with persistent apoptosis in tumor cells (108). Endostatin is in preclinical studies, with clinical trials in patients with AIDS-related KS in the planning stages.

III. ANTIVIRAL THERAPY FOR KAPOSI'S SARCOMA

Clearly, HIV plays a role in the development of KS. Numerous clinical studies have demonstrated that the introduction of highly active antiretroviral therapy, including the novel protease inhibitors, results in a decreased rate of development of KS. Similar to the original zidovudine trials, spontaneous remission of KS in patients treated with potent protease inhibitor-containing regimens occurs. However, trials of protease inhibitors as treatment for KS have been largely ineffective (130).

The identification of KSHV has heralded a renewed focus on viral pathogens in the development of opportunistic malignancies. Antiherpes medications reduced the incidence of KS in three retrospecitve studies (75–78). Both foscarnet and ganciclovir appear to have preventative activity with a greater than 50% reduction in the odds ratio. Acyclovir, at doses used clinically, is ineffective (73,74).

Antiherpes medications are effective against KSHV in vitro. Antiherpes medications inhibit both latent virus induction with sodium butyrate or phorbol esters(73) and transmission to new cells (74). The most potent of these agents appears to be lobucavir. The retrospective analysis and in vitro data suggest that the use of antiherpes medications as prophylaxis for the development of KS should be successful. A variety of serological assays for the detection of KSHV infection are available. Although the sensitivity and specificity of these assays are unclear (74), they are sufficiently sensitive to warrant their use in screening populations who might be at risk for the development of KS. A clinical trial is planned for the use of oral, daily, antiherpes medicines for the prophylaxis of KS in patients with HIV infection who have antibodies to KSHV.

IV. CONCLUSIONS

A tremendous amount is known about the pathogenesis of KS, including the critical role of human and viral cytokines, human viruses, and neoangiogenesis. A large number of potential therapeutic drugs exist that inhibit various aspects of these pathogenic mechanisms. The main problem with the clinical trials is that the agents used are minimally active against their target cytokine, or there is inadequate enrollment of patients. We have clearly reached a watershed era in the treatment of patients with KS. The possibility exists in the next few years to provide relatively nontoxic, antiangiogenic agents for the treatment of existing KS. Moreover, with the availability of oral antiherpes prophylaxis medications, the possibility exists that we may be able to prevent the development of Kaposi's sarcoma.

REFERENCES

1. Biggar RJ, Rabkin CS. The epidemiology of AIDS-related neoplasms. Hematol Oncol Clin North Am 10:997–1010, 1996.
2. Biggar RJ, Curtis RE, Cote TR, Rabkin CS, Melbye M. Risk of other cancers following Kaposi's sarcoma: relation to acquired immunodeficiency syndrome. Am J Epidemiol 139:362–368, 1994.
3. Rabkin CS, Biggar RJ, Horm JW. Increasing incidence of cancers associated with the human immunodeficiency virus epidemic. Int J Cancer 47:692–696, 1991.
4. Rabkin CS, Blattner WA. HIV infection and cancers other than non–Hodgkin lymphoma and Kaposi's sarcoma. Cancer Surv 10:151–160, 1991.
5. Albini A, Nakamura S, Poggi L, Gallo RC, Salahuddin SZ, Thompson EW. Cultured AIDS-related Kaposi's sarcoma cells (AIDS-KS) produce activators of endothelial cell chemotaxis and invasiveness. Int Conf AIDS 7:118, 1991.
6. Biberfield P, Nakamura S, Salahuddin ZS, Ensoli B, Gallo RC. Characteristics of in vitro culture of KS-derived cells. Int Conf AIDS 5:1989.
7. Buonaguro FM, Giraldo G, Nakamura Y, Vecchione R, Alessi E, Finzi AF, Safai B, Mueller N, Hatzakis A, Owili DM. Genetic mechanisms in Kaposi's sarcoma pathogenesis. Int Conf AIDS 7:117, 1991.
8. Ensoli B, Nakamura S, Salahuddin SZ, Biberfeld P, Larsson L, Beaver B, Wong-Staal F, Gallo RC. AIDS-Kaposi's sarcoma-derived cells express cytokines with autocrine and paracrine growth effects. Science 243:223–226, 1989.
9. Nakamura S, Salahuddin SZ, Biberfeld P, Ensoli B, Markham PD, Wong-Staal F, Gallo RC. Kaposi's sarcoma cells: long-term culture with growth factor from retrovirus-infected CD4+ T cells. Science 242:426–430, 1988.
10. Sakurada S, Nakamura S, Salahuddin SZ, Gallo RC. Cultured Kaposi's sarcoma-derived spindle cells express vascular permeability inducing activity. Int Conf AIDS 6:200, 1990.
11. Louie S, Cai J, Law R, Lin G, Lunardi-Iskandar Y, Jung B, Masood R, Gill P. Effects of interleukin-1 and interleukin-1 receptor antagonist in AIDS-Kaposi's sarcoma. J Acquir Immune Defic Syndr Hum Retrovirol 8:455–460, 1995.
12. Miles SA, Rezai AR, Logan D, Salazar-Gonzalez JF, Vander MM, Mitsuyasu RT, Taga T, Hirano T, Kishimoto T, Martinez-Maza O. AIDS Kaposi's sarcoma-derived cells produce and respond to interleukin 6. Int Conf AIDS 6:112, 1990.
13. Barillari G, Buonaguro L, Fiorelli V, Hoffman J, Michaels F, Gallo RC, Ensoli B. Effects of cytokines from activated immune cells on vascular cell growth and HIV-

1 gene expression. Implications for AIDS-Kaposi's sarcoma pathogenesis. J Immunol 149:3727–3734, 1992.

14. Buonaguro L, Barillari G, Chang HK, Bohan CA, Kao V, Morgan R, Gallo RC, Ensoli B. Effects of the human immunodeficiency virus type 1 Tat protein on the expression of inflammatory cytokines. J Virol 66:7159–7167, 1992.

15. Roth WK, Brandstetter H, Sturzl M. Cellular and molecular features of HIV-associated Kaposi's sarcoma [editorial]. [published erratum appears in AIDS 1992 Nov; 6:following 1410], AIDS 6:895–913, 1992.

16. Sturzl M, Brandstetter H, Roth WK. Kaposi's sarcoma: a review of gene expression and ultrastructure of KS spindle cells in vivo. AIDS Res Hum Retroviruses 8:1753–1763, 1992.

17. Sturzl M, Brandstetter H, Zietz C, Eisenburg B, Raivich G, Gearing DP, Brockmeyer NH, Hofschneider PH. Identification of interleukin-1 and platelet-derived growth factor-B as major mitogens for the spindle cells of Kaposi's sarcoma: a combined in vitro and in vivo analysis. Oncogene 10:2007–2016, 1995.

18. Sturzl M, Roth WK, Brockmeyer NH, Zietz C, Speiser B, Hofschneider PH. Expression of platelet-derived growth factor and its receptor in AIDS-related Kaposi sarcoma in vivo suggests paracrine and autocrine mechanisms of tumor maintenance. Proc Natl Acad Sci USA 89:7046–7050, 1992.

19. Ensoli B, Gendelman R, Markham P, Fiorelli V, Colombini S, Raffeld M, Cafaro A, Chang HK, Brady JN, Gallo RC. Synergy between basic fibroblast growth factor and HIV-1 Tat protein in induction of Kaposi's sarcoma. Nature 371:674–680, 1994.

20. Samaniego F, Markham PD, Gendelman R, Gallo RC, Ensoli B. Inflammatory cytokines induce endothelial cells to produce and release basic fibroblast growth factor and to promote Kaposi's sarcoma-like lesions in nude mice. J Immunol 158: 1887–1894, 1997.

21. Nakamura S, Murakami-Mori K, Rao N, Weich HA, Rajeev B. Vascular endothelial growth factor is a potent angiogenic factor in AIDS-associated Kaposi's sarcoma-derived spindle cells. J Immunol 158:4992–5001, 1997.

22. Corbeil J, Rapaport E, Richman D, Badel P, Looney DJ. Inhibition and killing of Kaposi's sarcoma cells by retinoids. Second Natl Conf Hum Retroviruses Relat Infect 1995, p 79.

23. Gill PS, Espina BM, Moudgil T, Kidane S, Esplin JA, Tulpule A, Levine AM. All-trans retinoic acid for the treatment of AIDS-related Kaposi's sarcoma: results of a pilot phase II study. Leukemia 8(suppl 3): S26–S32, 1994.

24. Guo WX, Gill PS, Antakly T. Inhibition of AIDS-Kaposi's sarcoma cell proliferation following retinoic acid receptor activation. Cancer Res 55:823–829, 1995.

25. Masood R, Lunardi-Iskandar Y, Jean LF, Murphy JR, Waters C, Gallo RC, Gill P, Inhibition of AIDS-associated Kaposi's sarcoma cell growth by DAB389-interleukin 6. AIDS Res Hum Retroviruses 10:969–975, 1994.

26. Murakami-Mori K, Mori S, Taga T, Kishimoto T, Nakamura S. Enhancement of gp 130-mediated tyrosine phosphorylation of STAT3 and its DNA-binding activity in dexamethasone-treated AIDS-associated Kaposi's sarcoma cells: selective syn-

ergy between dexamethasone and gp130-related growth factors in Kaposi's sarcoma cell proliferation. J Immunol 158:5518–5526, 1997.

27. Murakami-Mori K, Taga T, Kishimoto T, Nakamura S. The soluble form of the IL-6 receptor (sIL-6R alpha) is a potent growth factor for AIDS-associated Kaposi's sarcoma (KS) cells; the soluble form of gp130 is antagonistic for sIL-6R alpha-induced AIDS-KS cell growth Int Immunol 8:595–602, 1996.

28. Gill PS, Loureiro C, Bernstein-Singer M, Rarick MU, Sattler F, Levine AM. Clinical effect of glucocorticoids on Kaposi sarcoma related to the acquired immunodeficiency syndrome (AIDS). Ann Intern Med 110:937–940, 1989.

29. Justement JS, Poli G, Fauci AS. Glucocorticoids act synergistically with recombinant cytokines to induce HIV expression in chronically infected promonocyte cells. Int Conf AIDS 6:162, 1990.

30. Amaral MC, Miles S, Kumar G, Nel AE. Oncostatin-M stimulates tyrosine protein phosphorylation in parallel with the activation of p42MAPK/ERK-2 in Kaposi's cells. Evidence that this pathway is important in Kaposi cell growth. J Clin Invest 92:848–857, 1993.

31. Faris M, Ensoli B, Stahl N, Yancopoulos G, Nguyen A. Wang S, Nel AE. Differential activation of the extracellular signal-regulated kinase, Jun kinase and Janus kinase–Stat pathways by oncostatin M and basic fibroblast growth factor in AIDS-derived Kaposi's sarcoma cells. AIDS 10:369–378, 1996.

32. Albini A, Barillari G, Benelli R, Gallo RC, Ensoli B. Angiogenic properties of human immunodeficiency virus type 1 Tat protein. Proc Natl Acad Sci USA 92: 4838–4842, 1995.

33. Ensoli B. Vascular integrins in Kaposi's sarcoma pathogenesis. Third Conf Retro Viruses Opportun Infect 1996, p 177.

34. Fiorelli V, Gendelman R, Samaniego F, Markham PD, Ensoli B. Cytokines from activated T cells induce normal endothelial cells to acquire the phenotypic and functional features of AIDS-Kaposi's sarcoma spindle cells. J Clin Invest 95:1723–1734, 1995.

35. Barillari G, Gendelman R, Gallo RC, Ensoli B. The Tat protein of human immunodeficiency virus type 1, a growth factor for AIDS Kaposi sarcoma and cytokine-activated vascular cells, induces adhesion of the same cell types by using integrin receptors recognizing the RGD amino acid sequence Proc Natl Acad Sci USA 90: 7941–7945, 1993.

36. Buonaguro L, Buonaguro FM, Tornesello ML, Beth-Giraldo E, Del GE, Ensoli B, Giraldo G. Role of HIV-1 Tat in the pathogenesis of AIDS-associated Kaposi's sarcoma. Antibiot Chemother 46:62–72, 1994.

37. Ensoli B, Barillari G, Salahuddin SZ, Gallo RC, Wong-Staal F. Tat protein of HIV-1 stimulates growth of cells derived from Kaposi's sarcoma lesions of AIDS patients. Nature 345:84–86, 1990.

38. Ensoli B, Barillari G, Salahuddin SZ, Gallo RC, Wong-Staal F. HIV-1 Tat protein released during acute infection stimulates growth of spindle cells derived from AIDS-Kaposi's sarcoma. Int Conf AIDS 6:202, 1990.

39. Ensoli B, Buonaguro L, Barillari G, Fiorelli V, Gendelman R, Morgan RA, Wingfield P, Gallo RC. Release, uptake, and effects of extracellular human immunodefi-

ciency virus type 1 Tat protein on cell growth and viral transactivation. J Virol 67: 277–287, 1993.

40. Ensoli B, Buonaguro L, Barillari G, Gallo RC. Biological properties of *tat*, the transactivator gene of HIV-1. Int Conf AIDS 7:55, 1991.

41. Albini A, Soldi R, Giunciuglio D, Giraudo E, Benelli R, Primo L, Noonan D, Salio M, Camussi G, Rock W, Bussolino F. The angiogenesis induced by HIV-1 tat protein is mediated by the Flk-1/KDR receptor on vascular endothelial cells. Nat Med 2:1371–1375, 1996.

42. Huang YQ, Li JJ, Feiner DG, Zhang WG, Friedman-Kien AE. Coexpression of FGF3 (Int-2) and its receptor (a splice variant of FGFR2) in Kaposi's sarcoma tumors. Second Natl Conf Hum Retroviruses Relat Infect 1995, p. 79.

43. Huang YQ, Li JJ, Moscatelli D, Basilico C, Nicolaides A, Zhang WG, Poiesz BJ, Friedman-Kien AE. Expression of *int-2* oncogene in Kaposi's sarcoma lesions. J Clin Invest 91:1191–1197, 1993.

44. Li JJ, Huang YQ, Moscatelli D, Nicolaides A, Zhang WC, Friedman-Kien AE. Expression of fibroblast growth factors and their receptors in acquired immunodeficiency syndrome-associated Kaposi sarcoma tissue and derived cells. Cancer 72: 2253–2259, 1993.

45. Cornali E. Zietz C. Benelli R. Weninger W. Masiello L. Breier G. Tschachler E, Albini A, Sturzl M. Vascular endothelial growth factor regulates angiogenesis and vascular permeability in Kaposi's sarcoma. Am J Pathol 149:1851–1869, 1996.

46. Breen EC, Rezai AR, Nakajima K, Beall GN, Mitsuyasu RT, Hirano T, Kishimoto T, Martinez-Maza O. Infection with HIV is associated with elevated IL-6 levels and production. J Immunol 144:480–484, 1990.

47. Dourado I, Martinez-Maza O, Kishimoto T, Suzuki H, Detels R. Interleukin 6 and AIDS-associated Kaposi's sarcoma: a nested case control study within the Multicenter AIDS Cohort Study. AIDS Res Hum Retroviruses 13:781–788, 1997.

48. Dourado MC. Interleukin-6 (IL-6) and AIDS-Kaposi's sarcoma: a nested case–control study within the Multicenter AIDS Cohort Study (MACS). Diss Abstr Int [B.] 55:843, 1994.

49. Schoefer H, Roeder C, Ochsendorf FR, Hochscheid I. Kaposi's sarcoma (HIV+ and HIV−) in Caucasian women. Int Conf AIDS 9:397–1569, 1993.

50. Haverkos HW, Friedman-Kien AE, Drotman DP, Morgan WM. The changing incidence of Kaposi's sarcoma among patients with AIDS. J Am Acad Dermatol 22: 1250–1253, 1990.

51. Marmor M, Friedman-Kien AE, Zolla-Pazner S, Stahl RE, Rubinstein P, Laubenstein L, William DC, Klein RJ, Spigland I. Kaposi's sarcoma in homosexual men. A seroepidemiologic case–control study. Ann Intern Med 100:809–815, 1984.

52. Rosenberg ZF, Fauci AS. Immunopathogenesis of HIV infection. FASEB J 5: 2382–2390, 1991.

53. Ammann AJ, Palladino MA, Volberding P, Abrams D, Martin NL, Conant M. Tumor necrosis factors alpha and beta in acquired immunodeficiency syndrome (AIDS) and AIDS-related complex. J Clin Immunol 7:481–485, 1987.

54. Miles SA. Kaposi sarcoma: a cytokine-responsive neoplasia? Cancer Treat Res 63: 129–140, 1992.

55. Miles S, Rezai A, Gaynor R, Magpantay L, Kishimoto T, Martinez-Maza O. HIV-*tat* increases IL-6 production by and proliferation of AIDS-KS derived cells. Int Conf AIDS 7:55, 1991.

56. Petri V, Nishio CE, Nishio PA, Takizawa CM, Michalany NS. Leprosy and HIV coinfection in an endemic developing country: how to interpret occurrence of lepromatous leprosy in a HIV+ hemophiliac with no known contact with leprosy patients? Int Conf AIDS 11:103, 1996.

57. Ambrosino C, Ruocco MR, Chen X, Mallardo M, Baudi F, Trematerra S, Quinto I, Venuta S, Scala G. HIV-1 Tat induces the expression of the interleukin-6 (IL6) gene by binding to the IL6 leader RNA and by interacting with CAAT enhancer-binding protein beta (NF-IL6) transcription factors. J Biol Chem 272:14883–14892, 1997.

58. Benelli R, Adatia R, Ensoli B, Stetler-Stevenson WG, Santi L, Albini A. Inhibition of AIDS-Kaposi's sarcoma cell induced endothelial cell invasion by TIMP-2 and a synthetic peptide from the metalloproteinase propeptide: implications for an anti-angiogenic therapy. Oncol Res 6:251–257, 1994.

59. Chang Y, Cesarman E, Pessin MS, Lee F, Culpepper J, Knowles DM, Moore PS Identification of herpesvirus-like DNA sequences in AIDS-associated Kaposi's sarcoma [see comments]. Science 266:1865–1869, 1994.

60. Buonaguro FM, Beth-Giraldo E, Tornesello ML, Monaco M, Downing R, Biryahwaho B, Sempala SK, Giraldo G. HHV-8 and other DNA virus sequences in endemic (African), classic, iatrogenic epidemic Kaposi's sarcoma biopsies. Int Conf. AIDS, 11:215, 1996.

61. Li JJ, Friedman-Kien AE, Huang YQ, Zhang WG, Feiner D. Detection of HHV-8 in subsets of blood cells from patients with AIDS-related Kaposi's sarcoma. Int Conf AIDS 11:7, 1996.

62. Luppi M, Barozzi P, Maiorana A, Artusi T, Trovato R, Marasca R, Savarino M, Ceccherini-Nelli L, Torelli G. Human herpesvirus-8 DNA sequences in human immunodeficiency virus-negative angioimmunoblastic lymphadenopathy and benign lymphadenopathy with giant germinal center hyperplasia and increased vascularity. Blood 87:3903–3909, 1996.

63. Luppi M, Torelli G. The new lymphotropic herpesviruses (HHV-6, HHV-7, HHV-8) and hepatitis C virus (HCV) in human lymphoproliferative diseases: an overview. Haematologica 81:265–281, 1996.

64. Mendel I, Prevost M, Collandre H. Human herpes virus-like DNA in biopsy samples and PBMCs from patients with AIDS-associated Kaposi's sarcoma. Int Conf AIDS 11:97, 1996.

65. Mitsuishi T, Sata T, Matsukura T, Kawashima M. Human herpesvirus 8 DNA is rarely found in Bowen's disease of non-immunosuppressed patients [letter]. Br J Dermatol 136:803–804, 1997.

66. Moore PS. Kaposi's sarcoma-associated herpesvirus (KSHV/HHV8). Third Conf Retrovirus. Opportun Infect 1996, p 167.

67. Renne R, Zhong W, Herndier B, McGrath M, Abbey N, Kedes D, Ganem D. Lytic growth of Kaposi's sarcoma-associated herpesvirus (human herpesvirus 8) in culture. Nat Med 2:342–346, 1996.

68. Gao SJ, Kingsley L, Hoover DR, Spira TJ, Rinaldo CR, Saah A, Phair J, Detels

R, Parry P, Chang Y, Moore PS. Seroconversion to antibodies against Kaposi's sarcoma-associated herpesvirus-related latent nuclear antigens before the development of Kaposi's sarcoma. N Engl J Med 335:233–241, 1996.

69. Goedert JJ, Kedes DH, Ganem D. Antibodies to human herpesvirus 8 in women and infants born in Haiti and the USA [letter]. Lancet 349:1368, 1997.

70. Kedes DH, Ganem D, Ameli N, Bacchetti P, Greenblatt R. The prevalence of serum antibody to human herpesvirus 8 (Kaposi sarcoma-associated herpesvirus) among HIV-seropositive and high-risk HIV-seronegative women. JAMA 277:478–481, 1997.

71. Kedes DH, Operskalski E, Busch M, Kohn R, Flood J, Ganem D. The seroepidemiology of human herpesvirus 8 (Kaposi's sarcoma-associated herpesvirus): distribution of infection in KS risk groups and evidence for sexual transmission [see comments]. [published erratum Nat Med 1996; 2:1041]. Nat Med. 2:918–924, 1996.

72. Rabkin CS, Schulz T, Lennette ET, Browning PJ, Miles SA, Weiss R, Biggar RJ. Interlaboratory correlation of current HHV-8 serologic tests. Fourth Conf Retrovirus Opportun Infect, 1997.

73. Kedes DH, Ganem D. Sensitivity of Kaposi's sarcoma-associated herpesvirus replication to antiviral drugs. Implications for potential therapy. J Clin Invest 99:2082–2086, 1997.

74. Panyutich EA, Said JW, Miles SA. Detection of putative Kaposi's sarcoma herpesvirus (HHV-8) in human endothelial cells cocultivated with HHV-8 producing cell line. Fourth Conf Retrovirus Opportun Infect, 1997.

75. Glesby MJ, Hoover DR, Weng S, Graham NM, Phair JP, Detels R, Ho M, Saah AJ. Use of antiherpes drugs and the risk of Kaposi's sarcoma: data from the Multicenter AIDS Cohort Study. J Infect Dis 173:1477–1480, 1996.

76. Saillour M, Risbourg M, De TP, Valance A, Sarrazin E, Perronne C. Effects of anti-CMV agents on Kaposi's sarcoma (KS) in AIDS patients. Int Conf AIDS 11: 97, 1996.

77. Mocroft A, Youle M, Gazzard B, Morcinek J, Halai R, Phillips AN. Antiherpes virus treatment and risk of Kaposi's sarcoma in HIV infection. Int Conf AIDS 11: 27, 1996.

78. Jones JL, Hanson DL, Chu SY, Ward JW, Jaffe HW. AIDS-associated Kaposi's sarcoma [letter; comment]. Science 267:1078–1079, 1995.

79. Mocroft A, Youle M, Gazzard B, Morcinek J, Halai R, Phillips AN. Antiherpesvirus treatment and risk of Kaposi's sarcoma in HIV infection. Royal Free/Chelsea and Westminster Hospitals Collaborative Group. AIDS 10:1101–1105, 1996.

80. Moore PS, Boshoff C, Weiss RA, Chang Y. Molecular mimicry of human cytokine and cytokine response pathway genes by KSHV. Science 274:1739–1744, 1996.

81. Moore PS, Gao SJ, Dominguez G, Cesarman E, Lungu O, Knowle DM, Garber R, Pellet PE, McGeoch DJ, Chang Y. Primary characterization of a herpesvirus agent associated with Kaposi's sarcoma. J Virol 70:549–558, 1996.

82. Nicholas J, Ruvolo VR, Burns WH, Sandford G, Wan X, Ciufo D, Hendrickson SB, Guo HG, Hayward GS, Reitz MS. Kaposi's sarcoma-associated human herpesvirus-8 encodes homologues of macrophage inflammatory protein-1 and interleukin-6. Nat Med 3:287–292, 1997.

83. Boshoff C, Endo Y, Collins PD, Takeuchi Y, Reeves JD, Schweickart VL, Siani MA, Sasaki T, Williams TJ, Gray PW, Moore PS, Chang Y, Weiss RA. Angiogenic and HIV-inhibitory functions of KSHV-encoded chemokines. Science 278:290–294, 1997.

84. Cesarman E, Nador RG, Bai F, Bohenzky RA, Russo JJ, Moore PS, Chang Y, Knowles DM. Kaposi's sarcoma-associated herpesvirus contains G protein-coupled receptor and cyclin D homologs which are expressed in Kaposi's sarcoma and malignant lymphoma. J Virol 70:8218–8223, 1996.

85. Gao SJ, Boshoff C, Jayachandra S, Weiss RA, Chang Y, Moore PS. KSHV *ORF K9* (vIRF) is an oncogene that inhibits the interferon signaling pathway. Oncogene, 15:1979–1985, 1997.

86. Bais C, Santomasso B, Coso O, Arvanitakis L, Raaka EG, Gutkind, JS, Asch AS, Cesarman E. Gerhengorn MC, Mesri EA. G-protein-coupled receptor of Kaposi's sarcoma-associated herpesvirus is a viral oncogene and angiogenesis activator [see comments]. Nature 391:86–89, 1998.

87. Zimring JC, Goodbourn S, Offermann MK. Human herpesvirus 8 encodes an interferon regulatory factor (IRF) homolog that represses IRF-1-mediated transcription. J Virol 72:701–707, 1998.

88. Rettig MB, Ma HJ, Vesico RA, Pold M, Schiller G, Belson D, Savage A, Nishikubo C, Wu C, Fraser J, Said JW, Berenson JR. Kaposi's sarcoma-associated herpesvirus infection of bone marrow dendritic cells from multiple myeloma patients [see comments]. Science 276:1851–1854, 1997.

89. Whitby D, Boshoff C, Luppi M, Torelli G, Kaposi's sarcoma-associated herpesvirus infection and multiple myeloma [letter; comment]. Science 278:1971–1972, 1997.

90. Rabkin CS, Janz S, Lash A, Coleman AE, Musaba E, Liotta L, Biggar RJ, Zhuang Z. Monoclonal origin of multicentric Kaposi's sarcoma lesions. N Engl J Med 336: 988–993, 1997.

91. Popescu NC, Zimonjic DB, Leventon-Kriss S, Bryant JL, Lunardi-Iskandar Y, Gallo RC. Deletion and translocation involving chromosome 3 (p14) in two tumorigenic Kaposi's sarcoma cell lines. J Natl Cancer Inst 88:450–455, 1996.

92. Kaaya EE, Castanos-Velez E, Amir H, Lema L, Luande J, Kitinya J, Patarroyo M, Biberfeld P. Expression of adhesion molecules in endemic and epidemic Kaposi's sarcoma. Histopathology 29:337–346, 1996.

93. Wernert N, Raes MB, Lassalle P, Dehouck MP, Gosselin B, Vandenbunder B, Stehelin D. c-*est1* Proto-oncogene is a transcription factor expressed in endothelial cells during tumor vascularization and other forms of angiogenesis in humans. Am J Pathol 140:119–127, 1992.

94. Albini A, Mitchell CD, Thompson EW, Seeman R, Martin GR, Wittek AE, Quinnan GV. Invasive activity and chemotactic response to growth factors by Kaposi's sarcoma cells. J Cell Biochem 36:369–376, 1988.

95. Albini A, Fontanini G, Masiello L, Tacchetti C, Bigini D, Luzzi P, Noonan DM, Stetler-Stevenson WG. Angiogenic potential in vivo by Kaposi's sarcoma cell-free supernatants and HIV-1 *tat* product: inhibition of KS-like lesions by tissue inhibitor of metalloproteinase-2. AIDS 8:1237–1244, 1994.

96. Miles SA, Mitsuyasu R, LaFleur F, Ryback M, Kasden P, Suckow C, Groopman

J, Scadden D. Phase I/II trial of interleukin-4 in KS (ACTG 224). Int Conf AIDS 10:46, 1994.

97. Emilie D, Wijdenes J, Gisselbrecht C, Jarrousse B, Billaud E, Blay JY, Gabarre J. Gaillard JP, Brochier J, Raphael M. Administration of an anti-interleukin-6 monoclonal antibody to patients with acquired immunodeficiency syndrome and lymphoma: effect on lymphoma growth and on B clinical symptoms. Blood. 84: 2472–2479, 1994.

98. Friedman-Kien A, Dezube B, Lee J, Kaplan L, Groopman J, Saville W, Scadden D, Debruge J, Miles S, AMC 002 Team. Oral 9-*cis* retinoic acid is active in AIDS related Kaposi's sarcoma: AIDS Associated Malignancy Consortium Study 002 Krown SE, Paredes J, eds. Second National AIDS Malignancy Conf, 1998.

99. Polsky B, Pino MC, Agosti J, Phase I/II trial of soluble recombinant human interleukin-1 receptor (rhu IL-1R) in patients with human immunodeficiency virus-1 (HIV-1) infection [abstr]. Proc Annu Meet Am Assoc Cancer Res 14:A834, 1995.

100. Bilello JA, Stellrecht K, Drusano GL, Stein DS. Soluble tumor necrosis factor-alpha receptor type II (sTNF alpha RII) correlates with human immunodeficiency virus (HIV) RNA copy number in HIV-infected patients. J Infect Dis 173:464–467, 1996.

101. Walker RE, Spooner KM, Kelly G, McCloskey RV, Woody JN, Falloon J, Baseler M, Piscitelli SC, Davey RTJ, Polis MA, Kovacs JA, Masur H, Lane HC. Inhibition of immunoreactive tumor necrosis factor-alpha by a chimeric antibody in patients infected with human immunodeficiency virus type 1. J Infect Dis 174:63–68, 1996.

102. Alexander LN, Wilcox CM. A prospective trial of thalidomide for the treatment of HIV-associated idiopathic esophageal ulcers. AIDS Res Hum Retroviruses, 13: 301–304, 1997.

103. Little R, Welles L, Wyvill K, Pluda J, Figg W, Newcomb F, Tosato G, Yarchoan R. Preliminary results of a phase II study of oral thalidomide in patients with AIDS-related Kaposi's sarcoma. Second National AIDS Malignancy Conference, 1998.

104. Dezube BJ, Lederman MM, Spritzler JG, Chapman B, Korvick JA, Flexner C, Dando S, Mattiacci MR, Ahlers CM, Zhang L. High-dose pentoxiyfylline in patients with AIDS: inhibition of tumor necrosis factor production. National Institute of Allergy and Infectious Diseases AIDS Clinical Trials Group. J Infect Dis 171: 1628–1632, 1995.

105. Ockenga J, Rohde F, Suttman U, Herbarth L, Ballmaier M, Schedel I. Ketotifen in HIV-infected patients: effects on body weight and release of TNF-alpha. Eur J Clin Pharmacol 50:167–170, 1996.

106. Murata R, Nishimura Y, Hiraoka M. An antiangiogenic agent (TNP-470) inhibited reoxygenation during fractionated radiotherapy of murine mammary carcinoma. Int J Radiat Oncol Biol Phys 37:1107–1113, 1997.

107. Dezube BJ, VonRoenn JH, Holde-Wiltse J, Cheung TW, Remick SC, Cooley TR, Moore J, Sommadossi J-P, Shriver SK, Suckow CW, Gill PS. Fumagillin analog in the treatment of Kaposi's sarcoma. J Clin Oncol 16:1444–1449, 1998.

108. O'Reilly MS, Boehm T, Shing Y, Fukai N, Vasios G, Lane WS, Flynn E, Birkhead JR, Olsen BR, Folkman J. Endostatin: an endogenous inhibitor of angiogenesis and tumor growth. Cell 88:277–285, 1997.

109. Sim BK, O'Reilly MS, Liang H, Fortier AH, He W, Madsen JW, Lapcevich R,

Nacy CA. A recombinant human angiostatin protein inhibits experimental primary and metastatic cancer. Cancer Res 57:1329–1334, 1997.

110. Krown SE. Acquired immunodeficiency syndrome-associated Kaposi's sarcoma. Biology and management. Med Clin North Am 81:471–494, 1997.

111. Miles SA, Wang HJ, Cortes E, Carden J, Marcus S, Mitsuyasu RT. beta-Interferon therapy in patients with poor-prognosis Kaposi sarcoma related to the acquired immunodeficiency syndrome (AIDS). A phase II trial with preliminary evidence of antiviral activity and low incidence of opportunistic infections. Ann Intern Med 112:582–589, 1990.

112. Martinez-Maza O, Mitsuyasu RT, Miles SA, Giorgi JV, Heitjan DF, Sherwin SA, Fahey JL. gamma-Interferon-induced monocyte major histocompatibility complex class II antigen expression individuals with acquired immune deficiency syndrome. Cell Immunol 123:316–324, 1989.

113. Marfaing-Koka A, Aubin JT, Grangeot-Keros L, Portier A, Benattar C, Merrien D, Agut H, Aucouturier P, Autran B, Wijdenes J. In vivo role of IL-6 on the viral load and on immunological abnormalities of HIV-infected patients. J Acquir Immune Defic Syndr Hum Retrovirol 11:59–68, 1996.

114. Wallis RS, Nsubuga P, Whalen C, Mugerwa RD, Okwera A, Oette D, Jackson JB, Johnson JL, Ellner JJ. Pentoxifylline therapy in human immunodeficiency virus-seropositive persons with tuberculosis: a randomized, controlled trial. J Infect Dis 174:727–733, 1996.

115. Alexander LN, and Wilcox CM. A prospective trial of thalidomide for the treatment of esophageal ulcers. AIDS Res Hum Retrovirus 13:301–304, 1997.

116. James JS. Thalidomide for wasting syndrome: progress toward compromise. AIDS Treat News pp 1–5, 1995.

117. Klausner JD, Makonkawkeyoon S, Akarasewi P, Nakata K, Kasinrerk W, Corral L, Dewar RL, Lane HC, Freedman VH, Kaplan G. The effect of thalidomide on the pathogenesis of human immunodeficiency virus type 1 and *M. tuberculosis* infection. J Acquir Immune Defic Syndr Hum Retrovirol 11:247–257, 1996.

118. Reyes-Teran G, Sierra-Madero JG, Martinez DC, Arroyo-Figueroa H, Pasquett A, Calva JJ, Ruiz-Palacios GM, Effects of thalidomide on HIV-associated wasting syndrome: a randomized, double-blind, placebo-controlled clinical trial. AIDS 10: 1501–1507, 1996.

119. Kreuzer KA, Dayer JM, Rockstroh JK, Sauerbruch T, Spengler U. The IL-1 system in HIV infection: peripheral concentrations of IL-1 beta, IL-1 receptor antagonist and soluble IL-1 receptor type II. Clin Exp Immunol 109:54–58, 1997.

120. Brooks PC, Clark RA, Cheresh DA. Requirement of vascular integrin alpha$_v$beta$_3$ for angiogenesis. Science 264:569–571, 1994.

121. Brooks PC, Stromblad S, Klemke R, Visscher D, Sarkar FH, Cheresh DA. Antiintegrin alpha$_v$beta$_3$ blocks human breast cancer growth and angiogenesis in human skin [see comments]. J Clin Invest 96:1815–1822, 1995.

122. Brooks PC, Stromblad S, Sanders LC, Von ST, Aimes RT, Stetler-Stevenson WG, Quigley JP, Cheresh DA. Localization of matrix metalloproteinase MMP-2 to the surface of invasive cells by interaction with integrin alpha$_v$beta$_3$. Cell 85:683–693, 1996.

123. Haraguchi M, Okamura M, Konishi M, Konishi Y, Negoro N, Inoue T, Kanayama

Y, Yoshikawa J. Anti-angiogenic compound (TNP-470) inhibits mesangial cell proliferation in vitro and in vivo. Kidney Int 51:1838–1846, 1997.

124. Koyama H, Nishizawa Y, Hosoi M, Fukumoto, S, Kogawa K, Shioi A, Morii H.
      The fumagillin analogue TNP-470 inhibits DNA synthesis of vascular smooth mus-
      cle cells stimulated by platelet-derived growth factor and insulin-like growth factor-
      I. Possible involvement of cyclin-dependent kinase 2. Circ Res 79:757–764, 1996.

125. Yamaoka M, Yamamoto T, Ikeyama S, Sudo K, Fujita T. Angiogenesis inhibitor
      TNP-470 (AGM-1470) potently inhibits the tumor growth of hormone-independent
      human breast and prostate carcinoma cell lines Cancer Res. 53:5233–5236, 1993.

126. Kakeji Y, Teicher BA. Preclinical studies of the combination of angiogenic inhibi-
      tors with cytotoxic agents. Invest New Drugs 15:39–48, 1997.

127. Figg WD, Pluda JM, Lush RM, Saville MW, Wyvill K, Reed E, Yarchoan R. The
      pharmacokinetics of TNP-470, a new angiogenesis inhibitor. Pharmacotherapy 17:
      91–97, 1997.

128. O'Reilly MS, Holmgren L, Shing Y, Chen C, Rosenthal RA, Cao Y, Moses M,
      Lane WS, Sage EH, Folkman J. Angiostatin: a circulating endothelial cell inhibitor
      that suppresses angiogenesis and tumor growth. Cold Spring Harb Symp Quant
      Biol 59:471–482, 1994.

129. Cao Y, Ji RW, Davidson D, Schaller J, Marti D, Sohndel S, McCance SG, O'Reilly
      MS, Llinas M, Folkman J. Kringle domains of human angiostatin. Characterization
      of the anti-proliferative activity on endothelial cells. J Biol Chem 271:29461–
      29467, 1996.

130. Carr A, Milliken S, Lewis C, Mitsuyasu R, Miles S, Newell M, Cooper DA. A
      pilot phase II safety and activity study of ritonavir in the treatment of HIV-associ-
      ated cutaneous Kaposi's sarcoma. Fourth Conf Retro Virus Opportun Infect, 1997.

9

Non–Hodgkin's Lymphoma
Future Targets for Prevention and Therapy

David T. Scadden
*Massachusetts General Hospital and Harvard Medical School,
Boston, Massachusetts*

I. INTRODUCTION

Acquired immunodeficiency syndrome (AIDS)-related lymphoma (ARL) is the
most lethal complication of human immunodeficiency virus (HIV) infection (1).
Although the prevailing pessimism for individuals with AIDS has given way to
the successes of potent antiretroviral therapy, the outlook for those with ARL
remains distressingly poor. The improved prognosis for HIV-infected individuals
has highlighted the need to reduce the incidence, morbidity, and mortality of
prognosis-limiting complications such as ARL. Previous chapters have defined
developments in standard therapies for ARL. This chapter will discuss future
therapies and, in particular, therapies directed by underlying principles of pathogenesis.

II. PATHOGENIC MECHANISMS

The best-understood subtype of ARL is Epstein–Barr virus (EBV)-associated
lymphoma. The virtually ubiquitous nature of this infection in the general population is reflected in the fairly even risk of developing non–Hodgkin's lymphoma,
regardless of the risk group for HIV disease. Why some patients develop malignant transformation of B cells, while virtually all patients harbor persistent EBV-
infected B cells, remains unclear. However, the molecular mechanisms by which
EBV is capable of inducing this transformation have been gradually unraveled,

and the potential for using restoration of immune function as a therapeutic tool has entered clinical practice.

The molecular basis for at least some of the EBV-related lymphomas is the expression of the EBV latency membrane protein-1 (LMP-1) inducing the transformation of B cells. This integral membrane protein resembles members of the tumor necrosis factor receptor (TNFR) superfamily, which are known to regulate cell proliferation and apoptosis. TNFR molecules interact with TNF-associated factors (TRAF) and TNF death domain (TRADD) proteins as intermediate-signaling molecules. LMP-1 differs from other members of the TNFR superfamily in that it is capable of spontaneous aggregation in the absence of receptor ligand, resulting in molecular interactions with TRAFs and TRADDs (2). These interactions induce the expression of variety of activation antigens and induce the phenotypic changes of transformation. Although these molecular relations have been previously demonstrated in vitro in cell culture, there is now data to support similar interactions in primary tumor tissue (3). Structural components of LMP-1 necessary for the interaction with the TNF receptor pathway have been mapped to specific portions of the carboxy-terminus of LMP-1 (4). These structural motifs serve as areas of vulnerability that intracellular antibodies or small molecules could potentially exploit to interrupt this pathway.

The pattern of latent gene expression of EBV in patients with primary central nervous system (CNS) lymphoma and a subset of systemic lymphomas closely resembles that of B cells transformed in vitro by EBV. These data suggest the direct relations of EBV to development of at least a portion of ARL. However, the presence of EBV within systemic lymphomas is not uniform, and there are variable patterns of EBV latent gene expression. A subset of EBV-positive tumors express only EBNA-1 among the nine EBV latency proteins, raising the possibility of an EBV-independent mechanism of transformation, or of a unique, EBV-related mechanism of transformation of B cells. In addition, the large number of EBV-negative tumors must evolve by independent processes. The recent association of Kaposi's sarcoma associated herpesvirus (KSHV) with a small subset of tumors arising as primary effusions or of the bowel (5) suggest that this other member of the gamma herpesvirus family may participate in the malignant process.

The genetic analysis of tumors from patients with AIDS-related lymphoma have clearly demonstrated several molecular characteristics segregated by tumor subtype. These associations, defined by the work of Della-Favera and Knowles, suggest a role for mutagenic events participating in at least some of these tumors (6). Specifically, c-*myc* rearrangements and p53 gene mutations are associated with the small noncleaved histology and alterations of *bcl-6* are found in approximately 20% of large-cell histological-type tumors. Mutations of the regulatory region of the transcriptional repressor *bcl-6*, and reduction in *bcl-6* levels are often seen in the large-cell tumors (7). A model then emerges of abnormal B-cell regulation induced either directly by HIV itself or in the cytokine context of progressive HIV-induced immunosuppression, perhaps fueled by EBV-induced proliferation. This proliferative state may then be followed by mutational events occurring in the B cells, eventually resulting in the emergence of cell transformation. As immune suppression proceeds during the course of HIV disease, the ability for immune recognition and suppression of proliferating cells is compromised. The balance of reactive cytolytic cells to proliferating cells is then tipped and tumor may emerge. Each of these mechanisms participating in the emergence of tumors may be envisioned to serve as a point of attack for therapy. Monitoring correlates of these phenomena such as viral load or specifically reactive lymphocytes may ultimately provide insight into potential risk.

III. PATHOGENIC-DRIVEN THERAPIES

A. Interruption of Viral Cofactors

The role of viruses in ARL may be approached therapeutically by several routes. The first is in direct interruption of the life cycle of herpesviruses. The potential for nucleoside therapeutics to prevent KSHV-related tumors is evident from the retrospective analyses of patients who are receiving ganciclovir or foscarnet for cytomegalovirus (CMV) disease, in whom a lower incidence of Kaposi's sarcoma (KS) has been noted (8,9). Testing the potential for these medications in established KS is underway and a trial to determine their prophylactic potential in KSHV-seropositive individuals is under development. Whether such approaches can be applied to the small subset of KSHV-positive ARL is still unclear. However, some preliminary results using antiviral approaches in ARL have been intriguing. There has been a report of several cases of multiply relapsed large-cell ARL responding to foscarnet (10), and several patients with small noncleaved cell (SNCC) ARL responding to interferon alfa and zidovudine (AZT) before receiving cytotoxic chemotherapy (11). Furthermore, in vitro data have indicated that hydoxyurea may be capable of interfering with the maintenance of EBV episomal DNA and, therefore, may reduce the transforming capacity of the virus (12). Whether any of these preliminary observations can become meaningful therapeutics requires further clinical testing.

It has been hypothesized that through altered expression of EBV latency-inducing genes it may be possible to induce an antitumor effect. Specifically, if cells that expressed latent genes of EBV can be made to switch to the lytic phase of virus replication, the effect on the tumor cell may indeed be that of cell lysis. Therefore, there has been an effort to manipulate cells to induce such a change using agents such as arginine butyrate or bryostatin (13).

By similar mechanisms, the virus thymidine kinase (TK) can be induced, causing cells to become sensitive to the toxic effects of nucleoside analogues, such as ganciclovir. The potential for using arginine butyrate or bryostatin in vivo has been shown in other clinical contexts and may be entering clinical trial for patients with EBV-related ARL. In independent trials, patients with ARL will receive either bryostatin or arginine butyrate and ganciclovir by infusion. For patients with primary CNS ARL who are the target populations for the bryostatin protocol, a standard radiation therapy treatment program will also be administered. Therefore, patients will be receiving a conventional therapy which has a high rate of failure (XRT) to which will be coupled a novel, biologically based approach.

1. Chemotherapy Plus Intensive Retroviral Therapy

Another approach that is virus-directed focuses on the potential to enhance immune function in HIV-positive patients by suppression of HIV-1 replicative activity. It has been widely noted that retroviral suppression using triple antiretroviral therapy that combines protease inhibitors and dual nucleoside analogues can result in marked increases in CD4 cell counts and improvements in functional status. With nucleoside analogues other than zidovudine (AZT), there has generally been minimal myelosuppression, and the neurotoxicity seen with these agents has generally not been additive or synergistic with the vinca alkaloids. It has been feasible, therefore, to use nucleoside analogues in conjunction with chemotherapy for ARL (14).

The highly potent anti-HIV protease inhibitors have effects on the cytochrome P-450 systems of drug metabolism. Concerns have been raised about these compounds altering the metabolism of the anthracyclines or vinca derivatives. There is an ongoing trial through the AIDS Malignancy Consortium (AMC) to evaluate both the potential for pharmacokinetic interactions of intensive antiretroviral therapy and a standard chemotherapy regimen and the ability of such a combination to enhance the overall outcome for patients. Patients received the modified cyclophosphamide, doxyrubicin (hydroxydaunorubicin), vincristine (Oncorin), prednisone (CHOP) chemotherapy program and the combination of d4T (stavudine), 3TC (lamivudine), and indinavir (Crixivan). In addition to pharmacokinetics, secondary endpoints are to determine whether the antiviral and potential immune-enhancing effect of antiviral therapy can effect an alteration in tumor control. Preliminary results suggest that drug-drug interactions are minimal with analysis of tumor outcomes still pending.

B. Enhancing Immune Reactivity

1. Interleukin-2 Following Chemotherapy

The lymphotropic cytokines and their secondary alteration in cell-mediated immunity have been hypothesized to participate in the pathophysiological process of progressive HIV disease. Alterations in the T-helper-1 (TH-1), or cell-mediated, versus T-helper-2 (TH-2) or antibody-mediated, responses indirectly regulate susceptibility to opportunistic disease, including neoplasm. It is hypothesized that the TH-2 response may result in chronic B-cell stimulation, ultimately providing a proliferating substrate of cells in which mutational events lead to cell transformation. The use of interleukin-2 (IL-2) a TH-1 cytokine, has thus been proposed as a mechanism of altering the immune imbalance. In animal models, EBV-related proliferative disease has been abrogated by the use of low dose IL-2 (15). Doses comparable with those administered in the animal model are achievable in humans and have been tolerated in patients with AIDS malignancies (16). Ten patients received 17 courses of IL-2 therapy following preliminary treatment of their NHL or KS. There were no adverse effects on HIV RNA, and patient tolerance was quite favorable. CD4 and CD8 cell populations did not change; however, there was an increase in natural killer (NK) cell numbers by approximately twofold for patients receiving doses higher than or equal to 0.9×10^6 IU/m^2 per day. The NK cell population is a strong producer of the TH-1 cytokine, interferon gamma (IFN-γ) thereby potentially enhancing CTL activity in the TH-1 response. These changes, at least theoretically, may provide benefit for patients with immunodeficiency tumors. There is currently an active clinical trial to test this potential benefit in patients who have had a partial response (PR) to their induction chemotherapy for ARL. Patients will have received either CHOP or m-BACOD (Cytoxan, doxorubicin Adriamycin), vincristine, bleomycin, dexamethasone, methotrexate, folinc acid) induction therapy. They will then receive daily IL-2, 1.0×10^6 U/m^2 per day by subcutaneous injection for a maximum of 1 year or until disease progression. Patients will undergo extensive phenotypic analysis of B cells, T cells, and NK cells at regular intervals as well as evaluation of cytokine production by CD4 and CD8 cell subsets and production of IFN-γ by NK cells. HIV RNA will be sequentially evaluated. The endpoints of this study are to define the response and survival of patients with PR following induction chemotherapy. In addition, this study intends to define how low-dose IL-2 effects the expansion of the CD3−, CD56+ NK population and to evaluate the incidence of secondary opportunistic infections in patients with ARL receiving IL-2. The study is being conducted under the sponsorship of the Cancer and Leukemia Group B (CALGB), with participation of the (AMC), both are NCI cooperative groups in the United States.

A different approach using IL-2 is being tested in patients with relapsed ARL following chemotherapy. IL-2 will be administered in a different manner to take advantage of observations by Kovacs and colleagues, who found a CD4 increase in HIV-positive patients (with entry CD4 cell counts of more than 200/mm^3) using an intermediate-dose level of IL-2 given intermittently (17). Patients receiving an average dose of IL-2 of 9 million U/day for 5 days every 8 weeks, attained a 50% increase in CD4$^+$ cells after 1 year of therapy. These patients demonstrated an improvement in their response to tetanus toxoid and mitogens when their peripheral blood lymphocytes (PBLs) were evaluated in vitro. Patients generally tolerated this regimen reasonably well and, when given in conjunction with intensive antiretroviral therapy, did not show any evidence of sustained alterations in their circulating levels of HIV.

Other studies using subcutaneous IL-2 twice daily, administered every 8 weeks resulted in reasonable tolerance (18). The ability for patients to receive this medication and the theroretical ability to enhance CD8 + T–cell-mediated cell lysis make intermittent IL-2 an appealing regimen in patients with ARL. A phase II trial testing its ability to delay relapse and improve survival is under development.

2. Interleukin-12 Following Chemotherapy

Laboratory studies suggest that IL-12 may have therapeutic effect, in that they have demonstrated IL-12 to be a potent inducer of NK cell and CD8 + CTL cytotoxic activity. This heterodimeric glycoprotein can increase the generation and the cytotoxic activity of cytotoxic T lymphocytes CTL; 19). It enhances the production of IFN-γ at nanomolar concentrations and can do so from either resting T or NK cells independently of proliferation (20). IL-12 appears to alter T-cell differentiation to favor TH-1, development, counterbalancing the effects of IL-4, which enhances TH-2 cell generation (21).

Interleukin-12 improves the depressed NK cytotoxic activity observed in HIV-seropositive patients in vitro (22). It also restores PBL responses to HIV peptides or recall antigens in vitro (23) and is currently in the process of being clinically tested for HIV-positive patients.

In the context of non–Hodgkin's lymphoma or other tumors, IL-12 has been hypothesized to be useful because of its ability to enhance cell-mediated immune responses through NK activity. In animal models, IL-12 markedly reduces metastasis formation and growth of transplanted tumors and delays death (24). In the setting of AIDS-related lymphoma, it has been hypothesized that overexpression of IL-10 by tumor cells impairs IL-12 production and CD8-mediated cytoxicity. Addition of IL-12 to mixed populations of cells activates CD8 cells and results in cytoxicity against autologous HIV-associated B-cell lymphomas.

Interleukin-12 will be tested in several contexts for ARL. An NCI intramural trial is using IL-12 twice weekly for patients achieving a CR after initial EPOCH chemotherapy or in patients failing initial therapy. The AMC will test IL-12 in a randomized phase II study following response to a salvage regimen of ifosfamide–etoposide for patients who relapsed after initial therapy. Both the IL-12 and the IL-2 trials are intended to gain some indication of whether immune modulation can alter disease outcome: difficult to gauge in the context of noncytotoxic agents for a highly aggressive tumor. The trials are designed with extensive laboratory components to try to define immunological parameters that might correlate with improved outcome, seeking guideposts for the development of future such agents.

C. Anti-EBV Immune Reactivity

1. 5-Azacytidine Therapy

It has been noted that EBV is associated with 30–60% of systemic AIDS lymphomas, and among these, the expression of EBV latent genes varies considerably. There is a subpopulation of these tumors that do not express EBNA-2 the predominant epitope target for CTL activity. Rather, there is a pattern of EBNA-1 expression exclusively in about half of the systemic EBV-positive lymphomas. EBNA-1 has not been shown to be a CTL target and, indeed, it may have suppressive effects through perturbation of antigen presentation in conjunction with class I major histocompatibility complex (MHC) on professional antigen-presenting cells (25). Decreased expression of particular portions of the EBV genome is regulated through nucleotide methylation (26), which may be modified through the administration of agents such as 5-azacytidine. In vitro treatment of EBV-positive tumors with this agent has demonstrated the enhanced expression of latent genes and, in particular, the up-regulation of EBNA-2 expression (27). Therefore, it has been hypothesized that in patients who have EBV-positive, EBNA-2-negative tumors, the use of 5-azacytidine may result in increased surface expression of EBNA-2, rendering the cells sensitive to the potential cytolytic effect of anti-EBV CTLs.

A clinical trial has been initiated by ECOG and the AMC to evaluate ARL tumors in relapse by in situ PR and, if the expression profile is appropriate, to then begin a 5-day outpatient infusion of 5-azacytidine. Biopsies will be taken sequentially tumors to assess both expression of EBNA-2 and for the infiltration of tumor by reactive lymphocytes. Biological endpoints and tumor response are primary objectives for this study.

2. Allogeneic Transfer of Cells

In the setting of hematological malignancies it has been noted that allogenic peripheral blood mononuclear cells (PBMC) may be capable of inducing marked reductions in tumor mass. This has been best defined in the posttransplant setting for CML where patients who have essentially no other therapeutic options have received allogenic PBMC and had responses that have been both clinically meaningful and dramatic (28). Although the experience is limited in other hematological malignancies there are data suggesting clinical responses (29). A major complication of this type of approach is the induction of graft-versus-host disease (GVHD), which can be severe, but is titratable according to the dose of infused cells (30). The potential for this type of approach being useful depends on several features, including the ability of the transferred cells to recognize foreign epitopes on the tumor cells, the ability of these cells to expand in the host, and the balance of GVHD and graft versus malignancy (GVL). In the context of HIV disease, there has not been a documented increase in the incidence of transfusion-associated GVHD, suggesting that there is no unusual risk of GVHD in this patient population. In addition, the frequent association of lymphoma with the foreign antigens EBV or KSHV in AIDS suggests this type of approach has substantial clinical potential for these patients. Clinical trials have been undertaken at several sites to address this issue. Donor leukocytes from HLA-matched relatives are being infused into patients at variable levels of cell numbers, with or without supplemental interferon alfa or host pretreatment with immunosuppressives.

3. EBV-Specific CTLs

There have been several reports of dramatic regression of tumors with the use of allogeneic or autologous EBV-specific reactive lymphocytes (31–34). In studies by Rooney and colleagues, retroviral transduction of the subsequently infused cells has permitted evaluation of their persistence and expansion in the host. Infused cells have been documented to persist for over 18 months in patients after bone marrow transplantation, with expansion of the transduced subpopulation following entry into the host (35). The cells, when used therapeutically, have resulted in marked antitumor effects (36), and they are now being tested as prophylatic treatment in patients with a high-risk of lymphoproliferative disease in the postmismatched bone marrow transplantation setting. This approach is in development for AIDS-related lymphomas, and early pilot studies have suggested that EBV-specific CTLs can be derived from HIV-infected patients. Efforts to expand the cells ex vivo are underway with preliminary data suggesting the feasibility of this approach (Clay Smith, personal communication Duke University, Durham, North Carolina).

IV. ENHANCEMENT OF CYTOXICITY

The effort in approaching ARL has generally been to avoid highly intensive chemotherapy regimens in the HIV-positive population because of adverse experiences early in the epidemic. One alternative approach to try to improve tumor control is to use agents that have mechanisms of action independent from chemotherapy with nonoverlapping toxicities. In particular, there has been an effort to use monoclonal antibodies directed against pan–B-cell antigens and a number of clinical trials have indicated that monoclonal antibodies alone have activity against AIDS-related lymphomas (14,37,38). A clinical trial has recently been completed that indicates that the modified m-BACOD chemotherapy regimen may indeed be given in conjunction with the continuous infusion of the monoclonal antibody anti-B4, coupled to a modified ricin cytotoxin, anti-B4-blocked ricin (anti-B4bR; 39). In this trial, the chemotherapy dose did not need to be adjusted for the effects of the antibody, and patients were able to tolerate the combined therapy quite well. There subsequently has been development of various antibodies that have increased potency against non–Hodgkin's lymphomas of other types (40). In particular, the humanized monoclonal anti-CD20 has induced B-lymphoma cell line destruction by both complement-mediated cell lysis and antibody-dependent cellular cytotoxicity (ADCC). Although this antibody has been primarily tested in low-grade lymphomas, its response rates of approximately 50% in patients heavily treated with antibody therapy alone and 100% when given in combination with chemotherapy for therapy-naive patients, make it a highly attractive monoclonal to test in more aggressive lymphomas such as ARL. The antibody generally is well tolerated and, therefore, a clinical trial is ongoing that will address whether antibody plus CHOP chemotherapy provides any advantage over CHOP alone in previously untreated ARL.

The now open-ended prognosis for patients with HIV disease responding to antiviral therapy has both improved the tolerance for chemotherapy and highlighted the need for more aggressive anti-lymphoma strategies in a subset of patients. The use of autologous transplantation using protocols similar to the non-HIV infected population has now entered clinical trial. These offer a unique opportunity to not only evaluate the impact of intensive therapy on ARL, but also to assess the potential for stem-cell-based gene therapy approaches and the impact of cytotoxic therapy on virus reservoirs. Recent advances in the use of minimally myeloablative allogeneic transplantation have suggested their potential in treatment of lymphoma and are currently under development for ARL.

V. GENE THERAPY APPROACHES

A. Genetically Modified Tumor Reactive CTLs

An approach, which at this point remains theoretical, but is in the process of being tested in another context, is to transduce cells with a receptor that enables them to be highly specific for tumor cells. This concept is derived from the molecular alteration of the T-cell receptor zeta chain (TCR-ζ). TCR-ζ is the portion of the T-cell receptor capable of triggering downstream-signaling events. By coupling the intracellular domains of this portion of the TCR to extracellular and transmembrane regions of other molecules, such as monoclonal antibodies, or other cell surface receptors, the cells are rendered specific for the epitope recognized by the monoclonal antibody or for the ligand interacting with the receptor, independently of MHC (41). In particular, this has now been used in the context of HIV infection by using the extracellular and transmembrane portion of CD4 cells coupled to the TCR-ζ, creating a so-called universal receptor for HIV. In so doing, cells that express this chimeric molecule become highly reactive to the

HIV envelope (gp120) that is expressed by infected cells. Retroviral transduction of peripheral blood mononuclear cells has resulted in the generation of a population of cells that is specifically reactive to HIV gp120. This method is now being clinically tested in the context of HIV infection. It is hypothesized to be potentially useful in the setting of malignant disease; in particular, in the setting of malignant disease associated with viral infection. Generating EBV- or KSHV-specific CTLs through the use of similarly engineered molecules employing EBV- or KSHV-specific monoclonal antibodies linked to the TCR-ζ is a highly feasible approach.

B. Tumor-Specific Suicide Gene Therapy

The potential for genetic manipulation of cells thereby causing them to become sensitive to chemotherapeutic agents has been shown in animal models. The EBV latent gene EBNA-2 acts as a transcription factor and is capable of enhancing the expression of genes from various promoters and particularly the *BamC* promoter of the EBV genome (42). A *BamC* promoter has been used to drive a suicide gene (thymidine kinase) in a tumor model for ARL (43). Animals bearing EBNA-2-positive EBV-related tumors containing this construct have had established tumors regress and not recur following a single 5-day course of ganciclovir. The model suggests that it may be possible to induce tumor-specific cytotoxicity of ganciclovir with a similar genetic construct. Delivering such a construct remains a major impediment to this type of approach, but progress in the field of gene therapy has already brought similar strategies to clinical trials (44).

VI. CONCLUSION

The current optimism in caring for the patient with AIDS can realistically be similarly applied to patients with AIDS-related tumors. An era of new standard therapies has emerged, providing the basis for the evolution of new approaches with considerable potential for improving the outcome for this patient population.

REFERENCES

1. Chaisson RE, Gallant JE, Keruly JC, Moore RD. Impact of opportunistic disease on survival in patients with HIV infection. AIDS 12:29–33, 1998.
2. Mosialos G, Birkenbach M, Yalamanchilli R, VanArsdale T, Ware C, Kieff E. The Epstein–Barr virus transforming protein LMP1 engages signaling proteins for the tumor necrosis factor receptor family. Cell 80:389–399, 1995.

3. Liebowitz D, Olopade O. Evidence for signal transduction through the TNF receptor pathway in post-transplant lymphoproliferative disorders. J Acquir Immune Defic Syndr Hum Retrovirol 14:A139, 1997.

4. Devergue O, Iaumi DM, Kaye KM, Kleijnen MF, Kieff E, Mosialos G. Association of TRAF1, TRAF2, and TRAF3 with an Epstein–Barr virus LMP1 domain important for B-lymphocyte transformation: role in NF-kappaB activation. Mol Cell Biol 16:7098–7108, 1996.

5. DePond W, Tasaka T, deVos S, Kahn D, Cesarman E, Knowles DM, Koeffler H. Kaposi's sarcoma-associated herpesvirus and human herpesvirus 8 (KSHV/HHV8)-associated lymphoma of the bowel. Am J Surg Pathol 21:719–724, 1997.

6. Knowles DM. Etiology and pathogenesis of AIDS-related non–Hodgkin's lymphoma. Hematol Oncol Clin North Am 10:1081–1109, 1996.

7. Gaidano G, Gloghini A. Genetic alterations and expression of bcl-6 in AIDS-related lymphomas: relationship with EBV infection and identification of distinct molecular pathways in AIDS-lymphomagenesis. First National AIDS Malignancy Conference, Bethesda, Maryland [abstr 114]. J Acquir Immune Defic Syndr Hum Retrovirol 14: A44, 1997.

8. Youle M, Mocroft A, Gazzard B, Morcinek J, Halai R, Phillips AN. Anti-herpesvirus treatment and risk of Kaposi's sarcoma in HIV infection. Royal Free/Chelsea and Westminster Hospitals Collaborative Group. AIDS 10:1101–1105, 1996.

9. Glesby MJ, Weng S, Graham NM, Phair JP, Detels R, Ho M, Saah AJ. Use of antiherpes drugs and the risk of Kaposi's sarcoma: data from the Multicenter AIDS Cohort Study. J Infect Dis 173:1477–1480, 1996.

10. Schneider U, Delecluse H, Huhn D. Treatment of EBV-associated lymphoprolifera-tive disorders in HIV-infected patients with foscarnet. J Acquir Immune Defic Syndr Hum Retrovirol 14:A97, 1997.

11. Cabral L, Harrington WJ, Cai JP, Chan A, Wood C. Azothymidine and interferon-alpha are active in AIDS-associated small non-cleaved cell lymphoma but not large-cell lymphoma. Lancet 348:833, 1996.

12. Slobod KS, Belgaumi A., et al. Reversal of malignant cell growth phenotype by hydroxyurea-induced loss of Epstein–Barr virus episomes. First National AIDS Malignancy Conference, Bethesda, Maryland [Abstr 146]. J Acquir Immune Defic Syndr Hum Retrovirol 14:A53, 1997.

13. Saemundsen AK, Kalin B, Klein G. Effect of n-butyrate on cellular and viral DNA synthesis in cells latently infected with Epstein–Barr virus. Virology 107:557–561, 1980.

14. Levine AM, Espina B, Boswell W, Buckley J, Rasheed S, Stain S, Parker J, Nath-wani B, Gill PS. Low-dose methotrexate, bleomycin, doxorubicin, cyclophospha-mide, vincristine, and dexamethasone with zalcitabine in patients with acquired im-munodeficiency syndrome-related lymphoma. Effect on human immunodeficiency virus and serum interleukin-6 levels over time. Cancer 78:517–526, 1996.

15. Baiocchi RA. Low dose IL-2 prevents the development of Epstein–Barr virus-asso-ciated lymphoproliferative disease in the hu-PBL-SCID mouse model. Proc Natl Acad Sci USA 91:5577–5581, 1994.

16. Bernstein ZP, Gould M, et al. Prolonged administration of low-dose interleukin-2 in human immunodeficiency virus-associated malignancy results in selective expan-

sion of innate immune effectors without significant clinical toxicity. Blood 86:3287–3294, 1995.

17. Kovacs JA, Vogel S, Albert JM, Falloon J, Davey RT, Walker RE, Polis MA, Spooner K, Metcalf JA, Baseler M, Fyfe G, Lane HC. Controlled trial of interleukin-2 infusions in patients infected with the human immunodeficiency virus. N Engl J Med 335:1350–1360, 1996.

18. Davey RT, Chaitt DG, Piscitelli SC, Wells M, Kovacs JA, Walker RE, Falloon J, Polis MA, Metcalf JA, Masur H, Fyfe G, Lane HC. Subcutaneous administration of interleukin-2 in human immunodeficiency virus type 1-infected persons. J Infect Dis 175:781–790, 1997.

19. Bloom ET. Cellular and molecular mechanisms of the IL-12-induced increase in allospecific murine cytolytic T cell activity. Implications for the age-related decline in CTL. J Immunol 152:4242, 1994.

20. Kobayashi M, Ryan M, Hewick RM, Clark SC, Shan S, Loudon R, Sherman F, Perussia B, Trinchieri G. Indentification and purification of natural killer cell stimulatory factor (NKSF), a cytokine with multiple biologic effects on human lymphocytes. J Exp Med 170:827, 1989.

21. Manetti R, Giudizi MG, Piccinni M-P, Maggi E, Trinchieri G, Romagnani S. Natural killer cell stimulatory factor (NKSF/IL-12) induces Th1-type specific immune responses and inhibits the development of IL-4 producing Th cells. J Exp Med 177:1199, 1993.

22. Chehimi J, Frank I, Rengaraju M, Jackson SJ, Llanes C, Kobayashi M, Perussia B, Young D, Nickbarg E, Wolf SF, Trinchieri G. Natural killer cell stimulatory factor (NKSF) increases the cytotoxic activity of NK cells from both health donors and HIV-infected patients. J Exp Med 175:789, 1992.

23. Clerici M, Berzofsky JA, Pinto LA, Wynn TA, Blatt SP, Dolan MJ, Hendrix CW, Wolf SF, Shearer GM. Restoration of HIV-specific cell-mediated immune responses by interleukin-12 in vitro. Science 262:1721, 1993.

24. Brunda MJ, Warrier RR, Wright RB, Hubbard BR, Murphy M, Wolf SF, Gately MK. Antitumor and antimetastatic activity of interleukin 12 against murine tumors. J Exp Med 178:1223, 1993.

25. Levitskaya H, Coram M, Levitsky V, Imreh S, Stelgerwald-Mullen P, Klein G, Kurilla M, Masucci M. Inhibition of antigen processing by the internal repeat region of the Epstein–Barr virus nuclear antigen-1. Nature 375:685–688, 1995.

26. Robertson KD, Ling PD, Samid D, Ambinder RF. Transcriptional activation of the Epstein–Barr virus latency C promoter after 5-azacytidine treatment: evidence that demethylation at a single CpG site is crucial. Mol Cell Biol 15:6150–6159, 1995.

27. Masucci MG, Contreras-Salazar B, Ragnar E, Falk K, Minarovits J, Ernberg I, Klein G. 5-Azacytidine up regulates the expression of Epstein–Barr virus nuclear antigen 2 (EBNA-2) through EBNA-6 and latent membrane protein in the Burkitt's lymphoma line Rael. J Virol 63:3135–3141, 1989.

28. Porter DL, McGarigle C, Ferrara JLM, Antin JH. Induction of graft-versus-host disease as immunotherapy for relapsed chronic myeloid leukemia. N Engl J Med 330:100, 1994.

29. Collins RH, Shpilberg O, Drobyski W, et al. Donor leukocyte infusions in 140

patients with relapsed malignancy after allogeneic bone marrow transplantation. J Clin Oncol 15:433–444, 1997.

30. Mackinnon S, Papadopoulos EB, Carabasi MH, et al. Adoptive immunotherapy evaluating escalating doses of donor leukocytes for relapse of chronic myeloid leukemia after bone marrow transplantation: separation of graft-versus-leukemia responses from graft-versus-host disease. Blood 86:1261–1268, 1995.

31. Heslop HE, Rooney CM. Donor T cells to treat EBV-associated lymphoma. N Engl J Med 331:679–680, 1994.

32. Heslop HE, Li C, Smith CA, Loftin SK, Krance RA, Brenner MK, Rooney CM. Long-term restoration of immunity against Epstein–Barr virus infection by adoptive transfer of gene-modified virus-specific T lymphocytes. Nat Med 2:551–555, 1996.

33. Rooney CM. Use of gene-modified virus-specific T lymphocytes to control Epstein–Barr virus-related lymphoproliferation. Lancet 345:9–13, 1995.

34. Rooney C, Roskrow M, et al. Immunotherapy for EBV-associated lymphoproliferative disease. First National AIDS Malignancy Conference, Bethesda, Maryland [abstr S18]. J Acquir Immune Defic Syndr Hum Retrovirol 14:A15, 1997.

35. Papadopoulos EB, Emanuel D, Mackinnon S, et al. Infusion of donor leukocytes to treat Epstein–Barr virus-associated lymphoproliferative disorders after allogeneic bone marrow transplantation. N Engl J Med 330:1185–1192, 1994.

36. Kaplan LD, Kahn JO, et al. Phase 1 trial of anti-CD22 ricin-A-chain immunotoxin for treatment of AIDS-lymphoma. First National AIDS Malignancy Conference, Bethesda, Maryland [abstr 90]. J Acquir Immune Defic Syndr Hum Retrovirol 14: A38, 1997.

37. Kaplan LD, Testa MA, VonRoenn J, Dezube BJ, Cooley TP, Herndier B, Northfelt DW, Huang J, Tulpule A, Levine AM, the National Institute of Allergy and Infectious Diseases AIDS Clinical Trials Group. Low-dose compared with standard-dose m-BACOD chemotherapy for non–Hodgkin's lymphoma associated with human immunodeficiency virus infection. N Engl J Med 336:1641–1648, 1997.

38. Straus SE, Chen JI, Tosato G, Meier J. Epstein–Barr virus infections: biology, pathogenesis, and management. Ann Intern Med 118:45, 1993.

39. Scadden DT, Bernstein Z, Luskey B, Doweiko J, Tulpule A, Esseltine D, Levine A. Combined immunotoxin and chemotherapy for AIDS-related non–Hodgkin's lymphoma. Cancer 83:2580–2587, 1998.

40. McLaughlin P, Czuczman M, Link B, Levy R, Dillman R, Ho A. Preliminary report on a phase III pivotal trial of the anti-CD20 antibody (MAB) IDEC-C2B8 in patients with relapsed low-grade or follicular lymphoma. Proc Am Soc Cancer Oncol 15: 417, 1996.

41. Romeo C, Amiot M, Seed B. Sequence requirements for induction of cytolysis by the T cell antigen/Fc receptor zeta chain. Cell 68:889–897, 1992.

42. Wang F, Kikutani H, Tsang S, Kishimoto T, Kieff E. Epstein–Barr virus nuclear protein 2 transactivates a cis-acting CD23 DNA element. J Virol 65:4101-4106, 1991.

43. Franken M, Estabrooks A, Cavacini L, Sherburne B, Wang F, Scadden DT. Epstein–Barr virus-driven gene therapy for EBV-related lymphomas. Nat Med 2:1379–1382, 1996.

44. Culver KW, et al. In vivo gene transfer with retroviral vector-producer cells for treatment of experimental brain tumors. Science 256:1550–1552, 1992.

10

HPV-Related Neoplasia in HIV Infection
Proposed Mechanisms for Development of Malignancy

Cathy W. Critchlow and Nancy B. Kiviat
University of Washington, Seattle, Washington

I. INTRODUCTION

Despite the dramatic decrease in cervical cancer incidence that has occurred since the introduction of routine cytological screening, cervical cancer remains, globally, an important cause of female mortality. Even before the onset of the acquired immunodeficiency syndrome (AIDS) epidemic, cervical cancer was the second most common cancer among women worldwide, accounted for the greatest number of new cancer cases in developing countries, and was the major cause of cancer mortality among women in many parts of the developing world (1). There is now very strong evidence that specific high-risk types of human papillomavirus (HPV), for example HPV-16 and HPV-18 (based on the frequency with which those types have been identified in invasive cancer specimens; 2), are the probable etiologic agents of most cervical cancers and cervical precancer lesions. These precancer lesions are termed cervical intraepithelial neoplasia grade 1–3, or low- and high-grade cervical intraepithelial neoplasia (CIN 1 and CIN 2–3, respectively). It is estimated that from 35 to 50% of CIN 2–3 lesions, which are those thought to be most likely to develop into invasive cancers (3–6), would progress to invasive disease if not ablated (6).

It has now become apparent that women throughout the world are at increasing risk for infection with human immunodeficiency virus (HIV)-1 or in West Africa with HIV-2, that women acquiring HIV also are likely to be infected with HPV (7–19), and that coinfection with these two viruses increases risk for squamous cell intraepithelial neoplasia (13–23). Invasive cervical cancer is now designated an AIDS-defining illness among HIV-infected women. However, there has been no dramatic increase in the cervical cancer incidence rate, even in populations with a high risk of AIDS (24,25). Cumulatively, 558 (0.6%) of the 96,075 women with AIDS, reported through June 1997, have had invasive cervical cancer (26). On the basis of studies linking AIDS and cancer registry data, the rate of cervical cancer is about fourfold higher than the expected rate among age- and race-matched women in the general population (27). In industrialized countries, it is likely that significant increases in cervical cancer incidence associated with HIV infection have not occurred for the following reasons: First, HIV infection among women is rare. Second, only a small proportion of women have been infected with HIV for periods sufficient to develop invasive cervical cancer. Lastly, most women with high-grade intraepithelial neoplasia are identified by cytological screening and treated to prevent progression to invasive disease. In developing countries where HPV infection, cervical cancer, and HIV infection are common, increases in cervical cancer incidence may be occurring, but be difficult to detect because the cause of death is generally unknown. In addition, the lack of tumor registries in these countries hinders the detection of such a trend. Additionally, it is possible that most HIV-infected women die of other HIV-related diseases before development of cervical cancer. However, the evidence from epidemiological studies of associations between HIV infection, detection of HPV, and presence and persistence of cervical precancer lesions (see Chapter 7) suggest that HIV may be associated with development of cervical cancer. In this chapter, we will describe possible mechanisms by which HIV may be associated with an increased risk of these HPV-associated squamous cell tumors.

II. CLASSIFICATION AND DESCRIPTION OF HPV

Papillomaviruses, which constitute one of the two genera of the family Papovaviridae, are small, nonenveloped viruses with icosahedral symmetry, 72 capsomeres, 45–55 nm in diameter, and a double-stranded supercoiled circular DNA genome of approximately 8000 base pairs (28). The open-reading frames (ORFs), which are the potential protein-coding regions, are located on one strand. The viral genome is divided into three regions. The early region (ORFs E6, E7, E1, E2, and E4) encodes proteins necessary for viral DNA replication and transformation. The late region (ORFs L1 and L2) encodes viral structural proteins, including the major capsid proteins necessary for productive viral replication. The regulatory region (located between L1 and E6) contains the origin of replication and many of the control elements for transcription and replication (28,29). More than

70 human papillomavirus types have been described. HPVs are classified as being of the same or different type based on the amount of shared DNA homology. According to criteria adopted by the Papillomavirus Nomenclature Committee, *types* are defined as having less than 90% homology of the E6, E7, and L1 aggregate open-reading frame DNA sequences (or equivalently, greater than 10% sequence divergence). HPV *subtypes* have between 2 and 10% sequence divergence, and *variants of a specific type* have less than 2% divergence. Although it is clear that different HPV types vary in biological behavior (2), it remains to be seen whether subtypes or variants also have distinctly different biological properties.

III. HPV AND ONCOGENESIS

Human papillomavirus is one of the most common sexually transmitted agents (30–32). HPV infects stratified squamous, metaplastic squamous, and columnar epithelium. Many HPV types primarily infect genital tract epithelium. The virus appears to gain initial access to the lower portion of the epithelium in areas of local trauma, and there it infects basal epithelial cells (33,34). Although most HPV infections are self-limited (31), reexpression of virus has been noted to occur in areas of epithelial trauma, such as areas adjacent to sites that have been treated surgically to remove papillomavirus-associated lesions (35–37). Such reexpression is likely to be frequent and clinically significant in HIV-seropositive persons, particularly if they are latently infected with one or more of the HPV types associated with development of cervical (2) or anal carcinoma (38,39). The most common high-risk HPV types (i.e., types that predispose to development of anogenital tract carcinoma) include HPV types 16, 18, 45, and 56. HPV types 31, 33, and 35 are referred to as intermediate-risk types. HPV-6, 11, 42, 43, 44 are considered low-risk types because they are infrequently associated with malignancy in an immunocompetent individual (2). Although most studies evaluating the risk of invasive or in situ carcinoma associated with HPV infection have been case–control studies, cohort studies examining the risk of development of high-grade intraepithelial neoplasia in relation to detection of specific HPV types have been reported (40–42). However, the lack of a serological assay has made it difficult to estimate the true risk of malignancy conferred by infection with specific HPV types.

To see how HPV and HIV might act together to increase the risk of neoplasia, it is important to understand how HPV infection predisposes to development of neoplasia. HPV-associated cancers are characterized by retention and expression of E6 and E7, which play a major role in cellular transformation (43). The E6 and E7 gene products of high-, but not low-risk HPV types efficiently bind and inactivate the cell regulatory proteins of the p53 and retinoblastoma (Rb) genes, respectively (44,45). Each of these two processes results in inactivation of host tumor suppressor functions and dysregulation of cellular growth control. The binding of HPV E6 protein to p53 leads to degradation of p53 by ubiquitin-dependent proteolysis (44), and the binding of HPV E7 protein to Rb protein leads to release of the cellular transcription factor E2F-1, which promotes progression into the S phase of the cell cycle (46). These processes result in an increase in the number of dividing cells, which are susceptible to genetic alterations that may lead to development of cancer. Therefore, although development of cervical cancer involves a series of events initiated by HPV infection, including HPV E6/E7-mediated disturbance of tumor suppressor functions, such events are insufficient to assure progression to cancer (47). The role of HPV in the pathogenesis of invasive cervical cancer appears to involve facilitation of the development of genetic mutation resulting from exposure to other cofactors (e.g., constituents of cigarette smoke) or maintenance of cells with genetic mutations. Consistent with this notion are the long latency periods between first HPV exposure and development of invasive disease, the fact that only a few HPV-infected individuals eventually develop cancer (6), and observations of cytogenetic changes (not directly owing to E6/E7 expression) in invasive cervical tumors (48,49).

IV. MECHANISMS BY WHICH HIV MAY BE ASSOCIATED WITH INCREASED RISK OF HPV-RELATED NEOPLASIA

The malignancies that are associated with HIV infection are induced primarily by viruses that have established persistent infections, with Epstein–Barr virus, human herpesvirus type 8, and human papillomavirus being associated with lymphoma, Kaposi's sarcoma, and anogenital tract squamous cell cancers, respectively (Table 1). Although it is commonly thought that HIV-induced alterations of both systemic and local cell-mediated immunity result in uncontrolled expression of previously or newly acquired HPV infection (50–54), the specific immune functions involved in the control of HPV that are disrupted by HIV, are unknown. Among homosexual men, the presence of cell-associated HIV in the anal canal is associated with persistent HPV detection independent of generalized immunosuppression as measured by the CD4 cell count (55). This lends further support to the hypothesis that local immune dysfunction is important in development of epithelial neoplasia. The large numbers of germinal centers within lymphoid follicles commonly present in the submucosa of the lower rectum (56) normally contain antigen-presenting cells. These aggregates of lymphoid tissue within the anal canal are likely to be the initial site of HIV infection in many homosexual men, with many of the antigen-presenting cells probably infected early in the course of HIV infection. The decreased presence of Langerhans cells, which is associated with HIV infection (57–59), is also correlated with the increased presence and severity of HPV-related lesions (60–63). Langerhans cells are the principal antigen-presenting (dendritic) cells in the squamous epithelium of the anus and lower genital tract. When they are expressing HIV, they are unable to present other antigens to effect T-cell activation (58,64). Although it would be of interest to compare the cytotoxic T-lymphocyte response directed against HPV among HIV-seropositive and HIV-seronegative individuals, such data are not yet available.

Active HIV gene expression may affect the development of squamous cell cancer and its precursor lesions by acting directly on HPV, resulting in increased HPV expression and increased prevalence of squamous intraepithelial lesions. An in vitro study by Vernon et al. (65) examined the hypothesis that HIV might directly up-regulate HPV by studying the effect of HIV-1 Tat protein on gene expression directed by the HPV upstream regulatory region (URR) of HPV-16. They reported that HPV-16 URR-directed chloramphenicol acetyltransferase (CAT) expression, driven by the HPV-16 promoter (P_{97}) was increased in the presence of HIV-1 Tat protein and that this protein reversed E2-mediated repression of P_{97}-directed CAT expression. Furthermore, in vitro studies have shown that intracellular HIV-1 *tat* mRNA can transactivate HPV-16 E6 and E7 (66), which is important in the development of squamous cell cancers. Thus, it is possible that extracellular Tat migrates from Langerhans cells or other HIV-infected mononuclear cells that abut HPV-infected epithelial cells and up-regulate HPV.

Although HIV might increase risk of squamous cell neoplasia by maintaining or prolonging expression of HPV by one of the foregoing mechanisms, HIV is independently associated with risk of high-grade anal neoplasia, after adjusting for CD4 cell count and other factors associated with both development of anal neoplasia and immunosuppression (e.g., level and specific type of HPV present; 50). This suggests that the effect of HIV on neoplasia risk is not entirely explained by the presence of immunosuppression or by increased expression of HPV. The effect of HIV on risk of intraepithelial neoplasia and invasive cancer may be partly mediated by increased HPV expression, but also by other HPV-related factors, such as the type of HPV-16 variants present, or the occurrence of specific genomic changes resulting from exposure to relevant cofactors.

Given that only few women infected with HPV-16 go on to develop cervical cancer, there has been considerable speculation that different HPV-16 variants might have differing biological behaviors. The first HPV-16 to be cloned (from a cervical cancer in Germany) has been denoted the HPV-16 prototype variant. This variant is commonly used in molecular studies of HPV. Comparison of the long control region (LCR) of the prototype HPV-16 genome to HPV-16s identified in samples from approximately 700 women (most of whom had cancer) from

Table 1 Role of HIV in the Development of Malignancy

Malignancy	Viral etiologic agent	Proposed mechanism of viral pathogenesis	Proposed role of HIV in development of neoplasia		
			HIV-transactivating gene (*tat*)	Immune activation	Compromised immunological surveillance
Lymphoma					
Large cell lymphoma	EBV (minority of cases)	Promotion and maintenance of uncontrolled B-cell growth and differentiation p53 and BCL6 mutations ⇒ alterations in tumor suppressor functions ⇒ increased genomic instability and changes in cell cycle interactions Activation of the *c-myc* oncogene		Stimulation of monocytes and macrophages by HIV ⇒ cytokine release contributing to chronic (uncontrolled) B-cell proliferation	Disregulation of cell-mediated and humoral immunity ⇒ enhanced EBV replication ⇒ polyclonal stimulation and immortalization of B-cell clones subject to *c-myc* gene rearrangements ⇒ fully transformed EBV-containing monoclonal B-cell lymphoma
Primary CNS lymphoma	EBV	Expression of latent EBV genes with transforming potential			Defect in T-cell immunity to EBV
Body-cavity-based lymphoma	HHV-8				Disregulation of cell-mediated and humoral immunity

Kaposi's sarcoma	HHV-8		Tat protein ⇒ initial endothelial cell activation ⇒ cytokine up-regulation and angiogenesis	Cytokines produced by activated immune cells ⇒ production of intra- and extracellular cytokines ⇒ interruption of HIV-1 latency ⇒ increased tat gene expression	Disregulation of cell-mediated and humoral immunity
Squamous cell cervical, anal carcinomas	HPV	HPV E6 and E7 form complexes with p53 and Rb proteins, respectively ⇒ cellular genetic alterations	*tat* gene, with HPV 16 E2 protein ⇒ transactivation of HPV URR ⇒ increased HPV gene expression	Cytokine up-regulation ⇒ chronic proliferation of HPV-containing cells	Disregulation of cell-mediated and humoral immunity, reduced numbers of CD4 and Langerhans cells in the skin ⇒ enhanced HPV replication

various geographic regions throughout the world shows that multiple HPV-16 variants exist and occur in varying frequency among all populations thus far examined (67–70). Several attempts have been made to classify these variants into groups, including assignment to one of five geographically based distinct phylogenetic branches (68,69). Data suggesting that certain HPV variants may alter risk of clinical disease (71–75), include reports of an association between an HPV-16 variant with a base pair change at nucleotide 350 and persistence of detection of HPV DNA (71), and existence of an HPV-18 subtype with apparently decreased oncogenic potential (72). Additionally, HIV-seronegative men and women infected with certain HPV-16 non–prototype-like as compared with prototype-like variants are at greater risk for development of high-grade intraepithelial neoplasia (76,77). Therefore, it may be that differences in certain amino acid sequences might have functional importance for biological properties related to development of malignancy. It is possible, although as yet unproved, that such HPV-16 variants are more common among those with HIV infection, or alternatively, they are selectively up-regulated in the presence of HIV infection. Presently, few published data exist concerning the frequency of variants of HPV-16 in women or men with and without intraepithelial neoplasia or invasive cervical or anal cancer, respectively, either with or without HIV infection.

V. SUMMARY AND CONCLUSIONS

It is likely that HIV contributes to the development of squamous cell cancers and their precursor lesions by mechanisms similar to those involved in the development of the other known HIV-associated malignancies, non–Hodgkin's lymphoma, and Kaposi's sarcoma (summarized and compared in Table 1). For those neoplasias that are associated with oncogenic human viruses, the role of HIV most probably involves an immunosuppressive effect and interference with immune-mediated tumor surveillance, resulting in the unopposed proliferation of virus-infected cells. However, one cannot rule out that HIV-1, through its regulatory protein Tat, might also have a direct promoting effect on some lesions, particularly Kaposi's sarcoma or squamous cell carcinoma. In addition, further studies are required to investigate intriguing preliminary data suggesting that certain variants of oncogenic HPV types, particularly HPV-16, which may also be associated with HIV infection, are characterized by genomic changes that are related to development of malignancy. Given the recent observed increases in the survival time of patients following an AIDS diagnosis, the incidence of AIDS-related malignancies, including cervical cancer, would be expected to increase. As our knowledge of the pathogenesis of these malignancies increases, it is hoped that increasingly effective therapeutic strategies will be developed.

ACKNOWLEDGMENT

Supported by grants from the National Cancer Institute (CA-50738, CA-55488).

REFERENCES

1. Parkin DM, Laara E, Muir CS. Estimates of the worldwide frequency of sixteen major cancers in 1980. Int J Cancer 41:184–197, 1988.
2. Lorincz AT, Reid R. Jenson AB, Cullen A, Greenberg MD, Lancaster WD, Kurman RJ. Human papillomavirus infection of the cervix: relative risk associations of fifteen common anogenital types. Obstet Gynecol 79:328–337, 1992.
3. zur Hausen H. Human genital cancers: synergism between two virus infections or synergism between a virus infection and initiating events? Lancet 2:1370–1372, 1982.
4. zur Hausen H. The role of papillomaviruses in anogenital cancer. Scand J Infect Dis 69:107–111, 1990.
5. zur Hausen H. Human papillomaviruses in the pathogenesis of anogenital cancer. Virology 184:9–13, 1991.
6. Kiviat NB, Critchlow CW, Kurman RJ. Reassessment of the morphologic continuum of cervical intraepithelial lesions: does it reflect different stages in the progression to cervical carcinoma? In: Munoz N, Bosch FX, eds. Human Papilloma Virus and Cervical Cancer. Lyons: IARC, 1992:59–66.
7. ter-Meulen J, Eberhardt HC, Luande J, Mgaya HN, Chang-Claude J, Mtiro H, Mhina M, Kashaija P, Ockert S, Yu X, Meinhardt G, Gissmann L, Pawlita M. Human papillomavirus (HPV) infection, HIV infection and cervical cancer in Tanzania, East Africa. Int J Cancer 51:515–521, 1992.
8. Johnson JC, Burnett AF, Willet GD, Young MA, Doniger J. High frequency of latent and clinical human papillomavirus cervical infections in immunocompromised human immunodeficiency virus-infected women. Obstet Gynecol 79:321–327, 1992.
9. St Louis ME, Icenogle JP, Manzila T, Kamenga M, Ryder RW, Heyward WL, Reeves WC. Genital types of papillomavirus in children of women with HIV-1 infection in Kinshasa, Zaire. Int J Cancer 54;181–184, 1993.
10. Sun X-W, Kuhn L, Ellerbrock TV, Chiasson MA, Bush TJ, Wright TC. Human papillomavirus infection in women infected with the human immunodeficiency virus. N Engl J Med 337:1343–1349, 1997.
11. Sun X-W, Ellerbrock TV, Lungu O, Chiasson MA, Bush TJ, Wright TC Jr. Human papillomavirus infection in human immunodeficiency virus seropositive women. Obstet Gynecol 85(5 pt 1):680–686, 1995.
12. Van Doornum GJ, Van den Hoek JA, Van Ameijden EJ, Van Haastrecht HJ, Roos MT, Henquet CJ, Quint WG, Coutinho RA. Cervical HPV infection among HIV-infected prostitutes addicted to hard drugs. J Med Virol 41:185–190, 1993.

13. Williams AB, Darragh TM, Vranizan K, Ochia C, Moss A, Palefsky JM. Anal and cervical epithelial abnormalities in human immunodeficiency virus-infected women. Obstet Gynecol 82:205–211, 1994.
14. Coll-Seck A, Awa Faye M, Critchlow CW, Mbaye AD, Kuypers J, Woto-Gaye G, Langley C, Benga De E, Holmes KK, Kiviat NB. Cervical intraepithelial neoplasia and human papillomavirus infection among Senegalese women seropositive for HIV-1 or HIV-2 or seronegative for HIV. Int J Sex Transm Dis AIDS 5:189–193, 1994.
15. Kreiss JK, Kiviat NB, Plummer FA, Roberts PL, Waiyaki P, Ngugi E, Holmes KK. Human immunodeficiency virus, human papillomavirus, and cervical intraepithelial neoplasia in Nairobi prostitutes. Sex Transm Dis 19:54–59, 1992.
16. Laga M, Icenogle JP, Marsella R, Monoka AT, Nzila N, Ryder RW, Vermund SH, Heyward WL, Nelson A, Reeves WC. Genital papillomavirus infection and cervical dysplasia—opportunistic complications of HIV infection. Int J Cancer 50:45–48, 1992.
17. Vermund SH, Kelley KF, Klein RS, Feingold AR, Schreiber K, Munk G, Burk RD. High risk of human papillomavirus infection and cervical squamous intraepithelial lesions among women with symptomatic human immunodeficiency virus infection. Am J Obstet Gynecol 165:392–400, 1991.
18. Feingold AR, Vermund SH, Burk RD, Kelley KF, Schrager LW, Schreiber K, Munk G, Friedland GH, Klein RS. Cervical cytologic abnormalities and papillomavirus in women infected with human immunodeficiency virus. J Acquir Immune Defic Syndr 3:896–903, 1990.
19. Spinillo A, Tenti P, Zappatore R, Barbarini G, Maccabruni A, Carrata L, Guaschino S. Prevalence, diagnosis and treatment of lower genital neoplasia in women with human immunodeficiency virus infection. Eur J Obstet Gynecol Reprod Biol 43:235–241, 1992.
20. Rellihan MA, Dooley DP, Burke TW, Berkland ME, Longfield RN. Rapidly progressing cervical cancer in a patient with human immunodeficiency virus infection. Gynecol Oncol 36:435–438, 1990.
21. Smith JK, Kitchen VS, Botcherby M, Hepburn M, Wells C, Gor D, Forster SM, Harris JR, Steer P, Mason P. Is HIV infection associated with an increase in the prevalence of cervical neoplasia? Br J Obstet Gynaecol 100:149–153, 1993.
22. Langley CL, Benga-De E, Critchlow CW, Ndoye I, Mbengue-Ly MD, Kuypers J, Woto-Gaye G, Mboup S, Bergeron C, Holmes KK, Kiviat NB. HIV 1, HIV 2, human papillomavirus infection and cervical neoplasia in high risk African women. AIDS 10:413–417, 1996.
23. Wright TC Jr, Ellerbrock TV, Chiasson MA, Van Devanter N, Sun XW. Cervical intraepithelial neoplasia in women infected with human immunodeficiency virus: prevalence, risk factors, and validity of Papanicolaou smears. Obstet Gynecol 84:591–597, 1994.
24. Rabkin CS, Biggar RJ, Baptiste MS, Abe T, Kohler BA, Nasca PC. Cancer incidence trends in women at high risk of human immunodeficiency virus (HIV) infection. Int J Cancer 55:208–212, 1993.
25. Grant AD, Djomand G, De Cock KM. Natural history and spectrum of disease in adults with HIV/AIDS in Africa. AIDS 11(suppl B):S43–S54, 1997.

26. Centers for Disease Control and Prevention. HIV/AIDS Surveillance Report. 9:12–17, 1997.
27. Goedert JJ, Coté TR, Virgo P, Scoppa SM, Kingma DW, Gail MH, Jaffe ES, Biggar RJ. Spectrum of AIDS-associated malignant disorders. Lancet 351:1833–1839, 1998.
28. Shah KV, Howley PM. Papillomaviruses. In: Fields BN, Knipe DM, Howley PM, Chanock RM, Melnick JL, Monath TP, Roizman B, Straus SE, eds. Fields Virology. 3rd ed. Philadelphia: Lippincott–Raven, 1996:2077–2109.
29. Howley PM. Papillomavirinae: the viruses and their replication. In: Fields BN, Knipe DM, Howley PM, Chanock RM, Melnick JL, Monath TP, Roizman B, Straus SE, eds. Fields Virology. 3rd ed. Philadelphia: Lippincott Raven, 1996:2045–2076.
30. Koutsky L. Epidemiology of genital human papillomavirus infection. Am J Med 102:3–8, 1997.
31. Ho GY, Bierman R, Beardsley L, Chang CJ, Burk RD. Natural history of cervicovaginal papillomavirus infection in young women. N Engl J Med 338:423–428, 1998.
32. Burk RD, Kelly P, Feldman J, Bromberg J, Vermund SH, DeHovitz JA, Landesman SH. Declining prevalence of cervicovaginal human papillomavirus infection with age is independent of other risk factors. Sex Transm Dis 23:333–341, 1996.
33. Ferenczy A. Epidemiology and clinical pathophysiology of condylomata acuminata. Am J Obstet Gynecol 172(4 suppl):1331–1339, 1995.
34. Fletcher S, Norval M. On the nature of the deep cellular disturbances in human papillomavirus infection of squamous cervical epithelium. Lancet 2:546–549, 1983.
35. Schoenfeld A, Ziv E. Levavi H, Samra Z, Ovadia J. Laser versus loop electrosurgical excision in vulvar condyloma for eradication of subclinical reservoir demonstrated by assay for 2'5' oligosynthetase human papillomavirus. Gynecol Obstet Invest 40:46–51, 1995.
36. Bauman NM, Smith RJ. Recurrent respiratory papillomatosis. Pediatr Clin North Am 43:1385–1401, 1996.
37. Luchtefeld MA. Perianal condylomata acuminata. Surg Clin North Am 74:1327–1338, 1994.
38. Frisch M, Glimelius B, van den Brule AJC, Wohlfahrt J, Meijer CJLM, Walboomers JMM, Goldman S, Svensson C, Adami H-O, Melbye M. Sexually transmitted infection as a cause of anal cancer. N Engl J Med 337:1350–1358, 1997.
39. Daling JR, Sherman KJ. Relationship between human papillomavirus infection and tumours of anogenital sites other than the cervix. In: Munoz N, Bosch FX, Shah KV, Meheus A, eds. The Epidemiology of Human Papillomavirus and Cervical Cancer (IARC Scientific Publications No. 119). Lyon: IARC, 1992:223–241.
40. Chua KL, Hjerpe A. Persistence of human papillomavirus (HPV) infections preceding cervical carcinoma. Cancer 77:121–127, 1996.
41. Koutsky LA, Holmes KK, Critchlow CW, Stevens CE, Paavonen J, Beckmann AM, DeRouen TA, Galloway DA, Vernon D, Kiviat NB. Incidence of cervical intraepithelial neoplasia grade 2 or 3 among a cohort of women with negative cervical cytologic smears: role of human papillomavirus infection and other risk factors. N Engl J Med 327:1272–1278, 1992.
42. Remmink AJ, Walboomers JM, Helmerhorst TJ, Voorhorst FJ, Rozendaal L, Risse EK, Meijer CJ, Kenemans P. The presence of persistent high-risk HPV genotypes

in dysplastic cervical lesions is associated with progressive disease: natural history up to 36 months. Int J Cancer 61:306–311, 1995.

43. Munger K, Phelps WC, Bubb V, Howley PM, Schlegel R. The E6 and E7 genes of the human papillomavirus together are necessary and sufficient for transformation of primary human keratinocytes. J Virol 63:4417–4421, 1989.

44. Scheffner M, Werness BA, Huibregtse JM, Levine AJ, Howley PM. The E6 oncoprotein encoded by human papillomavirus 16 and 18 promotes the degradation of p53. Cell 63:1129–1136, 1990.

45. Dyson N, Howley PM, Munger K, Harlow E. The human papillomavirus-16 E7 oncoprotein is able to bind the retinoblastoma gene product. Science 243:934–937, 1989.

46. Scheffner M, Romanczuk H, Munger K, Huibregtse JM, Mietz JA, Howley PM. Functions of human papillomavirus proteins. Curr Top Microbiol Immunol 186:83–99, 1994.

47. McDougall JK. Immortalization and transformation of human cells by HPV. Curr Top Microbiol Immunol 186:101–119, 1994.

48. Atkin NB, Baker MC. Non-random chromosome changes in carcinoma of the cervix uteri. I. Nine near diploid tumors. Cancer Genet Cytogenet 7:209–222, 1982.

49. Teyssier JR. The chromosomal analysis of human solid tumors: a triple challenge. Cancer Genet Cytogenet 37:103–125, 1989.

50. Critchlow CW, Surawicz CM, Holmes KK, Kuypers J, Daling JR, Hawes SE, Goldbaum GM, Sayer J, Hurt C, Dunphy C, Kiviat NB. Prospective study of high grade anal squamous intraepithelial neoplasia in a cohort of homosexual men: influence of HIV infection, immunosuppression and human papillomavirus infection. AIDS 9:1255–1262, 1995.

51. Array I, Tyring SK. Status of local cellular immunity in interferon-responsive and nonresponsive human papillomavirus-associated lesions. Sex Transm Dis 23:475–480, 1996.

52. McArdle JP, Mueller K. Quantitative assessment of Langerhans cells in human cervical extraepithelial neoplasia and wart virus infection. Am J Obstet Gynecol 154:509–515, 1986.

53. Koutsky LA, Galloway DA, Holmes KK. Epidemiology of genital human papillomavirus infection. Epidemiol Rev 10:122–163, 1988.

54. Schneider A. Pathogenesis of genital HPV infection. Genitourin Med 69:165–173, 1993.

55. Critchlow CW, Hawes SE, Kuypers JM, Goldbaum GM, Holmes KK, Surawicz CM, Kiviat NB. Effect of HIV infection on the natural history of anal human papillomavirus infection. AIDS 12:1177–1184, 1998.

56. Quinn TC, Goodell SE, Mkrtichian E, Schuffler MD, Wang SP, Stamm WE, Holmes KK. *Chlamydia trachomatis* proctitis. N Engl J Med 305:195–200, 1981.

57. Kanitakis J, Misery L, Nicolas JF, Lyonnet S, Chouvet B, Haftek M, Faure M, Claudy A, Thivolet J. Disseminated superficial porokeratosis in a patient with AIDS. Br J Dermatol 131:284–289, 1994.

58. Knight SC, Macatonia SE, Patterson S. HIV-1 infection of dendritic cells. Int Rev Immunol 6:163–175, 1990.

59. Weier S, Muller H, Stutte HJ, Kapps R, Berger S, Shah PM. Lymphocytes, Langer-

hans cells and CD-68-positive monocytes/macrophages in the skin of HIV-infected patients and normal controls. Verh Dtsch Ges Pathol 75:114–118, 1991.

60. Spinillo A, Tenti P, Zappatore R, DeSeta F, Silini E, Guaschino S. Langerhans' cell counts and cervical intraepithelial neoplasia in women with human immunodeficiency virus infection. Gynecol Oncol 48:210–213, 1993.

61. Lehtinen M, Rantala I, Toivonen A, Luoto H, Aine R, Lauslahti K, Yla Outinen A, Romppanen U, Paavonen J. Depletion of Langerhans cells in cervical HPV infection is associated with replication of the virus. APMIS 101:833–837, 1993.

62. Tay SK, Jenkins D, Maddox P, Campion M, Singer A. Subpopulations of Langerhans' cells in cervical neoplasia. Br J Obstet Gynaecol 94:10–15, 1987.

63. Hughes RG, Norval M, Howie SE. Expression of major histocompatibility class II antigens by Langerhans' cells in cervical intraepithelial neoplasia. J Clin Pathol 41: 253–259, 1998.

64. Knight SC, Macatonia SE, Patterson S. Infection of dendritic cells with HIV-1: virus load regulates stimulation and suppression of T-cell activity. Res Virol 144:75–80, 1993.

65. Vernon SD, Hart CE, Reeves WC, Icenogle JP. The HIV-1 tat protein enhances E2-dependent human papillomavirus 16 transcription. Virus Res 27:133–145, 1993.

66. Tornesselo ML, Buonguro FM, Beth Giraldo E, Giraldo G. Human immunodeficiency virus type 1 tat gene enhances human papillomavirus early gene expression. Intervirology 36:57–64, 1993.

67. Xi LF, Demers GW, Koutsky LA, Kiviat NB, Kuypers J, Watts DH, Holmes KK, Galloway DA. Analysis of human papillomavirus type 16 variants indicates establishment of persistent infection. J Infect Dis 172:747–55, 1995.

68. Ho L, Chan S, Burk RD, Das BC, Fujinaga K, Icenogle JP, Kahn T, Kiviat N, Lancaster W, Mavromara P, Mitrani-Rosenbaum S, Norrild B, Pillai MR, Stoerker J, Syrjaenen K, Syrjaenen S, Tay S, Villa LL, Wheeler CM, Williamson A, Bernard H. The genetic drift of human papillomavirus type 16 is a means of reconstructing prehistoric viral spread and the movement of ancient human populations. J Virol 67:6413–6423, 1993.

69. Chan SY, Ho L, Ong CK, Chow V, Drescher B, Durst M, ter Meulen J, Villa L, Luande F, Mgaya HN, Bernard HU. Molecular variants of human papillomavirus type 16 from four continents suggest ancient pandemic spread of the virus and its coevolution with humankind. J Virol 66:2057–2066, 1992.

70. Yamada T, Manos M, Peto J, Greer CE, Munoz N, Bosch FX, Wheeler CM. Human papillomavirus type 16 sequence variation in cervical cancers: a worldwide perspective. J Virol 71:2463–2472, 1997.

71. Londesborough P, Ho L, Terry G, Cuzick J, Wheeler C, Singer A. Human papillomavirus genotype as a predictor of persistence and development of high grade lesions in women with minor cervical abnormalities. Int J Cancer 69:364–368, 1996.

72. Hecht JL, Kadish S, Jiang G, Burk RD. Genetic characterization of the human papillomavirus (HPV) 18 E2 gene in clinical specimens suggests the presence of a subtype with decreased oncogenic potential. Int J Cancer 60:369–376, 1995.

73. Ellis JRM, Keating PJ, Baird J, Hounsell EF, Renouf DV, Rowe M, Hopkins MF, Duggan-Keen ME, Bartholomew JS, Young LS, Stern PL. The association of an

HPV-16 oncogene variant with HLA-B7 has implications for vaccine design in cervical cancer. Nat Med 1:464–470, 1995.

74. Bavin PJ, Walker PG, Emery VC. Sequence microheterogeneity in the long control region of clinical isolates of human papillomavirus type 16. J Med Virol 39:267–272, 1993.

75. May M, Dong XP, Stubenrauch F, Fuchs PG, Pfister H, The E6/E7 promoter of extrachromosomal HPV16 DNA in cervical cancers escapes from cellular repression by mutation of target sequences for YY1. EMBO J 13:1460–1466, 1994.

76. Xi L-F, Critchlow CW, Wheeler CM, Koutsky LA, Galloway DA, Kuypers J, Hughes JP, Hawes SE, Surawicz C, Goldbaum G, Holmes KK, Kiviat NB. Risk of anal carcinoma in situ in relation to human papillomavirus type 16 variants. Cancer Res 58:3839–3844, 1998.

77. Xi LF, Koutsky LA, Galloway DA, Kuypers J, Hughes JP, Wheeler CM, Holmes KK, Kiviat NB. Genomic variation of human papillomavirus type 16 and risk for high grade cervical intraepithelial neoplasia. J Natl Cancer Inst 89:796–802, 1997.

11

Non–AIDS-Defining Cancers in the HIV-Infected Patient

Emanuela Vaccher and Umberto Tirelli
Aviano Cancer Center, Aviano, Italy

I. INTRODUCTION

The full spectrum of human immunodeficiency virus (HIV)-induced malignancies has not been fully elucidated, but a large variety of cancers other than acquired immunodeficiency syndrome (AIDS)-defining tumors have been diagnosed in HIV-infected individuals (1–8).

Prospective epidemiological studies have recently demonstrated an increased risk of some non–AIDS-defining tumors, including Hodgkin's disease (HD), anal carcinoma, oropharyngeal malignancy, testicular carcinoma, multiple myeloma, and melanoma (7,8). The statistical power of these studies is low because of the small number of patients with cancer; thus, the evidence for a relation between these tumors and HIV infection is still a matter of controversy.

With the improved survival of patients with HIV infection as a result of advances in both antibiotic prophylaxis and antiretroviral therapy, it is likely that non–AIDS-defining tumors will occur with greater frequency (6). Regardless of epidemiology, however, the natural history of most non–AIDS-defining tumors is altered in the setting of HIV infection. Moreover, the diagnosis of a non–AIDS-defining malignancy may be very difficult in HIV-infected patients, because symptoms and radiologic abnormalities of cancer may coincide with those of more common opportunistic infections (OI) or HIV infection itself.

This chapter reviews the pathology, clinical features, and treatment of the most frequently reported non–AIDS-defining tumors (i.e., HD, testicular, and lung cancers).

II. HODGKIN'S DISEASE

Hodgkin's disease represents the second most common type of non–AIDS-defining tumor. More than 400 cases of HD in HIV-infected individuals have been reported; namely, from the European countries (i.e., Italy, Spain, and France) and, to a smaller extent, from the United States (7–18). All series have documented an unusually more aggressive tumor behavior than in the general population, including higher frequency of unfavorable histological subtypes, advanced stages, and poorer therapeutic outcome.

A. Pathology and Pathogenesis

In the pathological spectrum of HIV-uninfected HD, or non-HIV HD, four histological groups may be identified, based on the Rye modification of the Lukes and Butler classification (19): (1) a major subset, including nodular sclerosis (NS) subtype (50–60% of cases); (2) a second subset consisting of mixed cellularity (MC) subtype (20–25% of cases), along with the smaller group of lymphocytic depletion (LD) subtype (3–6% of cases); and (3) a minor subset, including lymphocyte prevalence subtype (LP; 6–10% of cases), which seems to be a phenotypically distinct disease. A high rate of misdiagnosis of LD subtype occurs because the precise border between LD and MC subtypes and some non–Hodgkin's lymphoma (NHL) is not easily defined (20).

Serraino et al. (21) documented, for the first time, a significant difference in the distribution of HD histological subtypes in HIV-infected patients as compared with "primary" HD. The Italian research team found that in HIV-infected patients, the frequency of the two main subsets (i.e., NS subtype and MC plus LD subtypes) is reversed. In particular, they documented a 4-fold higher frequency of MC subtype and approximately 12-fold higher frequency of LD subtype among HIV-infected patients (Table 1). In all series, however, there is a high prevalence of MC subtype, ranging from 41 to 100%, as well as LD subtype (4–22%), with a relative decrease in NS subtype (22–50%; 9–18). The relative excess of these two subtypes compared with NS disease, may either represent a shift to these histological types, or an absolute increase.

Histologically, HD is characterized by a polymorphous admixture of cytologically abnormal cells (i.e., Reed-Sternberg [RS] cells and their mononuclear variants) and by a variety of apparently normal reactive elements. Distinct nodules and collagen band formation is required for diagnosing NS subtype, whereas lymph node biopsies characterized by increased fibrohistiocytoid stromal cells arranged in bundles is classified as MC subtype. The occurrence of nonlymphoid stromal cells (i.e., fibrohistiocytoid cells) in place of depleting lymphocytes appears to be the distinctive morphological feature of HIV HD (14). Tumors are classified as LD subtype in the presence of diagnostic features for either diffuse

Table 1 Number of Observed and Expected Cases of Hodgkin's Disease According to Histological Subtype Among 89 Patients with HIV Infection

		Case series from Europe and US		Case series from Italy	
	Observed (O)	Expected (E)	O/E ratio (95% CI)	Expected (E)	O/E ratio (95% CI)
Histological subtypes					
Lymphocyte predominance	1	6.4	0.2 (0.0–0.5)	7.8	0.1 (0.0–0.4)
Nodular sclerosis	19	55.6	0.3 (0.2–0.5)	68.2	0.3 (0.2–0.4)
Mixed cellularity	49	24.2	2.0 (1.5–2.6)	12.2	4.0 (2.9–5.1)
Lymphocyte depletion	20	2.8	7.1 (4.0–10.3)	1.6	12.5 (7.0–18.0)

Source: Ref. 7.

fibrosis or reticular subtype (22). In immunogenotypical characteristics, HIV HD is similar to primary HD, because in both groups no uniform evidence of B- or T-cell clonal expansion has been demonstrated by Southern blot analysis (11).

The biological basis and the molecular genetics underlying the pathogenesis of HD are still unclear. However, a pathogenetic role of Epstein–Barr virus (EBV) has been supposed on the basis of the high frequency of EBV genome demonstration. Virological studies, by the combined use of immunohistochemical detection of EBV-encoded latent membrane protein-1 (LMP-1), in situ hybridization, and southern blot analysis show that HIV HD cases are more closely associated with EBV than are primary HD cases. In particular, a significantly higher frequency of cases with RS cells that are positive for LMP-1 expression was observed among HD tissue from HIV-infected patients compared with those in HIV-uninfected individuals (78 versus 25%, p < 0.001; Table 2; 11,22–25). However, the increase of EBV genome expression in HIV HD may be partly related to the higher frequency of the MC subtype in these individuals. EBV association is stronger with the aggressive MC and LD subtypes than with the other subtypes.

The possible etiologic role of EBV in the large majority of HIV HD cases is also supported by the detection of monoclonal EBV genomes in all EBV-positive cases analyzed. This finding indicates that a monoclonal expansion of EBV-carrying cells is present, which is probably responsible for the induction and the persistence of the disease in an active state (11).

Table 2 EBV Association as Detected by Immunohistochemistry
for Latent Membrane Protein-1 (LMP-1) Expression in Patients
with Hodgkin's Disease (18 with and 104 Without HIV Infection)

Histology	LMP-1+	
	HIV+	HIV−
Lymphocyte predominance	0/18	0/12
Nodular sclerosis	1/4	10/61
Mixed cellularity	4/4	16/29
Lymphocyte depletion	8/9	1/2
Unclassifiable	1/1	–
Total	14/18 (78%)	27/104 (25%)*

* $p < 0.001$
Source: Ref. 11.

Recently, two types of EBV, which show differences in the sequence en-
coding for EBV-encoded nuclear antigens 2, 3, 4, and 6, have been described
(26). A different distribution of EBV genotypes in HIV HD tissue compared with
primary EBV-positive HD tissue was found. Type 2 EBV, which has a reduced
transforming potential relative to type 1 EBV, was detected in 50% of HIV-
positive HD tissue, but in only 4% of EBV-positive, HIV-negative HD cases
(11). These findings indicate that in the setting of HIV infection, type 2 EBV
also may be pathogenetically involved in the induction of HD, as previously
reported for HIV-related non–Hodgkin's lymphoma (NHL).

In the general population HD may exhibit considerable morphological resemblance to CD30/Ki1-positive anaplastic large cell lymphoma (ALCL). Moreover, both conditions shared several phenotypic and genotypic features, and the
existence of a continuum between these two neoplastic lesions has been suggested. The overlapping phenotypic features of HD and ALCL include the expression of the CD30 molecule and of other activation antigens, the inconsistent expression of T- or B-lineage antigens, and the production of specific cytokines
such as interleukin-9 (IL-9). In addition, HIV HD shows a high frequency of
EBV association and EBV latent antigenic phenotype similar to that seen in HIV
CD30/Kil-positive ALCL. Therefore, both these lymphomas may represent a
continuum of a single, EBV-related disease process also in the HIV setting (22).

B. Clinical Features

One of the most peculiar features of HIV HD is the widespread extent of the
disease at presentation and the frequency of systemic ''B'' symptoms, including

fever, night sweats, and weight loss of more than 10% of the normal body weight. At the time of diagnosis 70–96% of the patients have B symptoms and 74–92% have advanced disease (state III–IV according to Ann Arbor staging classification), with frequent involvement of extranodal sites, the most common being bone marrow, liver and spleen (Table 3). These features are in sharp contrast to primary HD in which B symptoms and advanced stages are seen in approximately 30–60% and 20–50% of cases, respectively (9–18). In the Italian series (the largest published so far) 77 and 81% of HIV-infected patients had systemic symptoms and stage III–IV disease, respectively, as compared with 35 and 44% in a group of 104 patients with primary HD diagnosed at the same institution (11).

In HIV-uninfected patients, HD typically involves contiguous lymph node groups, and dissemination and infiltration of extranodal sites are late occurrences. In HIV-infected patients noncontiguous spread of tumor may be observed (i.e., liver involvement without spleen disease; lung involvement without mediastinal adenopathy), and extranodal disease has been described in approximately 60% of cases at presentation. Bone marrow involvement is common, occurring in 40–50% of patients, and it may be the first indication of the presence of HD in approximately 20% of cases (9–14,18,27). The liver involvement develops in 15–40% of the patients, whereas the spleen is involved in approximately 20% of the patients (9–14,18). In contrast with HIV NHL, in HIV HD unusual sites of disease are extremely rare, few case reports having central nervous system, skin, rectum, tongue, and lung involvement (18).

Another distinctive feature of HIV HD is the lower frequency of mediastinal adenopathy, as compared with primary HD. Overall, the absence of mediastinal disease ranges from 77 to 87% in HIV-infected patients versus only 29–42% of HIV-negative control cases (9–14). In the Italian series, this difference was significant in patients with NS subtype (27% in HIV-positive versus 80% in HIV-negative patients; $p < 0.001$), but it was not in patients with MC histology (11).

C. Diagnosis

Hodgkin's diseases tends to develop as early manifestation of HIV infection with a median CD4 cell count, ranging from 275 to 306/μL (9–14).

At the time of diagnosis most patients with HD have persistent generalized lymphadenopathy (PGL; 65% of cases in the Italian series), and in approximately 50% of cases the lymphoma may be concurrently present with PGL in the same lymph node group (11,28). Hodgkin's disease may be clinically confused with PGL, therefore an increase in size of a preexistent adenopathy in patients with PGL should be evaluated with a biopsy. In particular cases, the initial diagnostic workup may also require lymph node biopsies at multiple sites. On the other hand, clinicians should recognize the possibility that HIV-positive patients will be overstaged with computed tomography (CT) scan of the abdomen as well as

Table 3 Clinical Features of 265 Patients with Hodgkin's Disease and HIV Infection

Clinical features	Knowles (12) No. (%)	Ree (14) No. (%)	Ames (13) No. (%)	Rubio (9) No. (%)	Levy (10) No. (%)	Tirelli (11) No. (%)
No. of patients	13	24	23	46	45	114
B symptoms	11 (85)	24 (100)	16 (70)	38 (83)	36 (80)	78ᵃ(77)
Stage						
I–II	1	2	6	5	11 (24)	21 (18)
III–IV	12 (92)	21 (91)	17 (74)	41 (89)	34 (76)	87 (76)
Extranodal involvement	9 (69)	12 (50)	17 (74)	23 (50)	15 (33)	72 (63)
Bone marrow	8 (62)	12 (50)	12 (52)	19 (41)	12 (27)	45 (39)
Liver	2 (15)	2ᵇ	9 (39)	6 (13)	7 (16)	25 (22)
Spleen	—	4ᵇ	12 (52)	—	1	40 (35)
Other	1	—	2	—	(CNSᶜ)	—
	(Lung)		(Tongue/bone)			

ᵃ Referred to 101 patients.
ᵇ Referred to 4 patients.
ᶜ Central nervous system.

lymphogram, owing to the presence of PGL in retroperitoneal lymph nodes (29). The chest x-ray film in PGL patients is negative for hilar or mediastinal adenopathy (29,30).

The diagnosis of HD can be made only by histologically examination of the tissue obtained by incisional or excisional biopsy. Needle aspiration of lymph nodes is inadequate for diagnosis, because it is not usually possible to subclassify the disease among the lymphomas with the limited amounts of biopsy material provided. Staging evaluation of patients should include a bone marrow biopsy; CT of the chest, abdomen and pelvis; and other tests if clinically indicated.

Systemic symptoms are frequently associated with both advanced HIV infection and OI. Thus these symptoms mandate a careful evaluation to exclude other causes, including the presence of tuberculosis, cryptococcosis, or cytomegalovirus infection.

D. Prognosis

Primary HD is considered a potentially curable tumor, the disease-free survival (DFS) being more than 70% at 10 years (31). HIV HD shows a significantly poorer outcome, with overall survival ranging from 8 to 20 months (9–18). Nevertheless, in HIV setting some prognostic factors for survival have also been identified, and some patients can obtain long-term survival and possible cure with appropriate antineoplastic therapy (10,11).

The classic prognostic criteria of the general population (i.e., stage, bulky disease, bone marrow involvement, inguinal node involvement, older age [> 40 years], high lactate dehydrogenase [LDH] level, high erythrocyte sedimentation rate, and anemia; 32) have to be supplemented by host prognostic criteria in the HIV setting (i.e., low CD4 cell count and prior AIDS diagnosis, both of which reflect the underlying immunodeficiency). In the Italian series, statistically significant predictors for survival included achievement of a complete response (CR), absence of prior AIDS diagnosis, and CD4 cell count of more than 250/μL. The median survival of patients achieving a CR was 58 months, whereas median survival of the remaining patients was 11 months (p < 0.001). The median survival of patients without or with AIDS diagnosis was 20 and 7 months, respectively (p < 0.001). Patients with CD4 cell count of more than 250/μL had a median survival of 38 months, whereas, patients who had CD4 cell count of 250/μL or fewer had a median survival of 11 months (p < 0.002; 11).

E. Treatment

Optimal therapy for HIV HD has not yet been defined. Combination chemotherapy (CT), with or without radiation therapy (RT), is the standard treatment for advanced stages or bulky primary HD (31). The response of HIV HD to conventional CT regimens (i.e., MOPP [mechlorethamine, vincristine, procarbazine, and prednisone]), MOPP alternating or followed by ABVD (doxorubicin, bleomycin, vinblastine, and dacarbazine) with or without RT, remains poorer than that of primary HD. Moreover, the therapy of HIV HD, as well as of other HIV tumors, presents many problems. The main one is represented by immunosuppression, induced by antineoplastic treatment, that can further compromise immunocellular deficit of HIV-infected patients, and can facilitate the onset of OI or the evolution of the viral infection itself. Finally, leukopenia, frequently present in these patients owing to previous therapy with zidovudine or to HIV-related dysmyelopoiesis, often makes conventional dosage of CT difficult to administer.

Retrospective evaluation of 46 patients treated with MOPP, MOPP alternating or followed by ABVD (23 patients in both groups), with or without RT, was performed within the Italian Cooperative Group on AIDS and Tumors (GICAT). The findings of this study show a higher CR rate (68 versus 41%) and a lower OI rate during therapy and follow-up (38 versus 73%) in the patients treated with MOPP and ABVD compared with those treated with MOPP alone (Table 4; 11).

The first prospective treatment trial was reported by Errante et al. (33),

Table 4   Response to Standard Therapy in Patients with Hodgkin's Disease and HIV Infection

	MOPP[a] + RT		MOPP[a]–ABVD[b]	
	No.	%	No.	%
No. of assessable patients	17/23	74	19/23	83
No. of cycles				
Median	5		6	
Range	1–7		2–11	
Response				
CR	7/17	41	13/19	68
PR	10/17	59	6/19	32
Initial CD4+ count/µL				
Median	345		252	
Range	9–829		9–842	
OI follow-up	11/15	73	5/13	38
Median follow-up (mo)	10		12	

[a] Mechlorethamine (nitrogen mustard), vincristine, procarbazine, and prednisone.
[b] Doxorubicin, bleomycin, vinblastine, and dacarbazine.
Source: Ref. 11.

with a combination of EBV (epirubicin, bleomycin, and vinblastine), an ABVD-like regimen, and zidovudine. In this trial 17 consecutive patients were stratified in two groups based on the presence or absence of prognostic factors. Patients with an Eastern Cooperative Oncology Group performance status of 3 or more or previous OI were treated with a 50% reduced dose of EBV, whereas patients without these factors were eligible for full-dose CT. This study demonstrated the feasibility and the activity of the combined antineoplastic and antiretroviral therapy. Overall, CR was achieved in 53% of patients, and OI during CT or follow-up occurred in only 6% of cases. However, overall survival (median 11 months) was not satisfactory (33).

In an attempt to improve on these results the GICAT started a second trial consisting of full-dose EBV plus prednisone (EBVP regimen), concomitant antiretroviral therapy (zidovudine or didanosine), primary use of granulocyte colony-stimulatin factor (G-CSF), and *Pneumocystis carinii* pneumonia prophylaxis with sulfamethoxazole–trimethoprin (co-trimoxazole). Preliminary results of this trial, in which 35 patients were enrolled, show a CR rate of 74% and an OI rate during or after CT of 23% (median follow-up 16 months). Toxicity was moderate, with grade 3–4 leukopenia and thrombocytopenia in 29 and 9% of patients, respectively. Thirty-eight percent of patients who received CR relapsed. Overall, HD progression alone and in association with OI was the cause of death in 34 and in 20% of patients, respectively. The 2-year survival rate and the 2-year DFS was 40 and 58%, respectively. The combined treatment was feasible; however, relapse rate and overall survival rate were not satisfactory and need to be improved with better combined antineoplastic and antiretroviral approaches (34).

Levine et al. (35) have recently examined a regimen of ABVD in 21 HIV-infected patients with HD. Poor prognostic factors included stage IV disease (62%), systemic B symptoms (86%), and a median CD4 cell count of 128/µL. Of 15 evaluable patients, CRs were observed in 9, whereas a median survival of 78 weeks was noted for all patients. Toxicities were extensive with full-dose ABVD, including a nearly 50% incidence of grade 4 neutropenia despite G-CSF support.

In conclusion, our recommendations are to give conservative CT regimens (i.e., EBVP) in poor-risk categories. Alternative therapeutic strategies must be explored in good-risk patients.

III. TESTICULAR GERM CELL CANCERS

Testicular germ cell cancers are relatively rare and are among the most curable malignancies. However, testicular germ cell cancers are relatively common diseases in young men between 15 and 35 years of age, in whom HIV infection is also not an uncommon disease. Therefore, these malignancies should not be expected to be a rare event in young men with HIV infection. More than 110 cases of testicular tumors in HIV-infected patients have now been published in the literature (6,36–45). Moreover, recent cohort data from the Pittsburgh area Multicenter AIDS Cohort Study indicate that HIV-seropositive homosexual men have a significant increase in the incidence of testicular cancer (standardized incidence rate = 3.9), compared with that of the general male population (8). Current reports suggest that the natural history of these diseases in the HIV setting is remarkably similar to that in the general population.

The ratio of seminoma to nonseminoma germ cell tumors has varied in the reported series. In the GICAT's series (the largest published so far), 54% of patients had seminoma and 46% nonseminoma, a proportion similar to that reported in HIV-uninfected individuals with testicular cancer. The median CD4 cell count of 260/µL reported in this series of 26 patients, 60% of whom had asymptomatic HIV disease, suggests that the risk of testicular cancer is not directly related to the level of immune function (45). Overall, approximately 60–80% of patients have clinical stage I and II (i.e., disease confined to the testis and retroperitoneal lymph nodes), and only 20–30% have clinical stage II (i.e., disseminated disease above the diaphragm or visceral disease), again a proportion similar to that observed in the general population (6,38,43–45).

A testicular mass in a young man, with or without HIV infection, should be initially considered malignant. In most cases testicular tumors are painless, but approximately 30% of patients have moderate testicular pain. Cough (pulmonary metastases), abdominal pain (lymph node or retroperitoneal soft tissue metastases, hydronephrosis), or weight loss may all occur with testicular neoplasms.

The diagnosis of testicular germ cell cancer should be made by radical inguinal orchiectomy. Staging evaluations should include tumor marker studies (i.e., chorionic gonadotropin, alpha-fetoprotein, and lactic acid dehydrogenase), chest radiographs, and abdominal CT scan. As in HD, the presence of PGL should be considered, alerting clinicians to the danger of overstaging carcinoma by abdominal CT scan. In patients with normal serum markers and limited abdominal lymphadenopathy, PGL should be suspected and careful surveillance alone may be reasonable after orchiectomy.

Germ cell neoplasms are among the most sensitive to CT and RT, resulting in long-term DFS for patients in the general population of approximately 90% (44). Most HIV-infected patients with germ cell tumors reported in the literature tolerate standard therapy and achieve cure rate similar to that of HIV-uninfected patients (39–45). Survival of HIV-infected patients with testicular tumors closely parallels the natural history of HIV disease. One-year survival in the study by Bernardi et al. (45) was no different from that reported for HIV-infected patients without testicular tumors with similar CD4 cell count (85 versus 87%). In the report by Timmerman et al. (44), shorter survival was associated with advanced

HIV disease, but not with advanced tumor stage. The median survival times for patients without AIDS with CD4 cell count of 200/μL or more, versus those with AIDS or CD4 cell count of fewer than 200/μL were 40 months and 26 months, respectively. The median survival times for patients with limited- versus advanced-stage tumors were 42 months and 22 months, respectively.

For early-stage seminoma standard treatment is RT, whereas for advanced disease, it is combined treatment that includes CT (cisplatin, etoposide, and bleomycin [PEB] or cisplatin, vinblastine and bleomycin [PVB] and RT (46). In the Italian series, all patients affected by seminoma received standard treatment at the time of diagnosis according to the stage of disease and irrespective of HIV seropositivity. As far as patients affected by nonseminoma, all received postsurgical CT (PEB or PVB), also irrespective of HIV status. A 95% CR rate was observed in the 20 evaluable patients, approximately half of whom received CT and the other half irradiation (Table 5). Less than 50% of these patients experienced severe grade 3 and 4 hematological toxicity (45). As was true in the Italian study, all patients in the Timmerman's series also received standard therapy based on histology and stage, and among seven evaluable patients who received CT, five achieved CR (44). It is remarkable that in both these series investigators reported no OI occurring during the treatment.

Table 5 Therapy and Response to Treatment in 26 Patients with Germ Cell Cancers and HIV infection

	Response	
Therapy	No.	%
Surgery only	4/26 (1 S, 3 NS)	15
Chemotherapy only (PEB)	1[a]/26 (1 NS)	4
Surgery + chemotherapy (8 PEB, 1 PVB)	9/26 (1 S, 8 NS)	35
Surgery + radiotherapy	10/26 (10 S)	38
Surgery + chemotherapy (PEB) + radiotherapy	1/26 (1 S)	4
Unknown	1/26 (1 S)	4
No. of patients assessable for response	20/26 (11 S, 9 NS)	
CR	19/20 (11 S, 8 NS)	95
PR	1/20 (1 S)	5
PD	0	
Relapses	6/19 (4 S, 2 NS)	32

S, seminoma; NS, nonseminoma; PEB, cisplatin, etoposide, and bleomycin; PVB, cisplatin, vinblastine and bleomycin.
[a] Extranodal.
Source: Ref. 43.

In conclusion, patients with HIV infection affected by testicular cancer should be offered the standard therapeutic approach, because most can be cured of their tumor and have a good quality of life. Attention should be paid to effective therapeutic options for the underlying HIV infection and for OI prophylaxis.

IV. LUNG CANCER

In the general population, lung cancer is the second most common cancer in men and women, and it is the most common cause of cancer mortality for both sexes. Although more than 120 cases of lung cancer have been reported in HIV-infected patients (1,6,47–60), epidemiological data do not support the existence of an increased risk for the development of this tumor in the HIV setting. Population-based studies in San Francisco and New York have failed to detect any increase in the incidence of lung cancer attributable to HIV infection (5). Smaller studies, based in hospitals where large numbers of HIV-infected patients are cared for, have similarly failed to detect a significant effect of HIV in the incidence of lung cancer (55).

Many features of lung cancer in HIV-infected patients differ from the disease in the general population. The median age at diagnosis ranges from 38 to 47 years, compared with 55 to 70 years in the general population (Table 6).

Adenocarcinoma predominates as histopathological type, ranging from 30 to 100% of cases, whereas small cell histology is rare (approximately 10% of cases). This feature differs from the usual distribution of tumor type in most lung cancer series of the general population, from whom adenocarcinoma, squamous cell carcinoma, and small cell carcinoma each account for approximately one-third of cases. However, a larger percentage of adenocarcinoma has been reported in studies of lung cancer occurring in the subset of younger HIV-uninfected patients (61). These findings stress the need for case–control studies to compare the prevalence of adenocarcinoma in young age groups, with and without HIV infection.

Lung fibrosis is one of the most common risk cofactors for the development of adenocarcinoma in the general population. In one of the two largest published series of HIV-infected patients with lung cancer, a high (55%) association between tuberculosis infection (a fibrosing disease) and adenocarcinoma has been found (57). Severe immunodeficiency may not be a significant cofactor in the pathogenesis of lung cancer in these patients with median CD4 cell counts ranging from 120 to 288/μL. Overall, tobacco smoking appears to be the major carcinogen in HIV-infected patients, being present in more than 80% of cases, similar to the general population (50,54,57–59). More than 70% of HIV-infected patients presents with advanced (stages III–IV according to TNM classification) or inop-

Table 6 Clinical Features and Survival of 58 Patients with Lung Cancer (ca) and HIV Infection

	Braun (48) No. (%)	Sridhar (52) No. (%)	Vaccher (55) No. (%)	Gruden (56) No. (%)	Krap (57) No. (%)
No. of patients	6	19	19	7	7
Age (yrs) median (range)	40 (30–48)	47 (36–66)	38 (28–55)	42 (?)	38 (?)
CD4 cell count/μL median (range)	?	121 (13–628)	288 (13–617)	103 (7–468)	?
Histology					
Small cell carcinoma	—	1 (5)	3 (16)	1	—
Squamous cell carcinoma	2 (33)	6 (32)	2 (11)	2	—
Adenocarcinoma	4 (67)	8 (42)	11 (58)	2	7 (100)
Other	—	4 (21)	3 (16)	2	—
Stage					
III–IV	4 (67)	15 (79)	14 (100)	4 (67)	7 (100)
Survival (mo)	?	3	4	?	1

erable disease, including two-thirds with metastases at the time of diagnosis. Two studies, however, did not identify a difference in clinical stage between HIV-seropositive and HIV-indeterminated control subjects (54).

The typical symptoms of lung cancer (cough, chest pain, hemoptysis, dyspnea) do not distinguish HIV-infected from noninfected patients. However, diagnosis of lung cancer may be delayed in HIV-infected patients, because signs and symptoms of the disease may be similar to that of common thoracic OI.

Lung cancer must be in the differential diagnosis of an abnormal chest x-ray film, especially when one or more of the following features are present: a mass lesion in the lung, unilateral hilar adenopathy, rib destruction, Pancoast's syndrome, hard or fixed scalene lymphadenopathy, phrenic or left recurrent nerve paralysis, and paraneoplastic syndromes commonly associated with lung cancer. However, the syndrome of inappropriate secretion of antidiuretic hormone may occur in patients with infections or cancer of the lung. The neoplasia may also be found unexpectedly during bronchoscopy and bronchoalveolar lavage in the workup of OI.

The diagnosis of lung cancer should be made by sputum–bronchoalveolar lavage cytology or histologically examination of the tissue obtained by invasive procedures (i.e., bronchoscopy [brush or transbronchial biopsies], or transcutaneous transthoracic needle biopsy). Other diagnostic procedures may include thoracentesis, pleural biopsy, and mediastinoscopy. If indicated liver, brain, and bone scans should be also performed. Although bronchoalveolar lavage has high diagnostic yield for opportunistic organisms, the cytological examination of the lavage fluid has been disappointing in confirming malignancy. On the other hand, viral infections can produce cellular changes difficult to distinguish from malignancy, especially adenocarcinoma.

Lung cancer may be missed in some patients with HIV infection. Underdiagnosis may occur owing to the difficulty in performing invasive diagnostic procedures because of the poor general and respiratory status or because of patients noncomplicance (1,6,47–60). The available survival data suggest a very poor prognosis for HIV-seropositive patients with lung cancer, with no survivors beyond 1 year from diagnosis. In the five published series (total of 58 patients) the median survival is only 1–4 months, and most patients die of cancer progression (50,54,57–59).

There are few data to support specific treatment recommendations for HIV-infected patients with lung cancer. However, it is important that characteristics of the underlying HIV disease are not ignored. Therapy should be individualized based not only on tumor histology and stage, but also on the degree of HIV-related immunodeficiency. HIV infection is not a contraindication to surgery in patients with potentially resectable disease and absence of severe immunodeficiency. Unfortunately, the large majority of patients present with advanced inoperable disease and are candidates for palliative RT or CT. Careful attention must be paid to the patient's quality of life.

REFERENCES

1. S Monfardini, E Vaccher, G Pizzocaro, R Stellini, A Sinicco, S Sabbatani, M Maran-golo, R Zagni, M Clerici, R Foà, U Tirelli, F Gavosto. Unusual maligant tumors in 49 patients with HIV infection. AIDS 3:449–452, 1989.
2. M Hajjar, D Lacoste, G Brossard, P Morlat, M Dupon, LR Salami, F Dabis, Groupe d'Epidémiologie Clinique du SIDA en Aquitaine. Non-acquired immune deficiency syndrome-defining malignancies in a hospital-based cohort of human immunodefi-ciency virus-infected patients: Bordeaux, France, 1985–1991. J Natl Cancer Inst 84: 1593–1595, 1992.
3. A Gachupin-Garcia, PA Selwyn, N Salysbury Budner. Population-based study of malignancies and HIV infection among injecting drug users in a New York City methadone treatment program, 1985–1991. AIDS 6:843–848, 1992.
4. U Tirelli, E Vaccher, M Spina. Other cancers in HIV-infected patients. Curr Opin Oncol 6:508–511, 1994.
5. CS Rabkin, F Yellin. Cancer incidence in a population with a high prevalence of infection with human immunodeficiency virus type 1. J Natl Cancer Inst 86:1711–1716, 1994.
6. MD Volm, JH Von Roenn. Non–AIDS-defining malignancies in patients with HIV infection. Curr Opin Oncol 8:386–391, 1996.
7. D Serraino, P Pezzotti, A Cozzi-Lepri, E Grigoletto, U Tirelli, G Rezza, for the Italian Seroconverter Study Group. Incidence of Hodgkin's disease (HD) in a cohort of HIV seroconverters [abstr 847]. Proc Am Soc Clin Oncol p 304, 1996.
8. DW Lyter, LA Kingsley, CR Rinaldo, J Bryant. Malignancies in the Multicenter AIDS Cohort Study (MACS), 1984–1994 [abstr 852]. Proc Am Soc Clin Oncol 1996, p 305.
9. R Rubio, for the Cooperative Study Group of Malignancies Associated with HIV Infection of Madrid. Hodgkin's disease associated with human immunodeficiency virus infection. A clinical study of 46 cases. Cancer 73:2400–2407, 1994.
10. R Lévy, P Colonna, J-M Tourani, JA Gastaut, P Brice, M Raphaël, B Taillan, J-M Andrieu, for the French Registry of HIV-associated Tumors. Human immunodefi-ciency virus associated Hodgkin's disease: report of 45 cases from the French Regis-try of HIV-Associated Tumors. Leuk Lymphoma 16:451–456, 1995.
11. U Tirelli, D Errante, R Dolcetti, A Gloghini, D Serraino, E Vaccher, S Franceschi, M Boiocchi, A Carbone. Hodgkin's disease and human immunodeficiency virus in-fection: clinicopathologic and virologic features of 114 patients from the Italian Co-operative Group on AIDS and Tumors. J Clin Oncol 13:1758–1767, 1995.
12. DM Knowles, GA Chamulak, M Subar, JS Burke, M Dugan, J Wernz, C Slywotzky, P-G Pelicci, R Dalla Favera, B Raphael. Lymphoid neoplasia associated with the acquired immunodeficiency syndrome (AIDS). Ann Intern Med 108:744–753, 1988.

13. ED Ames, MS Conjalka, AF Goldberg, R Hirschman, S Jain, A Distenfeld, CE Metroka. Hodgkin's disease and AIDS. Twenty-three new cases and a review of the literature. Hematol Oncol Clin North Am 5:343–365, 1991.
14. HJ Ree, JA Strauchen, AA Khan, JE Gold, JP Crowley, H Kahn, R Zalusky. Human immunodeficiency virus-associated Hodgkin's disease. Clinicopathologic studies of 24 cases and preponderance of mixed cellularity type characterized by the occurrence of fibrohistiocytoid stromal cells. Cancer 67:1614–1621, 1991.
15. JA Gold, D Altarac, HJ Ree, A Khan, PP Sordillo, R Zalusky. HIV-associated Hodgkin's disease: a clinical study of 18 cases and review of the literature. Am J Hematol 36:93–99, 1991.
16. RJ Pelstring, RB Zellmer, LE Sulak, PM Banks, N Clare. Hodgkin's disease in association with human immunodeficiency virus infection. Pathologic and immunologic features. Cancer 67:1865–1873, 1991.
17. SR Newcom, M Ward, VM Napoli, M Kutner. Treatment of human immunodeficiency virus-associated Hodgkin disease. Is there a clue regarding the cause of Hodgkin disease? Cancer 71:3138–3145, 1993.
18. AM Levine. HIV-associated Hodgkin's disease. Biologic and clinical aspects. Hematol Oncol Clin North Am 10:1135–1148, 1996.
19. J Diebold, J Audouin. Maladie di Hodgkin. Une o plusieurs maladies? Ann Pathol 9:84–91, 1989.
20. DH Wright. Pathology of Hodgkin's disease: anything new? In: V Diehl, M Pfreunfshuh, M Loeffler, eds. New Aspects in the Diagnosis and Treatment of Hodgkin's Disease. Berlin: Springer-Verlag, 1989:3–13.
21. D Serraino, A Carbone, S Franceschi, U Tirelli, for the Italian Coperative Group on AIDS and Tumors. Increased frequency of lymphocyte depletion and mixed cellularity subtypes of Hodgkin's disease in HIV-infected patients. Eur J Cancer 29A: 1948–1950, 1993.
22. A Carbone, M Boiocchi, A Gloghini, V De Re, R Dolcetti, P De Paoli, L Barzan, G Bertola, C Rossi, S Morassut, M Valentini, M Sozzi, D Serraino, E Vaccher, S Franceschi, U Tirelli, S Monfardini. Can a specifically-aimed pathologic classification overcome the difficulties in defining HIV-associated lymphomas? Pathologica 87:4–13, 1995.
23. S Uccini, F Monardo, A Stoppacciaro, A Gradilone, AM Aglianò, A Faggioni, V Manzari, L Vago, G Costanzi, LP Ruco, CD Baroni. High frequency of Epstein–Barr virus genome detection in Hodgkin's disease of HIV-positive patients. Int J Cancer 46:581–585, 1990.
24. BJ Herndier, HC Sanchez, KL Chang, Y-Y Chen, LM Weiss. High prevalence of Epstein–Barr virus in the Reed–Sternberg cells of HIV-associated Hodgkin's disease. Am J Pathol 142:1073–1079, 1993.
25. A Carbone, R Dolcetti, A Gloghini, R Maestro, E Vaccher, D Di Luca, U Tirelli, M Boiocchi. Immunophenotypic and molecular analyses of acquired immune deficiency syndrome-related and Epstein–Barr virus-associated lymphomas: a comparative study. Hum Pathol 27:133–146, 1996.
26. MJ Boyle, E Vasak, M Tschuchnigg, JJ Turner, T Sculley, R Penny, DA Cooper, B Tindall, WA Sewell. Subtypes of Epstein–Barr virus (EBV) in Hodgkin's disease: association between B-type EBV and immunocompromise. Blood 81:468–474, 1993.

27. DS Karcher. Clinically unsuspected Hodgkin disease presenting initially in the bone marrow of patients infected with the human immunodeficiency virus. Cancer 71: 1235–1238, 1993.

28. S Monfardini, U Tirelli, E Vaccher, R Foà, F Gavosto, for the Gruppo Italiano Cooperativo AIDS e Tumori (GICAT). Hodgkin's disease in 63 intravenous drug users infected with human immunodeficiency virus. Ann Oncol 2(suppl 2):201–205, 1991.

29. U Tirelli, E Vaccher, A Carbone, P De Paoli, S Morassut. Lymphangiography and abdominal computerized tomography in persistent generalized lymphadenopathy. AIDS Res 2:149–153, 1986.

30. DI Abrams, LD Kaplan, HS McGrath, PA Volberding. AIDS-related benign lymphadenopathy and malignant lymphoma: clinical aspects and virologic interactions. AIDS Res 2:5131–5139, 1986.

31. RT Hoppe, AL Hanlon GE Hanks, JB Owen. Progress in the treatment of Hodgkin's disease in the US: 1973 versus 1983: the patterns of care study. Cancer 74:3198–3203, 1994.

32. B Coiffier. Prognostic factors in Hodgkin's and non–Hodgkin's lymphomas. Curr Opin Oncol 3:843–851, 1991.

33. D Errante, U Tirelli, R Gastaldi, D Milo, AM Nosari, G Rossi, G Fiorentini, A Carbone, E Vaccher, S Monfardini, for the Italian Cooperative Group on AIDS and Tumors. Combined antineoplastic and antiretroviral therapy for patients with Hodgkin's disease and human immunodeficiency virus infection. Cancer 73:437–444, 1994.

34. D Errante, J Gabarre, AC Ridolfo, G Rossi, AM Nosari, C Gisselbrecht, Y Kerneis, F Mazzetti, E Vaccher, R Talamini, A Carbone, U Tirelli. Hodgkin's disease in 35 patients with HIV infection: an experience with epirubicin, bleomycin, vinblastine and prednisone chemotherapy in combination with antiretroviral therapy and primary use of G-CSF. Ann Oncol 10:189–195, 1999.

35. AM Levine, T Cheung, J Huang, M Testa, for the oncology committee ACTG. Prospective, multicentre phase II trial of ABVD chemotherapy with G-CSF in HIV-infected patients with Hodgkin's disease (HD): AIDS clinical trials groups (ACTG) study 149 [abstr 194]. Proc Am Soc Clin Oncol 16:56a, 1997.

36. CJ Gunthel, DW Northfèlt. Cancers not associated with immunodeficiency in HIV-infected persons. Oncology 8:59–64, 1994.

37. CJ Logothetis, GR Newell, ML Samuels. Testicular cancer in homosexual men with cellular immune deficiency: report of 2 cases. J Urol 133:484–486, 1985.

38. AN Tessler, A Catanese. AIDS and germ cell tumors of testis. Urology 30:203–204, 1987.

39. L Damstrup, G Daugaard, J Gerstoft, M Rørth. Effects of antineoplastic treatment of HIV-positive patients with testicular cancer. Eur J Cancer Clin Oncol 25:983–986, 1989.

40. MC Palmer, DR Mador, PM Venner. Testicular seminoma associated with the acquired immunodeficiency syndrome and acquired immunodeficiency syndrome related complex: 2 case reports. J Urol 142:128–130, 1989.

41. CG Roehrborn, JT Worrell, EL Wiley. Bilateral synchronous testis tumors of different histology in a patient with the acquired immunodeficiency syndrome related complex. J Urol 144:353–355, 1990.

42. M Wilkinson, PR Carroll. Testicular carcinoma in patients positive and at risk for human immunodeficiency virus. J Urol 144:1157–1159, 1990.
43. WT Wilson, E Frenkel, F Vuitch, AI Sagalowsky. Testicular tumors in men with human immunodeficiency virus. J Urol 147:1038–1040, 1992.
44. JM Timmerman, DW Northfelt, EJ Small. Malignant germ cell tumors in men infected with the human immunodeficiency virus: natural history and results of therapy. J Clin Oncol 13:1391–1397, 1995.
45. D Bernardi, R Salvioni, E Vaccher, L Repetto, N Piersantelli, B Marini, R Talamini, U Tirelli, for the Italian Cooperative Group on AIDS and Tumors. Testicular germ cell tumors and human immunodeficiency virus infection: a report of 26 cases. J Clin Oncol 13:2705–2711, 1995.
46. LH Einhorn, JP Richie, WU Shipley. Cancer of the testis. In: VT De Vita, S Hellman, SA Rosenberg, eds. Cancer. Principles and Practice of Oncology. Philadelphia: JB Lippincott, 1993:1126–1151.
47. JE Groopman, K Mayer, T Zipoli, S Wallach, B Fallon, J Clark. Unusual neoplasms associated with HTLV-III infection [abstr 14]. Proc Am Soc Clin Oncol 1986, p 4.
48. D Lake-Lewin, YS Arkel. Spectrum of malignancies in HIV positive individuals, [abstr 20]. Proc Am Soc Clin Oncol, 1988, p 5.
49. ER Heitzman. Pulmonary neoplastic and lymphoproliferative disease in AIDS: a review. Radiology 177:347–351, 1990.
50. MA Braun, DA Killam, SC Remick, JC Ruckdeschel. Lung cancer in patients seropositive for human immunodeficiency virus. Radiology 175:341–343, 1990.
51. AE Fraire, RJ Awe. Lung cancer in association with human immunodeficiency virus infection. Cancer 70:432–436, 1992.
52. PM Broussier, MJ Postal, B Dautzenberger, F Antoun. Cancer bronchique au cours du SIDA. Presse Med 19:1638, 1990.
53. SM Lichtman, M Kaplan, L Donahue, B Farber, D Shepp, W Hall, J Samuels, M Epstein. HIV associated malignancy (HAM). Report of single institution experience with 1591 HIV positive patients [abstr 14]. Proc Am Soc Clin Oncol, 1992, p 47.
54. KS Sridhar, MR Flores, WA Raub, M Saldana. Lung cancer in patients with human immunodeficiency virus infection compared with historic control subjects. Chest 102:1704–1708, 1992.
55. TK Chan, CP Aranda, WN Rom. Bronchogenic carcinoma in young patients at risk for acquired immunodeficiency syndrome. Chest 103:862–864, 1993.
56. MF Tenholder, HD Jackson. Bronchogenic carcinoma in patients seropositive for human immunodeficiency syndrome. Chest 104:1049–1053, 1993.
57. E Vaccher, U Tirelli, M Spina, D Errante, I Crosato, S Sabbatani, A Sinicco, S Monfardini, for the Italian Cooperative Study Group on AIDS and Tumors (GICAT). Lung cancer in 19 patients with HIV infection. Ann Oncol 4:85–86, 1993.
58. JF Gruden, JS Klein, WR Webb. Percutaneous transthoracic needle biopsy in AIDS: analysis in 32 patients. Radiology 189:567–571, 1993.
60. J Karp, G Profeta, PR Marantz, JP Karpel. Lung cancer in patients with immunodeficiency syndrome. Chest 103:410–413, 1993.
61. SD Aaron, E Warner, JD Edelson. Bronchogenic carcinoma in patients seropositive for human immunodeficiency virus. Chest 106:640–642, 1994.
62. World Health Organization. The WHO histological typing of lung tumors. Am J Pathol 77:123–136, 1982.

12
Pediatric Malignancies

Brigitta U. Mueller and Philip A. Pizzo
*Children's Hospital and Harvard Medical School,
Boston, Massachusetts*

I. INTRODUCTION AND EPIDEMIOLOGY

As of December 1998, a total of 8461 children younger than 13 years of age have had a diagnosis of acquired immunodeficiency syndrome (AIDS) in the United States. During 1988–1993, before the successful reduction of the transmission rate, from mother to child, through the use of zidovudine during pregnancy, at delivery, and in the neonatal period (1), an estimated 1000–2000 children were infected each year in the United States (2). Worldwide, the Joint United Nations Programme on AIDS (UNAIDS) estimates that 460,000 new infections occurred in 1997, and that currently 1.2 million children are living with human immunodeficiency virus (HIV) infection or AIDS (ref: UNAIDS Web site). It has been estimated that in 1998 alone, 5.8 million adults and 590,000 children were newly infected with HIV-1 (16,000 new cases per day), and 2.5 million adults and 510,000 children younger than the age of 15 years have died of HIV-related complications.

Since 1995, the decrease in the perinatal transmission rate, increases in rate and duration of survival of HIV-infected children have changed the appearance of the epidemic in the United States. However, as infected children survive longer, many with impaired immune function, they may be prone to the development of neoplastic or preneoplastic diseses. Furthermore, despite the advances in industrialized countries, the epidemic affecting children and adults continues unabated in developing nations.

The revised classification of pediatric AIDS issued in 1994 by the Centers for Disease Control and Prevention (CDC), lists (as in adults) primary brain lymphomas, small noncleaved cell (SNCC; Burkitt's) non–Hodgkin's lymphomas, immunoblastic or large cell lymphoma of B-cell or unknown immunological phenotype, as well as Kaposi's sarcoma as AIDS-defining events (category C; 3). Leiomyosarcomas are included in category B as a sign of a moderately symptomatic stage. This classification has several problems. First, only the initial AIDS-defining event is listed. Thus, if a child has an initial diagnosis of another category C symptom (for example *Pneumocystis carinii* pneumonia; PCP), the occurrence of a tumor will not be registered. This precludes an exact estimate of the incidence of tumors in HIV-infected children. Second, it has become clear over the last few years, that HIV-infected children can develop many different kinds of non–Hodgkin's lymphomas (NHL), including tumors of T-cell phenotype. Thus, simple or restricted categorizations might miss important new tumors. Third, lymphoproliferative disorders are clearly part of the spectrum of pediatric HIV disease and potentially represent a preneoplastic disorder. However, only lymphadenopathy (category A) and lymphoid interstitial pneumonia (LIP; category B) are currently included in the CDC definition.

Through December 1997, 162 of 8086 (2%) children with AIDS have had a tumor diagnosed as their AIDS-defining event. Fifty-two children had a Burkitt's NHL, 51 an immunoblastic NHL, 31 a primary NHL of the central nervous system (CNS), and 28 Kaposi's sarcoma. In 1997, Kaposi's sarcoma was diagnosed in none of 473 children, compared with 1500 cases among 60,161 newly diagnosed adults (2.3%) (4). However, this underestimates the discrepancy, because in adults, the majority (65%) of diagnoses of AIDS are based on a low CD4 cell count, a criteria not consistently applicable as an AIDS indicator in children. A survey conducted by the Children's Cancer Group and the National Cancer Institute (NCI) identified 57 HIV-infected children with diagnoses of cancer between July 1982 and January 1997. Twenty-five of these children would not have been captured through the current CDC classification system (5).

In developing countries, the incidence rate for HIV-associated tumors might be different. There have now been several reports of an increased incidence of Kaposi's sarcoma in children from Zambia and Uganda, but also a trend to an increase in the numbers of retinoblastomas, nasopharyngeal carcinomas, and rhabdomyosarcomas, tumors not commonly associated with immunodeficiency states (6,7). A prospective and detailed epidemiological study is clearly indicated in these epicenters of the AIDS epidemic.

The interrelation between the immune system and cancer risk is notable, but complicated. Presumably, the risk of developing a cancer is higher with a weakened immune system (8). The absolute CD4 cell count alone is not a sufficient measure to stage the integrity of a child's immune system, for we and others have seen HIV-infected children develop a tumor while their CD4 cell count was only moderately depressed. On the other hand, we have also cared for children with very low numbers of CD4 cells, who had a tumor diagnosed and were successfully treated, only to develop a histologically different tumor at a later time.

Thus, immunological disruption can alter the risk for primary as well as secondary malignancies.

II. NON–HODGKIN'S LYMPHOMA

Infection with HIV is often associated with lymphadenopathy, hepatosplenomegaly, and on occasion, impairment of the function of the CNS. It is not uncommon that the diagnosis of a NHL is delayed in a child with HIV disease because of the similarity of symptoms associated with an infectious or a neoplastic disorder. Furthermore, not every HIV-infected child with a NHL will experience the rapid progression associated with this malignancy in non–HIV-infected children. One explanation may be that, although small noncleaved tumors with a high growth fraction are common, the more indolent anaplastic large cell lymphomas occur with equal frequency in HIV-infected children. Small noncleaved tumors are of B-cell origin, whereas large cell lymphomas can have either B- or T-cell phenotype, and they are often characterized by the CD30 marker (Ki-1), which was originally found on Reed–Sternberg cells of Hodgkin's disease (9). As in adults, lymphomas of the CNS are generally high-grade tumors, mainly of B-cell origin and commonly associated with Epstein–Barr virus (EBV; 10–14).

Although CNS and systemic NHL can occur in children with relatively well-preserved immune systems, measured by CD4 cell counts, the risk of developing a NHL increases with the depth and duration of very low CD4 counts. Furthermore, indolent tumors, such as mucosa-associated tumors (MALT) of both the pulmonary or gastric mucosa, can be either a manifestation of advanced disease, or the very first symptom of HIV infection (15–18).

A. Systemic Non–Hodgkin's Lymphoma

The clinical profile and modes of presentation of systemic NHL in the HIV-infected child is different from tumors seen in HIV-infected adults, but also from NHLs in noninfected children. The incidence of large cell lymphomas appears to be higher in HIV-infected children than in noninfected age-matched controls. In one study, 43% of NHLs were of large cell (LC) histological type (immunoblastic [IBLC] diffuse, or anaplastic [ALC]), whereas roughly 20% of childhood NHLs are large cell lymphomas in non–HIV-infected children (19). Similar to the general pediatric population, the majority of HIV-infected children present with high-grade, predominantly B-cell lymphomas, but more commonly affecting extranodal sites. The gastrointestinal tract and CNS are common extranodal sites for both adults and children with HIV infection. Nonspecific complaints such as fatigue, loss of appetite; and night sweats are common, and patients can have marked variability in age, CD4 cell count at diagnosis, and sites of presentation

(5). At the Pediatric Branch of the National Cancer Institute we diagnosed NHL in 14 children (out of over 450 children with HIV infection) between 1986 and 1996. Table 1 shows the variability in age, CD4 cell counts at diagnosis, and sites of presentation. Extranodal involvement (including lungs, liver, bones, or meninges) was common and resulted in vague and difficult to evaluate symptoms, such as refusal to walk, pleural pain, or hepatomegaly.

Because these symptoms can also be caused by either HIV infection itself or an opportunistic infection, such as *Mycobacterium avium* complex (MAC) bacteremia, a heightened index of suspicion must be sustained to discriminate between infectious and neoplastic etiologies. When cancer is suspected, a careful staging should include radiologic studies with computer assisted tomography (CT) or magnetic resonance imaging, (MRI), a gallium and bone scan, a bone marrow examination, and a lumbar puncture. HIV disease often results in multiorgan problems, and it is important to assess hepatic, peripheral neurological, renal, bone marrow, and cardiac function as best as possible before intervention, because HIV disease can affect these and other organ systems, thereby adding to the consequences of the administration of cytotoxic chemotherapy. Although NHL can be treated successfully in an HIV-infected child, it is imperative that every attempt be made to prevent or treat potential infectious complications and that the prospect for organ toxicity related to antiretroviral or cancer treatment be fully considered.

The treatment of choice for pulmonary MALT is surgical excision, and we have cared for two children who remain disease-free more than 3 years after surgery alone (20). Gastric MALT is often associated with *Helicobacter pylori* infection, and an empirical trial of antibiotic therapy with amoxicillin and metronidazole is indicated (21,22). We also treated one patient with refractory and very painful gastric MALT with oral cyclophosphamide, which resulted in endoscopic disappearance of the lesions and resolution of pain (23).

There are currently no published studies comparing the response rate and treatment-associated toxicities in children with NHL and concurrent HIV infection with those in uninfected children. Because of the preexisting organ dysfunctions (most commonly bone marrow), impaired immune system, possible opportunistic infections, and the need for multiple drugs to treat HIV infection, it is assumed that HIV-infected children are less likely to tolerate standard chemotherapy. However, although this might be true for prolonged intensive treatment modalities, it may be possible to successfully treat them with short, but dose-intensive, regimens. A protocol at the National Cancer Institute successfully employed a dose-intensive regimen of cyclophosphamide and methotrexate given for three cycles (24). For the aforementioned reasons, this regimen did not include doxorubicin (because of concerns of cardiotoxicity), vincristine (because neuropathy can be a problem owing to overlapping toxicity with some antiretroviral agents), or steroids (because of added immunosuppression). The strength of this approach

Table 1 Lymphomas Diagnosed in 14 HIV-Infected Children[a] Between 1986 and 1996 (National Cancer Institute, Bethesda)

Age (yr)	Sex	Site of presentation	Histology	Phenotype	CD4 cells/mm
9.5	Female	Central nervous system	"High-grade"	?	2
2	Female	Central nervous system	Large cell	?	7
3.5	Male	Bone, disseminated	Burkitt-like	B cell	68
3	Male	Cervical lymph nodes, mediastinum	Plasmacytoid	B cell	256
13	Male	Cervical lymphadenopathy	Small, noncleaved cell	B cell	323
11	Female	Infratemporal area	Small, noncleaved cell	B cell	1
4	Male	Inguinal lymphadenopathy	Large cell, immunoblastic	B cell	14
14[b]	Male	Multiple lung nodules	Large cell, immunoblastic	B cell	9
12[b]	Male	Retropharynx	Burkitt-like	B cell	9
15	Male	Solitary lung nodule	MALT	B cell	148
7	Female	Solitary lung nodule	MALT	B cell	606
18	Male	Gastric mucosa	MALT	B and T cell	36
13	Female	Mandible	Anaplastic, large cell, Ki-1+	nonB–nonT cell	22
1	Male	Initially scalp lesion, then multiple skin nodules, later mandibular tumor	Anaplastic, large cell, Ki-1+	T cell	1988
4	Female	Systemic lymphadenopathy	Anaplastic, large cell, Ki-1+	T cell	354

[a] One child had two different tumors.
[b] Same patient.
MALT, mucosa-associated lymphoid tumor.

is related to dose-intensity, with three consecutive cycles being given as soon as the absolute neutrophil count (with concurrent granulocyte colony-stimulating factor [G-CSF] therapy) approaches 500/mm^3. Other important supportive care modalities included prophylaxis for PCP biweekly infusions of intravenous immune globulin, acyclovir for herpes simplex prophylaxis, and continued antiretroviral therapy with an approved regimen (currently zidovudine and didanosine or zidovudine and lamivudine, and perhaps the protease inhibitor ritonavir). Nine patients (age 1–14 years) with ten tumors have so far been treated (three SNCC, three ALC, three IBLC NHL, and one plasmacytoid NHL). Seven patients achieved a complete response (CR), one a partial response, and two showed no response. The regimen was fairly well tolerated and the median duration of neutropenia was 3 days (range 0–14) during each cycle. The three partial or nonresponders were subsequently treated with a relapse regimen consisting of ifosfamide and cytarabine, and two of them achieved a CR. Survival ranged from 5–45 months (median 21 months) and five of the nine patients remain alive, all of them in CR. Four patients have died: two of HIV-related complications, one of PCP, and one of progressive disease with NHL. None of the deaths occurred during chemotherapy (24).

Some patients present with "slowly growing" NHL, tumors that clearly have a monoclonal phenotype, may exhibit atypical mitoses, but clinically do not behave like the typical NHL of childhood. These tumors are often large cell anaplastic NHL, commonly CD30 (Ki-1)-positive and can be of B- or T-cell phenotype. We have seen one child with such a tumor in the jaw, who remained stable without chemotherapeutic intervention for more than 6 months, and a second child with multiple skin lesions that were clinically reminiscent of lymphomatoid papulosis with a spontaneously waxing and waning course.

B. Lymphomas of the CNS

Although CNS NHL appear to be more common in adults with low CD4 cell counts, we and others have treated children with relatively well-preserved immune status who developed a CNS tumor. The symptoms are similar to adults, with cranial nerve deficits, seizures, and hemiparesis being the most common. In adolescents, infection with *Toxoplasma gondii* has to be considered in the differential diagnosis, but in younger children it is more likely that the intracranial lesion represent a malignancy or lymphoproliferative process. However, because brain tumors (of nonlymphoid origin) are the second most common cancers in non–HIV-infected children (25), it is likely that they will be seen more often in HIV-infected children who survive longer. Unlike adults, in whom CNS toxoplasmosis is not uncommon, this is rare in children. The approach of using empirical antiparasitic therapy as the first intervention in a patient with a brain lesion is less well defined in children.

Only case reports are available describing the treatment outcome of HIV-infected children with CNS lymphomas. In the very young child, chemotherapy alone is preferable becasue of concerns about including developmental delays, but in the older child (more than 3 years of age), radiotherapy is probably indicated in conjunction with intrathecal and systemic chemotherapy. In adults, the prognosis for patients with CNS NHL is extremely guarded.

III. HODGKIN'S DISEASE

In industrialized countries, the epidemiology of Hodgkin's disease (HD) shows a first peak in incidence in mid- to late adolescence and, therefore, does not currently represent a major problem in HIV-infected children (26). However, in developing countries, HD occurs at an earlier age, and some cases of HD in HIV-infected children have been observed in unusually young children. At the National Cancer Institute we treated one child, a 3.8-year-old boy with a very aggressive, lymphocyte-depleted form of HD, with the primary site in the liver. Unfortunately, the child did not show any response, despite very aggresive chemotherapy, not unlike the experience in adults.

IV. LYMPHOPROLIFERATIVE DISORDERS

Lymphoproliferative disorders (LPD) are an interesting entity that could well represent the link between increased proliferation and overt malignancy (27,28). The spectrum of manifestations includes the following presentations:

1. Lymphadenopathy with hypergammaglobulinemia is very common in HIV-infected children, especially at the early stages of disease. The disease process is polyclonal and the lymph node architecture is preserved, but typically shows follicular hyperplasia (27,28). This form of LPD usually responds to antiretroviral interventions.
2. A diffuse infiltrative lymphocytosis syndrome (DILS; 29,30), consisting of bilateral parotid enlargement, cystic enlargement of the salivary or lacrimal glands, is closely related to the lymphoid interstitial pneumonitis (LIP), which is a typical feature of childhood HIV infection (31–33). Both DILS and LIP can become clinically problematic, either because of location and size or because of the development of oxygen-dependency. Histologically, both B and T cell have been implicated, and the role of EBV remains to be determined. Several cases of pulmonary MALT (20) have been associated with LIP, and a pathogenetic link is currently being investigated. The recently described pa-

tients with multiple cystic lesions in their grossly enlarged thymus may also belong into this same group (34). The treatment approach for these manifestations include optimization of antiretroviral therapy, steroid therapy in the case of lung disease (lymphocytic interstitial pneumonitis; LIP) with oxygen-dependency, possibly surgical excision (in the case of MALTs), or more experimental approaches as described later.

3. Diffuse polyclonal and polymorphic infiltrates of lymph nodes, kidneys, or lungs; effacing the normal architecture have been mainly associated with B-cell phenotype. No atypical mitoses are seen, but often a characteristic eosinophilic infiltrate is present, and the tumors can evolve into an oligoclonal process. Therapy consists of optimization of antiretroviral therapy, possibly steroids, or innovative, but experimental, treatments as described later.

It is currently not known whether LPDs can develop into an overt malignancy, but they themselves can be life-threatening. Prognosis varies with the different manifestations. Many children will become clinically asymptomatic with optimization of their antiretroviral therapy and suppression of viral replication. Surprisingly, the children with large cystic mediastinal masses were completely asymptomatic and the diagnosis was made incidentally during a routine radiologic evaluation (34). However, LPDs can become a therapeutic challenge, either because of location, size, or continued growth. At the National Cancer Institute we cared for one child with an intracranial LPD (similar to posttransplant situation), who died of the disease before any therapy was initiated.

Because of the potential for malignant transformation and clinically significant problems in some children, we evaluated a therapeutic approach with interferon alfa and all-*trans*-retinoic acid for children with clinically significant LPD (e.g., no response to optimized antiretroviral therapy; large mass; or steroid-dependent LIP), and preliminary results indicate that this therapy is relatively well tolerated and, in some cases, will lead to marked reduction of tumor size (35). Further evaluation of this therapy, including in patients who develop an LPD after transplant or as part of a congenital immunodeficiency, is planned.

A. Smooth-Muscle Tumors

Leiomyosarcomas are rare tumors in children, representing less than 2% of all childhood cancers (36). An increased number of leiomyomas and leiomyosarcomas have been described in HIV-infected children (37–42), which led to their inclusion as a category B symptom in the revised 1994 classification of pediatric HIV disease (3). In our survey of the cases reported to the Children's Cancer Study Group and the National Cancer Institute, we noted eight cases (14% of all reported tumors) of leiomyomas or leiomyosarcomas (5). Although most commonly found in the gastrointestinal tract (43,44), unusual localizations, such as spleen, pleural space, adrenal glands, and lungs have been described in HIV-infected children. Of interest is the recent finding of EBV by in situ hybridization and quantitative polymerase chain reaction (PCR), which appears to be unique to tumors from HIV-infected patients (45). The course of disease is highly variable with indolent tumors (more likely leiomyomas), that probably do not necessitate intervention, in some children, and very aggressive, disseminated tumors in others. Unfortunately, smooth-muscle tumors are in general not very sensitive to chemotherapy or radiotherapy and in non–HIV-infected children, local excision is the first line of therapy (36).

V. KAPOSI'S SARCOMA

Although Kaposi's sarcoma (KS) is a very common feature of HIV infection in adults, it is rarely diagnosed in children from the United States, with the exception of vertically infected children from Haiti or older adolescents (46–50). In the United States, KS is the AIDS-defining illness in less than 1% of children younger than 13 years of age and only 3% of adolescents between 13 and 19 years of age (4). However, the incidence increases to 9% in young adults between 20 and 24 of years of age, and to 13% in adults older than 25 years of age (4,51). Recently, there have been several reports about a significant increase in the incidence of KS in children from African countries (6,52). In Zambia, KS now constitutes almost 20% of all childhood cancers, compared with 6% before 1986. The male/female ratio has changed from 3:1 before the AIDS epidemic to about 1.7:1 and the peak incidence occurred in children younger than 5 years of age.

Kaposi sarcoma is rarely the first presentation of HIV disease in children. Most will have had a history of hepatosplenomegaly, failure to thrive, or recurrent infections (6). Three distribution patterns were observed among 100 childhood KS cases in Uganda: an orofacial distribution (in 79 patients), with regional (86%) or generalized (60%) lymphadenopathy and variable skin involvement (39%); an inguinal–genital distribution (in 13 children), with inguinal lymphadenopathy (100%), skin (57%), and anogenital (14%) involvement; and a less common pattern with solitary tumors in the extremities or visceral organs (8%) (6). A trend toward more common occurrence of the nonlymphadenopathic form in HIV-infected children compared with non–HIV-associated pediatric cases was noted, but did not reach statistical significance (7).

Herpesvirus type 8 (HHV-8) was demonstrated in eight of eight archival samples from pediatric KS cases in Uganda. This age distribution and that HHV-8 is found in the lesions raises the possibility of an endemic presence of this viral infection in African countries, affecting children at an early age. Also intriguing is that KS is a vascular tumor and that one of the most common vascular tumors of childhood, hemangioma, exhibits a rapid growth phase in early infancy. This generates not only questions about pathogenesis, but also the potential for a therapeutic approach with angiogenesis inhibitors, some of which (e.g., thalidomide) are currently undergoing clinical trials for the treatment of both KS and hemangiomas.

VI. OTHER TUMORS

Over the last few years, several miscellaneous tumors have been reported to occur in HIV-infected children, including leukemia, Ewing's sarcoma, rhabdomyosarcoma, and ependymoblastoma (53–58). Although the incidence for anyone of these tumors does not appear to be increased, some children have developed distinctly unusual tumors, such as a small cell carcinoma located between the esophagus and trachea, a papillary carcinoma of the thyroid (59), or a fibrosarcoma of the liver (54).

In HIV-infected adults, there also has been an increase in the incidence of anal and cervical neoplasias. Because many adolescents are sexually active, it is important for the pediatrician to be aware of this increased risk and to actively rule out such malignancies in sexually active patients. The prevalence of cervical dysplasia has increased in adolescents, and human papilloma virus (HPV) infection, a risk factor for cervical dysplasia, has a prevalence of 15–38% in this age group (60).

Zidovudine given during gestation is incorporated into the DNA of newborn mice and monkeys, as well as into the nuclear DNA of cord blood samples drawn from children whose mothers had been treated with the drug. Studies of the offsprings of mice who had been treated with zidovudine during the last trimester, revealed an increased risk to develop liver and lung tumors as well as tumors of the reproductive organs (61). A panel organized by the National Institutes of Health acknowledged the validity of the findings, but also recognized that the benefit of preventing transmission of HIV disease in the vast majority of children currently outweighs the potential concerns of carcinogenicity. These data nonetheless emphasize the importance of careful long-term follow-up of *all* children exposed in utero to antiretroviral therapy, including those who are not HIV-infected.

VII. SUMMARY AND OUTLOOK

Whether other factors (such as a lymphoproliferative disorder or therapies used to treat HIV infection) can increase the risk for the development of a neoplastic disease in HIV-infected children should be kept in mind with a growing population of long-term survivors. Furthermore, as children are being exposed in utero to antiretroviral agents, careful surveillance of infected and uninfected children for the occurrence of malignancies is mandatory. Importantly, even in the event of successful treatment of the underlying tumor, the HIV-infected child remains at risk to develop a new malignancy or to die of the complications of his or her underlying disease. A combined treatment approach by pediatric oncologists and infectious disease specialists is, therefore, important to provide optimal care for these children. Children with HIV disease who also develop cancer can both respond to and tolerate the effects of multimodal treatment regimens, making it important to employ appropriate treatment interventions in children who may benefit from them.

REFERENCES

1. Connor EM, Sperling RS, Gelber R, et al. Reduction of maternal–infant transmission of immunodeficiency virus type 1 with zidovudine treatment. N Engl J Med 331: 1173–1180, 1994.
2. Centers for Disease Control and Prevention. AIDS among children–United States, 1996. MMWR Morbid Mortal Wkly Ref 45:1005–1010, 1996.
3. Centers for Disease Control and Prevention. Revised classification system for human immunodeficiency virus infection in children less than 13 years of age. MMWR Morbid Martal Wkly Ref 43:1–12, 1994.
4. Centers for Disease Control and Prevention. US HIV and AIDS cases reported through December 1998. HIV/AIDS Surv Rep. [year-end edition] 9:1–44, 1998.
5. Granovsky MO, Mueller BU, Nicholson HS, Rosenberg PS, Rabkin CS. Cancer in human immunodeficiency virus-infected children: a case series from the Children's Cancer Group and the National Cancer Institute. J Clin Oncol 16:1729–1735, 1998.
6. Ziegler JL, Katongole-Mbidde E. Kaposi's sarcoma in childhood: an analysis of 100 cases from Uganda and relationship to HIV infection. Int J Cancer 65:200–203, 1996.
7. Athale UH, Patil PS, Chintu C, Elem B. Influence of HIV epidemic on the incidence of Kaposi's sarcoma in Zambian children. J Acquir Immune Defic Syndr Hum Retrovirol 8:96–100, 1995.
8. Mueller BU, Pizzo PA. Cancer in children with primary or secondary immunodeficiencies. J Pediatr 126:1–10, 1995.
9. Shad A, Magrath IT. Malignant non-Hodgkin's lymphomas in children. In: Pizzo PA, Poplack DG, eds. Principles and Practice of Pediatric Oncology. Philadelphia: Lippincott-Raven, 1997:545–588.
10. Epstein LG, DiCarlo FJ, Joshi VV, et al. Primary lymphoma of the central nervous system in children with acquired immunodeficiency syndrome. Pediatrics 82:355–363, 1988.

11. Del Mistro A, Laverda A, Calabrese F, et al. Primary lymphoma of the central nervous system in two children with acquired immune deficiency syndrome. Am J Clin Pathol 94:722–728, 1990.
12. Neumann Y, Toren A, Mandel M, et al. Favorable response of pediatric AIDS-related Burkitt's lymphoma treated by aggressive chemotherapy. Med Pediatr Oncol 21:661–664, 1993.
13. Nadal D, Caduff R, Frey E, et al. Non–Hodgkin's lymphoma in four children infected with the human immunodeficiency virus. Cancer 73:224–230, 1994.
14. Guterman KS, Hair LS, Morgello S. Epstein–Barr virus and AIDS-related primary central nervous system lymphoma. Viral detection by immunohistochemistry RNA in situ hybridization, and polymerase chain reaction. Clin Neuropathol 15:79–86, 1996.
15. Chetty R. Parotid MALT lymphoma in an HIV positive child. Histopathology 29:195–197, 1996.
16. Joshi VV, Gagnon GA, Chadwick EG, et al. The spectrum of mucosa-associated lymphoid tissue lesions in pediatric patients infected with HIV: a clinicopathological study of six cases. Am J Clin Pathol 107:592–600, 1997.
17. Corr P, Vaithilinum M, Theipal R, Jeena P. Parotid MALT lymphoma in HIV infected children. J Ultrasound Med 16:615–617, 1997.
18. Berrebi D, Lescoeur B, Faye A, Faure C, Vilmer E, Peuchmaur M. MALT lymphoma of labial minor salivary gland in an immunocompetent child with a gastric *Helicobacter pylori* infection. J Pediatr 133:290–292, 1998.
19. Reiter A, Riehm H. Large-cell lymphomas in children. In: Magrath IT, ed. The Non–Hodgkin's Lymphomas. London: Arnold, 1997:829–851.
20. Teruya-Feldstein J, Temeck BK, Sloas MM, et al. Pulmonary malignant lymphoma of mucosa-associated lymphoid tissue (MALT) arising in a pediatric HIV–positive patient. Am J Surg Pathol 19:357–363, 1995.
21. Bayerdörffer E, Neubauer A, Rudolph B, et al. Regression of primary gastric lymphoma of mucosa-associated lymphoid tissue after cure of *Helicobacter pylori* infection. Lancet 345:1591–1594, 1995.
22. Savio A, Franzin G, Wotherspoon AC, et al. Diagnosis and posttreatment follow-up of *Helicobacter pylori*-positive gastric lymphoma of mucosa-associated lymphoid tissue: histology, polymerase chain reaction, or both? Blood 87:1255–1260, 1996.
23. Hammel P, Haioun C, Chaumette M-T, et al. Efficacy of single-agent chemotherapy in low-grade B-cell mucosa-associated lymphoid tissue lymphoma with prominent gastric expression. J Clin Oncol 13:2524–2529, 1995.
24. Shad A, Mueller BU, Adde M, et al. Results of a treatment protocol for children with HIV and non–Hodgkin's lymphomas (NHL). J Acquir Immune Defic Syndr Hum Retrovirol 14:A54, 1997.
25. Robison LL. General principles of the epidemiology of childhood cancer. In: Pizzo PA, Poplack DG, eds. Principles and Practice of Pediatric Oncology. Philadelphia: Lippincott–Raven, 1997:1–10.
26. Hudson MM, Donaldson SS. Hodgkin's disease. In: Pizzo PA, Poplack DG, eds. Principles and Practice of Pediatric Oncology. Philadelphia: Lippincott–Raven, 1997: 523–544.
27. Joshi VV, Kauffman S, Oleske JM, et al. Polyclonal polymorphic B-cell lymphopro-

liferative disorder with prominent pulmonary involvement in children with acquired immune deficiency syndrome. Cancer 59:1455–1462, 1987.

28. Joshi VV. Systemic lymphoproliferative lesions in children with AIDS. Pediatr AIDS HIV Infect Fetus Adolesc 1:44–48, 1990.
29. Soberman N, Leonidas JC, Berdon WE, et al. Parotid enlargement in children seropositive for human immunodeficiency virus: imaging findings. AJR Am J Radiol 157:553–556, 1991.
30. Kazi S, Cohen PR, Williams F, Schempp R, Reveille JD. The diffuse infiltrative lymphocytosis syndrome: clinical and immunogenetic features in 35 patients. AIDS 10:385–391, 1996.
31. Connor EM, Andiman WA. Lymphoid interstitial pneumonitis. In: Pizzo PA, Wilfert CM, eds. Pediatric AIDS. The Challenge of HIV Infection in Infants, Children, and Adolescents. Baltimore: Williams & Wilkins, 1994:467–482.
32. Pitt J. Lymphocytic interstitial pneumonia. In: Edelson PJ, ed. Childhood AIDS. Vol 38. Philadelphia: WB Saunders, 1991:89–96.
33. Sharland M, Gibb DM, Holland F. Respiratory morbidity from lymphocytic interstitial pneumonitis (LIP) in vertically acquired HIV infection. Arch Dis Child 76:334–336, 1997.
34. Kontny HU, Sleasman JW, Kingma DW, et al. Multilocular thymic cysts in children with human immunodeficiency virus infection. Clinical and pathological aspects. J Pediatr 131:264–270, 1997.
35. Walsek C, Edgerly M, Nelson RP, et al. The combination of retinoic acid and interferon-alpha for the treatment of lymphoproliferative disorders in children with immunodeficiency disorders, National AIDS Malignancy Conference, Bethesda, MD, April 28–30, 1997.
36. Miser JS, Triche TJ, Kinsella TJ, Pritchard DJ. Other soft tissue sarcomas of childhood. In: Pizzo PA, Poplack DG, eds. Principles and Practice of Pediatric Oncology. Philadelphia: Lippincott–Raven, 1997: 865–888.
37. Chadwick EG, Connor EJ, Guerra Hanson IC, et al. Tumors of smooth muscle origin in HIV-infected children. JAMA 263:3182–3184, 1990.
38. Sabatino D, Martinez S, Young R, Balbi H, Ciminera P, Frieri M. Simultaneous pulmonary leiomyosarcoma and leiomyoma in pediatric HIV infection. Pediatr Hematol Oncol 8:355–359, 1991.
39. McLoughlin LC, Nord KS, Joshi VV, DiCarlo FJ, Kane MJ. Disseminated leiomyosarcoma in a child with acquired immune deficiency syndrome. Cancer 67:2618–2621, 1991.
40. Mueller BU, Butler KM, Feuerstein IM, et al. Smooth muscle tumors in children with human immunodeficiency virus infection. Pediatrics 90:460–463, 1992.
41. Ross JS, Del Rosario A, Bui HX, Sonbati H, Solis O. Primary hepatic leiomyosarcoma in a child with the acquired immunodeficiency syndrome. Hum Pathol 23:69–72, 1992.
42. Orlow SJ, Kamino H, Lawrence RL. Multiple subcutaneous leiomyosarcomas in an adolescent with AIDS. Am J Pediatr Hematol Oncol 14:265–268, 1992.
43. Angerpointner TA, Weitz H, Haas RJ, Hecker WC. Intestinal leiomyosarcoma in childhood—case report and review of the literature. J Pediatr Surg 16:491–495, 1981.

44. Ranchod M, Kempson RL. Smooth muscle tumors of the gastrointestinal tract and retroperitoneum. A pathologic analysis of 100 cases. Cancer 39:255–262, 1977.
45. McClain KL, Leach CT, Jenson HB, et al. Association of Epstein–Barr virus with leiomyosarcomas in young people with AIDS. N Engl J Med 332:12–18, 1995.
46. Buck BE, Scott GB, Valdes-Dapena M, Parks WP. Kaposi sarcoma in two infants with acquired immune deficiency syndrome. J Pediatr 103:911–913, 1983.
47. Baum LG, Vinters HV. Lymphadenopathic Kaposi's sarcoma in a pediatric patient with acquired immune deficiency syndrome. Pediatr Pathol 9:459–465, 1989.
48. Bouquety JC, Siopathis MR, Ravisse PR, Lagarde N, Georges-Courbot MC, Georges AJ. Lympho-cutaneous Kaposi's sarcoma in an African pediatric AIDS case. Am J Trop Med Hyg 40:323–325, 1989.
49. Gutierrez-Ortega P, Hierro-Orozco S, Sanchez-Cisneros R, Montana LF. Kaposi's sarcoma in a 6-day-old infant with human immunodeficiency virus. Arch Dermatol 125:432–433, 1989.
50. Connor E, Boccon-Gibod L, Joshi V, et al. Cutaneous acquired immunodeficiency syndrome-associated Kaposi's sarcoma in pediatric patients. Arch Dermatol 126: 791–793, 1990.
51. Serraino D, Franceschi S. Kaposi's sarcoma and non-Hodgkin's lymphomas in children and adolescents with AIDS. AIDS 10:643–647, 1996.
52. Moore PS, Kingsley LA, Holmberg SD, et al. Kaposi's sarcoma-associated herpesvirus infection prior to onset of Kaposi's sarcoma. AIDS 10:175–180, 1996.
53. Scully RE, Mark RE, McNeely BU. Case records of the Massachusetts General Hospital. N Engl J Med 314:629–640, 1986.
54. Ninane J, Moulin D, Latinne D, et al. AIDS in two African children—one with fibrosarcoma of the liver. Eur J Pediatr 144:385–390, 1985.
55. DiCarlo FJ, Joshi VV, Oleske JM, Connor EM. Neoplastic diseases in children with acquired immunodeficiency syndrome. Prog AIDS Pathol 2:163–185, 1990.
56. Arico M, Caselli D, D'Argenio P, et al. Malignancies in children with human immunodeficiency virus type 1 infection. Cancer 68:2473–2477, 1991.
57. Lyall EGH, Langdale-Brown B, Eden OB, Mok JYQ, Croft NM. Ewing's sarcoma in a child with human immunodeficiency virus (type 1) infection. Med Pediatr Oncol 21:127–131, 1993.
58. Mandel M, Toren A, Hadani M, Engelberg I, Martinowitz U, Rechavi G. Ependymoblastoma in an HIV-positive hemophilic girl. Med Pediatr Oncol 23:441–443, 1994.
59. Diamond FB, Price LJ, Nelson RP Jr. Papillary carcinoma of the thyroid in a seven-year-old HIV-positive child. Pediatr AIDS HIV Infect Fetus Adolesc 5:232–235, 1994.
60. Stratton P, Ciacco KH. Cervical neoplasia in the patient with HIV infection. Curr Opin Obstet Gynecol 6:86–91, 1994.
61. Olivero OA, Anderson LM, Diwan BA, et al. AZT is a genotoxic transplacental carcinogen in animal models. J Acquir Immune Defic Syndr Hum Retrovirol 14: A29, 1997.

13

Attenuation of Chemotherapy Side Effects in AIDS-Associated Malignancies

Alice Reier, Fa-Chyi Lee, and Ronald T. Mitsuyasu
University of California, Los Angeles, Los Angeles, California

I. INTRODUCTION

Since the beginning of the AIDS epidemic, tumors have been known to occur in HIV-infected individuals. Kaposi's sarcoma (AIDS KS), non-Hodgkin's lymphomas (AIDS NHL), primary central nervous system (CNS) lymphoma, and cervical carcinoma are AIDS-defining diseases (1), and other malignancies, such as lung, rectal, breast, colon, head and neck, and testicular carcinoma, have been described in patients with HIV infection (2). AIDS KS and AIDS NHL tend to occur in patients with more severe immune deficiency, whereas other tumors may manifest at any level of CD4 cell counts. Treatment with chemotherapy to control these tumors should be based on clinical necessity and should not be withheld simply because of the patient's HIV status. Even patients with advanced-stage AIDS NHL may benefit from chemotherapy. An Italian group reported median survival of 42 months with intensive chemotherapy in a subgroup of AIDS NHL patients with the following characteristics: age younger than 30 years, CD4 cell counts of more than $100/mm^3$, and without B symptoms (3).

Nevertheless, side effects and toxicities of chemotherapy do occur in HIV-infected individuals and may influence outcome of treatment in these patients. Although direct comparison of the incidence of chemotherapy-related side effects in HIV-infected and uninfected patients is not available, HIV-infected patients do appear to suffer more frequent and more severe side effects from treatment. This may be due to their generally poor clinical status at the time they develop their tumors, the effects of other medications they are receiving for HIV or related diseases, or the potentiation of already existing symptoms by the chemotherapy drugs themselves (e.g., peripheral neuropathy).

In this chapter, we will discuss some of the commonly encountered side effects of chemotherapy in AIDS patients and their management. Aggressive prevention and treatment of opportunistic infections and the use of combination antiretroviral medications have resulted in longer survival for HIV-infected individuals (4), which has increased the likelihood of HIV patients developing a malignancy during their lifetime. Also, with the improved outcomes of therapy for AIDS malignancies, the quality of life of patients who receive these treatments takes on greater meaning. The benefits of chemotherapy in curing or in alleviating symptoms from these tumors need to be balanced against its side effects and its effects on the patient's quality of life. Minimization of side effects and treatment of drug-induced toxicities are major goals in the management of all patients with AIDS malignancies.

II. PRECHEMOTHERAPY APPROACHES

A. Initial Evaluation

Antiretroviral drugs and antibiotics to prevent opportunistic infections are themselves chemotherapeutic agents and have associated toxicities. Currently, all U.S. Food and Drug Administration (FDA)-approved antiretroviral medications have the potential to cause bone marrow suppression, although zidovudine (ZDV) is the most myelosuppressive of the antiretroviral drugs currently in use for HIV (5). Patients will also often be receiving several prophylactic medications, such as trimethoprim-sulfamethoxazole, acyclovir, and ganciclovir, which are also myelosuppressive. Several of the antiretroviral medications can also cause peripheral neuropathy (e.g., zalcitabine [ddC], didanosine [ddI], and stavudine [d4T]). Adjustment of medications to maintain good antiretroviral control and prophylaxis for opportunistic infections, while minimizing side effects, is an important part of the evaluation for patients in whom chemotherapy is being contemplated.

Other common HIV-associated infections, such as parvovirus B19, cytomegalovirus (CMV), *Mycobacterium tuberculosis* (MTB), and *Mycobacterium avium* complex (MAC), can also cause leukopenia (6) or anemia (7) in patients with HIV. Treatment of opportunistic infections (OIs) should be given, and the infections should be brought under optimal control before initiating chemotherapy in most situations. If this is not possible, such as in patients with rapidly progressing NHL, when a delay in chemotherapy can be life-threatening, simultaneous treatment of OIs and of the malignancy may be necessary. In these situations, close attention to minimizing side effects and toxicities of concurrent drug administration must be made. Polyradiculopathy and CNS symptoms associated with certain opportunistic infections (e.g., CMV) can be successfully treated if diagnosed early (8) and may lessen the likelihood of potentiation of these symptoms when chemotherapy is administered.

Hematological abnormalities can also occur without obvious offending medications or infections. Especially in patients with advanced HIV infection, cytopenia often occurs as a direct or indirect effect of HIV itself (9). HIV-infected individuals also have a high rate of neurological complications without definable insult. The cause for this neuropathy is believed to be autoimmune owing to HIV (10).

When correctable causes of cytopenia have been ruled out, the use of hematopoietic growth factors to maintain a more normal blood count has become a common practice. Available clinical data indicate that use of hematopoietic growth factors can effectively raise total neutrophil counts and hemoglobin levels in nonmalignant conditions associated with HIV infection (11). A concern in patients requiring chemotherapy is whether there may be long-term effects of extended hematopoietic growth factor use on bone marrow progenitor cells that may make patients more susceptible to the myelosuppressive effects of subsequent chemotherapy. Janit et al. (12) showed that prechemotherapy administration of granulocyte-macrophage colony-stimulating factor (GM-CSF) did not increase, but reduced the incidence of neutropenia in patients receiving topotecan (12). On the other hand, a study in breast cancer patients showed a significantly higher incidence of grade 3 and 4 thrombocytopenia and a trend toward more severe neutropenia in a group of patients receiving prechemotherapy granulocyte colony-stimulating factor (G-CSF) for neutropenia (13). Despite this concern, we continue to recommend appropriate use of hematopoietic growth factors to overcome severe cytopenia in HIV patients starting use, even before chemotherapy, to prevent infections and to allow administration of therapeutically important medications. In addition, myeloid hematopoietic growth factors can increase neutrophil functions and may be important in the host's immune response to a variety of infections and malignant diseases (14,15).

B. Selection of Chemotherapeutic Agent

Once the decision to proceed with chemotherapy has been made, the next step is the selection of the appropriate drugs to use. In addition to myelosuppression with almost all chemotherapeutic drugs, each agent has its own unique set of toxicities. Palmar–plantar syndrome, an acute erythematous painful swelling of the hands and feet, has been associated with liposomal doxorubicin (16) used in the treatment of AIDS KS. Alopecia and stomatitis, however, occur less frequently with liposomal daunorubicin (17) and liposomal doxorubicin (16) than with other chemotherapeutic drugs. Cardiac toxicity is extremely infrequent with either liposomal doxorubicin or liposomal daunorubicin (18,19). A recent comparison of combination chemotherapy with single-agent therapy has shown similar outcomes and fewer toxicities with single-drug therapy for AIDS KS with agents, such as liposomal doxorubicin (20), liposomal daunorubicin (21), and paclitaxel. The potential pulmonary toxicity of bleomycin and the neurotoxicity with vincristine may be avoided by using single-agent, rather than combination chemotherapy, in patients with KS who are receiving chemotherapy for the first time.

Combination regimens, however, remain the primary approach for treating AIDS NHL. No single regimen has been proven to be superior to others. The drugs used in the various chemotherapy regimens can exacerbate certain preexisting conditions. Methotrexate is part of the m-BACOD (methotrexate, bleomycin, doxorubicin, cyclophosphamide, vincristine [Oncovin], dexamethasone) regimen and may induce or exacerbate hepatic and renal toxicity. Cyclophosphamide is part of the CHOP (cyclophosphamide, doxorubicin, vincristine, prednisone) regimen and can worsen neutropenia in some patients and exacerbate preexisting hepatic abnormalities. Vincristine in both m-BACOD and CHOP can potentiate peripheral neuropathy in patients with AIDS. Gastrointestinal toxicity occurs with a variety of regimens.

Potential drug interactions between anti-HIV medications and chemotherapy drugs is an area that clearly requires greater investigation. Ritonavir has a high affinity for several cytochrome P-450 (CYP) isoenzymes, especially CYP3A, and can inhibit the metabolism of many drugs that are metabolized through this mechanism. Drugs metabolized by CYP3A will have significant increases in the area under the concentration versus time curve (AUC) in the presence of ritonavir. Some chemotherapeutic drugs, such as etoposide, prednisone, paclitaxel, tamoxifen, vinblastine, and vincristine, are metabolized through CYP3A, and close monitoring for side effects is necessary when ritonavir is part of the anti-HIV regimen in patients receiving these drugs. Indinavir and saquinavir are also metabolized by CYP3A4 and do not appear to have significant interactions with the commonly used chemotherapeutic agents in HIV-associated malignancies. There is little formal data on chemotherapeutic drug interactions with most of the nucleoside analogues and nonnucleoside reverse transcriptase inhibitors; however, concomitant use of ZDV and chemotherapy may cause significant bone marrow suppression. Studies using ddI or ddC with CHOP or ABV (doxorubicin, bleomycin, vincristine) have not shown increased risk of peripheral neuropathy in patients treated with these agents if they did not have underlying peripheral neuropathy from HIV or other causes. It is our belief that HIV-infected patients should continue their effective antiretroviral medications while receiving chemotherapy to reduce the risks associated with rapid increases in HIV replication.

III. HEMATOLOGICAL TOXICITY

Hematological toxicity remains the most frequently encountered dose-limiting side effect in HIV-infected patients undergoing chemotherapy. In most patients, manifestations are usually pancytopenia, neutropenia, or anemia. Thrombocytopenia has generally not been a major problem in HIV-infected patients with normal platelet counts before initiating chemotherapy. The extent of toxicity tends to be cycle- and dose-dependent (22). A few different approaches can be taken to lessen the extent of toxicity.

A. Myeloid Hematopoietic Growth Factors

The most common approach is to use hematopoietic growth factors. According to the guidelines of the American Society of Clinical Oncology (ASCO) (23,24), primary administration of myeloid colony-stimulating factors to prevent neutropenia in previously untreated patients is not recommended. Before the FDA approval of granulocyte colony-stimulating factor (G-CSF), clinical trials showed that HIV-infected individuals could tolerate multiple cycles of combination chemotherapy for AIDS KS (25,26,27) by applying dose reductions to manage hematological toxicity. Unfortunately, there has been no study specifically designed to evaluate the dose responsiveness of AIDS KS to chemotherapy. Liposomal doxorubicin (10–40 mg/m^2) (28), liposomal daunorubicin (20–60 mg/m^2) (29) and paclitaxel (100–135 mg/m^2) (30) were effective when given in 21-day cycles; however, one trial with liposomal daunorubicin showed that breakthrough lesions at 40 mg/m^2 responded to a higher dose of 60 mg/m^2 with G-CSF support for neutropenia (31). Other clinical studies have supported the use of GM-CSF (32) or G-CSF (33) to deliver full doses of chemotherapy on schedule for patients with AIDS KS. As treatment for most patients with AIDS KS is palliative and not curative, dose reduction remains a valid alternative approach for initial management of hematological toxicity, as long as the lower dose continues to show effectiveness in controlling KS lesions.

Experiences in patients with AIDS NHL are somewhat different. The French–Italian Cooperative Study Group showed that 21% of their study patients could tolerate only one cycle of low-dose chemotherapy (cyclophosphamide 300 mg/m^2, doxorubicin 25 mg/m^2, teniposide 30 mg/m^2 on day 1, followed by prednisone 20 mg/m^2 on days 1–5, vincristine 2 mg and bleomycin 10 units on day 15) because of bone marrow toxicity (34). A U. S. multicenter study of low-dose m-BACOD (cyclophosphamide 300 mg/m^2, doxorubicin 25 mg/m^2, vincristine 1.4 mg/m^2, with maximum 2 mg on day 1, dexamethasone 3 mg/m^2 on day 1–5, and methotrexate 200 mg/m^2 on day 15) given in 21-day cycles, found that only 7 of the 42 patients could tolerate more than six cycles of chemotherapy (35). The reason appears to be that patients with AIDS NHL, in general, have advanced HIV infection with low CD4 cell counts and poor bone marrow reserve at the time of diagnosis and are more susceptible to the myelosuppressive effects of the combination regimens used for AIDS NHL. Consequently, it is advisable to initiate G-CSF early in the course of treatment for AIDS NHL and for HIV-infected patients with Hodgkin's disease.

HIV-infected patients with squamous cell carcinoma of the anus treated with chemotherapy (flurouracil [5-FU] and mitomycin-C) and concurrent radiation experience a higher incidence of toxicity, local skin reaction, and bone marrow suppression, compared with non–HIV-infected patients, which requires either treatment interruption or dose reduction (36). Longer disease-free intervals may be achieved with this combined modality approach in patients with early (stage I/II) disease (37).

The natural history and response to treatment with orchiectomy, retroperitoneal lymph node dissection, radiation, and chemotherapy for malignant germ cell tumors in an HIV-infected patient is comparable to that seen in noninfected patients (38). In one study, patients received four cycles of either PEB (cisplatin, etoposide, bleomycin) or PVB (cisplatin, vinblastine, bleomycin) chemotherapy. Of the seven HIV-infected patients who completed treatment, six developed grade 4 toxicity (ANC < 500) during therapy, which was treated with G-CSF. None of the HIV-infected patients with malignant germ cell tumors died of their tumors. All deaths were due to HIV-related complications.

Although data on chemotherapy for other malignant tumors in HIV-infected patients are not readily available, the experiences in AIDS patients with anal carcinoma and malignant germ cell tumors support the following observations: (1) HIV-infected patients can respond to treatment; (2) long-term tumor-free survival is possible with appropriate treatment; and (3) use of G-CSF to support full-dose and on-schedule delivery of chemotherapy is advisable.

In vitro, GM-CSF enhances HIV replication, but also enhances the anti-HIV activity of ZDV (39). Therefore, it is recommended that all patients with HIV receiving GM-CSF be on an effective antiretroviral therapeutic regimen. GM-CSF used in either high or low doses (500 $\mu g/m^2$ or 250 $\mu g/m^2$), however, does not up-regulate p24 antigen in patients with AIDS KS treated with a combination of doxorubicin, bleomycin, and vincristine (40). Rare associations of GM-CSF with rapid progression of AIDS KS (41) and of G-CSF associated with the development of acute myelomonocytic leukemia (42) are yet to be confirmed by other studies. Both GM-CSF and G-CSF are effective in the management of neutropenia. There are no comparison trials to evaluate the superiority of G-CSF versus GM-CSF; therefore, the timing and duration of myeloid hematopoietic growth factor use as an adjunct to chemotherapy rests in the hands of the treating physician and should generally follow guidelines used in non–HIV-infected patients receiving chemotherapy.

Commonly used dosages for GM-CSF are 5 $\mu g/kg$ per day or 250 $\mu g/m^2$

per day (43). The recommended dose for G-CSF is 5–10 µg/kg per day or 300 µg per day. Both factors can be given intravenously or subcutaneously. As per ASCO guidelines, growth factor administration is generally started 24–72 hours after administering the chemotherapy, but a later starting date is reasonable if shorter duration of growth factor use can achieve adequate neutrophil recovery. Use of growth factor should continue until the absolute neutrophil cell count is at least 10,000/mm^3. For patients receiving myeloid growth factor before chemotherapy, growth factor should be discontinued at least 24 h before giving cytotoxic agents and resumed 24 h after treatment. Patients receiving liposomal anthracyclines may also benefit from starting administration of myeloid growth factors at 5–7 days after chemotherapy, as a delay in the nadir of the WBC has typically been seen with these agents.

B. Cytoprotective Agent

The use of hematopoietic growth factors hastens bone marrow recovery after the insult of cytotoxic drugs. The FDA recently approved agents that can protect end-organ toxicity from certain chemotherapeutic agents. Dexrazoxane was approved for protection against cardiac toxicity from doxorubicin; however, more severe myelosuppression has been observed when the dexrazoxane dose is higher than 1 g/m^2 with concurrent chemotherapy. The use of dexrazoxane in HIV patients may be limited because liposomal anthracyclines do not cause pronounced cardiac toxicity. The doxorubicin dose used in AIDS NHL has not been associated with any significant degree of cardiac toxicity.

Amifostine, formerly known as WR-2721, was recently approved by the FDA for renal protection in use with cisplatin. In mice after irradiation, amifostine enhances hematopoietic reconstitution in the presence of hematopoietic factors (44). When tested against breast and ovarian cancer cell lines, amifostine does not reduce the cytotoxic effects of chemotherapeutic agents (45). Pretreatment with amifostine in human subjects with various solid malignancies receiving cyclophosphamide at 1.5 g/m^2 protected against hematological toxicity by shortening the duration of neutropenia, 2.4 days versus 3.9 days, and by improving mean nadir neutrophil counts, 1247 versus 541/mm^3 (46). One trial using a combination of cyclophosphamide and cisplatin, with or without amifostine, for patients with advanced ovarian cancer, showed that amifostine reduced neutropenia-associated events by 53% and resulted in a significant decrease in days of hospitalization and days of antibiotic use without adverse effects on the antitumor response (47). Abstracts on the cytoprotective effect of amifostine against hematological toxicity induced by paclitaxel and doxorubicin were presented at the 1996 ASCO annual meeting (48,49).

Amifostine is a prodrug that requires dephosphorylation, catalyzed by plasma membrane-bound alkaline phosphatase, to the free-thiol, WR-1065 (50).

The neutral pH environment of normal tissue relative to tumor tissue favors activation of alkaline phosphatase in the normal tissue bed and facilitates uptake of the active drug, WR-1065, into normal cells through a carrier-mediated transport process (51). With the exception of the CNS, all major organs can potentially be protected by amifostine through increased intracellular free thiol (52). Amifostine appears to be an interesting compound that deserves further investigation for its application in HIV-infected patients receiving chemotherapy, as these patients appear to be more susceptible to the adverse side effects of many chemotherapeutic drugs.

C. Granulocyte Transfusion

Clinical trials in neutropenic patients (53) and in neonates (54) using allogeneic granulocyte transfusion, before the availability of G-CSF, have not demonstrated benefit in either infection control or survival. The short half-life of transfused granulocytes in circulation, and the small number of granulocytes that can be collected from donors, all contribute to the fading interest in granulocyte transfusion (55). The use of G-CSF to increase donor production of granulocytes has renewed some interest to reexplore the potential of granulocyte transfusion in neutropenic patients with life-threatening infections (56,57). This approach has not been reported in HIV-infected patients. Transfusion-related graft-versus-host disease (GVHD) is a potential problem with this approach in HIV-infected patients, although allogeneic red blood cell transfusion is a common event in HIV-infected patients receiving chemotherapy or in the late stages of HIV infection. Little GVHD has been seen in this situation (58). Because of the possibility of transmitting infections and other potentially life-threatening complications (59), granulocyte transfusion for HIV-infected patients from allogeneic donors cannot be recommended at the present time.

Autologous stem cell transfusion is another possibility for HIV-infected patients. G-CSF at 10 µg/kg per day for 5 days can mobilize functional CD34 cells in HIV-infected patients (60). Progenitor cells from the bone marrow of HIV-infected patients engrafted successfully after high-dose chemotherapy for hematological malignancies (61). In the future, autologous stem cells may be able to support continued chemotherapy in HIV-infected patients, or act as vehicles for gene therapy treatment approaches.

IV. NEUROPATHY

Some chemotherapeutic agents commonly used in AIDS malignancies cause or exacerbate peripheral neuropathy; however, global CNS dysfunction is rare. Vincristine is the most commonly used drug associated with peripheral neuropathy.

One trial in patients with AIDS KS showed that high-grade neurotoxicity occurred in one-third of the study subjects (62). In other studies, there was no increase in neuropathy among patients without preexisting neuropathy receiving vincristine as part of ABV chemotherapy with ddI and ddC. For patients with preexisting peripheral neuropathy, the best strategy may be to avoid using vincristine. If severe neurotoxicity develops while receiving chemotherapy, dose reduction or discontinuing vincristine is advisable.

Paclitaxel is another agent that causes a high incidence of neuropathy; however, when paclitaxel is administered to patients with AIDS KS, myelotoxicity usually overshadows the neurotoxicity (63). Once neuropathy develops with paclitaxel, it is advisable to switch the patient to another chemotherapeutic drug.

Peripheral neuropathy can cause profound morbidity. Reducing the dose or discontinuing the neurotoxic agent before irreversible nerve damage occurs is

Table 1 Nonsteroidal Anti-Inflammatory Drugs

Class	Generic name	Trade name(s)	Usual dose in mg and frequency in hour
Salicylates	Aspirin	Ecotrin	650–1000 Q 4–6
	Diflunisal	Dolobid	500–1000 Q 12
	Salicylic acid	Disalcid, Salsalate	1000–1500 Q 12
	Choline magnesium trisalicylate	Trilisate	500–2000 Q 12
Propionic acid	Ibuprofen	Motrin, Nurpin, Brufen, Advil, etc.	200–800 Q 8
	Naproxen	Naprosyn, Anaprox, Laraflex	250 Q 8
	Fenoprofen	Nalfon, Fenopron, Progesic	200 Q 4
	Flubiprofen	Anasaid, Froben	25–50 Q 4–6
	Ketoprofen	Orudis, Oruvail	50–75 Q 6–8
Acetic acids	Indomethacin	Indocin, Indocid	25–75 Q 8
	Ketorolac	Toradol	30–120 Q 24
	Diclofenac	Voltaren, Voltarol	75 Q 12
	Nabumetone	Relafen	1000–2000 Q 24
	Etodelac	Lodine	200–400 Q 8
	Sulindac	Clinoril	200 Q 4
	Tolmetin	Tolectin	400–600 Q 8
Anthranilic acid	Meclofenamate	Meclomen	100 Q 6
Oxicams	Piroxocam	Feldene	20 Q 24

the best approach (64). Medications used to treat peripheral neuropathy in AIDS are derived from experiences in treating patients with neuralgia and diabetic neuropathy. They include nonsteroidal anti-inflammatory drugs (NSAIDs), acetaminophen, antidepressants, anticonvulsive medications, and opioid analgesics, depending upon the degree of symptoms. The effectiveness of these medications in controlling symptoms is mixed, and a trial-and-error approach in finding the right medication for each individual may be required. Supplementation with vitamin B_{12} is controversial (65,66). Subjectiveness in grading the symptoms of neuropathy is one of the difficulties in fully evaluating a patient's response to any medical intervention. A strong placebo effect was documented in a trial with negative results using mexiletine in painful neuropathy (67). Nonhabit-forming agents should be tried before using opiates, although opiates should not be avoided when necessary to control symptoms. There is no data indicating superior results with combining agents with different modes of action.

NSAIDs constitute a large group of medications with a wide dose range (Table 1). Gastrointestinal irritation with a potential for gastrointestinal bleeding, platelet dysfunction with prolonged bleeding time, decreased renal function from

Table 2 Psychotropic Drugs

Class	Generic name	Trade name	Usual dose per day in mg
Tricyclics	Amitriptyline	Elavil	10–150
	Nortriptyline	Pamelor, Aventyl	10–150
	Imipramine	Tofranil	15.5–150
	Desipramine	Norpramin	10–150
	Clomipramine	Anafranil	10–150
	Doxepin	Sinequan	12–150
Heterocyclics and non-cyclics	Trazodone	Desyrel	125–300
	Maprotiline	Ludiomil	50–300
Serotonin re-uptake inhibitors	Fluoxetine	Prozac	20–80
	Paroxetine	Paxil	10–60
	Sertraline	Zoloft	50–200
Anticonvulsants	Carbamazepine	Tegretol	800–1600
	Clonazepam	Klonopin	0.5–4
	Phenytoin	Dilantin	200–600
	Valproic acid	Depakote, Depakene	1500–3000
	Gabapentin	Neurontin	900–3600

Table 3 Opiates

Class	Drug name	Usual dose in mg	Onset of action	Duration of action in hours	Other trade name or as in one of the active ingredients
Weak	Codeine	15–60	30–60 min	4–8	As in Robitussin A–C, Tylenol 3, Brontex, Dimetane-DC, Nucofed, Tussar DM, Tussar-2
	Propoxyphene	65–130	1–2 hours	3–6	As in Darvocet, Darvocet-N, Wygesic
Moderate	Dihydrocodeine	10–30	30 min	3–6	As in DHC Plus, Synalgas-DC
	Hydrocodone	5–10	60 min	4–6	As in Lorcet, Vicodin, Vicodin ES, Zydone
	Oxycodone	5–80	30–60 min	3–4	OxyContin, or as in Percocet, Tylox, Endocet, Endodan, Roxicet, Roxiprin
Strong	Morphine	10 and above	15–30 min	4–5	MS Contin
	Hydromorphone	2 and above	5–30 min	4–5	Dilaudid
	Methadone	10–20	30 min–4 h	24	Dolophine
	Levorphanol	2–4	10–60 min	6–8	Levo–Dromoran
	Meperidine	75–300	10–30 min	2–4	Demerol
	Fentanyl	0.01–0.1	2 h	48–72	Duragesic

papillary necrosis, and life-threatening bronchospasm are some of the severe side effects that can occur with these drugs.

Antidepressants appear to be useful for the burning component of neuropathic pain (Table 2). Common adverse side effects with these agents are dry mouth, constipation, urinary retention, sedation, orthostatic hypotension, and other anticholinergic effects.

Anticonvulsants tend to be the best agents for managing lancenating, hyperesthetic pain (see Table 2). Potential side effects include hepatotoxicity, especially with carbamazepine, idiosyncratic bone marrow suppression, and severe hypersensitivity reaction (Stevens–Johnson syndrome).

Opiates are potent narcotic analgesics (Table 3). When used properly, opiates offer the best soothing effects for pain management. Opiates are divided into weak, moderate, and strong according to their potency. As a group, opiates can cause severe nausea. Coadministering laxatives is necessary to prevent constipation. Skin reaction, manifested as pruritus, is common with opiates. Central nervous system side effects with opiates include sedation, confusion, hallucination, nightmares, and possible seizures at high doses. Developing tolerance after long-term use usually requires titrating up the dose or switching to another agent. Some treating physicians may mistake the need for a higher dose as addiction and leave the patients undertreated.

V. ORAL COMPLICATIONS

Painful oral mucositis, induced by chemotherapy or radiation therapy, is a common side effect encountered by at least 40% of cancer patients. It can be caused either by direct toxicity of the chemotherapeutic drug or indirectly, as a result of myelosuppression (68). In 1989, the National Institutes of Health determined that oral complications from anticancer chemotherapies affect 400,000 U.S. patients annually and can significantly affect morbidity, the patient's tolerance to treatment, and quality of life (69). In addition, chemotherapy-induced mucositis, by disrupting the mucosal barrier, can increase the risk for oral bacterial, viral and fungal infections.

Cancer patients with AIDS may also suffer concomitant xerostomia from salivary gland dysfunction caused by diffuse infiltrative lymphocytosis syndrome. Other AIDS-associated conditions, such as oral herpes simplex, cytomegalovirus infection, candidiasis, aphthous ulcers, periodontal or gingival disease, may predispose patients to nutritional deficits and further compromise the patient's quality of life beyond that caused by the side effects of chemotherapy.

There is no standardized practice for managing mucositis in patients receiving chemotherapy. Management in U.S. hospitals is heterogeneous and consists of a combination of topical agents, such as lip lubricants and mouthwashes, and parenteral pain medication (70). Swish-and-swallow or expectorate solutions consisting of viscous lidocaine, diphenhydramine, and an antacid such as Maalox, are often combined with a corticosteroid mixed in Orabase (70). Some hospitals use oral nystatin or parenteral prophylactic antibiotics when giving high-dose chemotherapy. Others use antimicrobials only for culture-proved infections (70). The oral complications of chemotherapy can be minimized by thorough pretherapy oral examinations, appropriate treatment of oral infections, and continued good oral hygiene during chemotherapy (68,69,71).

Effective antimicrobial management for AIDS-associated oral or esophageal infections is very important. Local or systemic treatment with antifungal agents have proved effective against oral candidiasis. Oral herpes simplex and varicella–zoster usually respond well to systemic acyclovir. Cytomegalovirus (CMV) infections require treatment with ganciclovir or foscarnet, which may increase the risk of bone marrow suppression and possible renal insufficiency. Careful monitoring during treatment is critical.

Periodontal disease, which has a prevalence of 16–52% in HIV-infected patients (72), can occasionally progress to necrotizing stomatitis. Oral radiation therapy is more closely associated with periodontal disease than is chemotherapy. Close attention to oral care and cooperation by the medical and dental specialists is key to preventing dental complications from chemotherapy. In patients who cannot use toothbrushes, oral hygiene maintenance with chlorhexidine-soaked foam brushes has proved to be an effective alternative (71). Chlorhexidine is a broad-spectrum antimicrobial with no reported systemic toxicity (71).

Recurrent oral aphthous ulcers (RAU) occur more frequently and with greater severity in HIV-infected patients than in noninfected individuals and may be exacerbated with chemotherapy. RAU can often be treated effectively with local oral steroids, such as fluocinonide (Lidex) 0.05% ointment, mixed with equal parts of Orabase, applied to the lesion up to six times per day; or clobestasol (Temovate), 0.05% mixed with Orabase, applied three times daily (73). Painful aphthous ulcers in HIV can affect any area of the gastrointestinal tract, and systemic therapy may be appropriate in many patients. Data from a multicenter, placebo-controlled trial of the AIDS Clinical Trial Group (ACTG 251) showed that 14 of 23 patients (61%) receiving thalidomide, 200 mg/day, as compared with 1 of 22 patients (4.5%) receiving placebo, healed their aphthous ulcers with treatment (74). Thalidomide is an inhibitor of tumor necrosis factor-α (75), and because it lacks the immunosuppressive effects of corticosteroids, it is an attractive drug for HIV-infected patients with aphthous ulcers, especially those undergoing chemotherapy. Thalidomide has, however, increased HIV viral load as much as one log in some patients (76).

Iatrogenic oral ulcers and mucositis can also be seen after the use of foscarnet, interferon, and zalcitabine, or from radiation therapy for mucosal KS or oral NHL. As in other cancer patients, radiation therapy should not be given concurrently with systemic chemotherapy in HIV-infected patients. Ice-cold mouth-washes have been used before and after chemotherapy with fluorouracil (5-FU) and with melphalan and appear to have some benefit in preventing mucositis (77). In a placebo-controlled study of 44 patients with non-AIDS-related malignancies requiring 5-FU chemotherapy, allopurinol mouthwashes were a cost-effective method for reducing 5-FU oral toxicity, resolving stomatitis in 40% of patients and diminishing toxicity in 10 more patients, as compared with placebo (77).

Idiopathic esophageal ulcerations in HIV-infected patients can also add to the discomfort of chemotherapy-associated oral mucositis. In a recent study of esophageal ulcers in non–HIV-infected patients, 35% of patients had no infectious or malignant diagnosis by endoscopic biopsy. In 33/35 of these patients, there was a complete clinical response when these patients were treated with prednisone, 40 mg daily, tapering to 10 mg/day or 40 mg daily for two weeks (78).

The pain caused by chemotherapy-induced mucositis is often underappreciated and undertreated by many physicians. Topical anesthetics, such as viscous lidocaine and dyclonine, are the most commonly used first-line treatments in U. S. hospitals, followed by systemic opioids (70). Topical anesthetics are short acting, and opioids, when given in adequate doses, often cause unwanted somnolence and constipation. Oral desensitization with capsaicin, a derivative of chili peppers, may be an effective treatment for painful mucositis in some patients. A recent study using a taffy candy containing cayenne pepper in patients with chemotherapy- or radiation therapy-induced mucositis of ECOG grades 1–4 showed that of 11 patients treated, the candy temporarily decreased or abolished the mucositis pain in all patients, with few adverse effects (79). This approach, with some modifications, may be an effective adjunct to the treatment of pain caused by mucositis. Physicians should aggressively treat HIV-infected patients with pain caused by chemotherapy-induced mucositis to maximize patient comfort and to minimize nutritional deficits caused by the inability to eat. When local anesthetics prove insufficient, appropriately scheduled systemic opioids should be prescribed, without undue hesitation.

VI. NAUSEA AND VOMITING

Nausea and dyspepsia are common symptoms in HIV-infected patients (80). Patients often receive a daunting, combination oral drug regimen consisting of three or four antiretroviral drugs and multiple prophylactic or therapeutic antibiotics. Many of the antiretroviral drugs, such as ritonavir, and to a lesser extent, saquinavir and indinavir, can cause gastrointestinal distress. DdI, ddC and d4T, all can cause pancreatitis, especially in patients who have a history of pancreatitis, drink alcohol, or take other medications that can induce pancreatitis (81). Additionally, GI tract infections, such as CMV, MAC, candida, or parasites, may cause dyspepsia, nausea, or diarrhea, as can stomach or small intestine involvement by KS or lymphoma (80). It is extremely important for HIV-infected patients taking antiretroviral drugs not to miss or lose doses through emesis, because erratic dosing is believed to be the primary cause of HIV drug resistance (82). Preventing emesis in the HIV-infected patient receiving chemotherapy, therefore, is critical, may be especially challenging, and may affect a patient's rate of developing antiretroviral drug resistance.

The fear of nausea and vomiting as a result of chemotherapy is also an important concern for most cancer patients. Advances in the prevention and treatment of chemotherapy-induced nausea and vomiting over the past decade, however, have made these uncomfortable symptoms unnecessary for most patients (83). In general, the same antiemetic regimens can be used in HIV-infected patients, with efficacy equal to that in other cancer patients undergoing chemotherapy. Drug interactions with some of the protease inhibitors, however, may preclude the use of some combination antiemetic regimens or may require adjustment in dosing.

Dopaminergic as well as histaminic and muscarinic receptors are involved in chemotherapy-induced nausea and vomiting; however, antagonists of these receptors can reduce these symptoms. One of the major mediators of chemotherapy-induced nausea and vomiting is serotonin, which is released by chemotherapy-damaged enterochromaffin cells of the gastrointestinal tract, activating 5-hydroxytryptamine ($5\text{-}HT_3$) receptors in vagal afferents of the upper gastrointestinal tract and in the nucleus tractus solitarius and area postrema (83,84,85). The widespread use of $5\text{-}HT_3$ receptor blockers, such as ondansetron and granisetron, has greatly improved the tolerability of moderately and highly emetogenic chemotherapy regimens; however, as only 50–60% of patients receiving highly emetogenic chemotherapy are completely protected by blocking $5\text{-}HT_3$ receptors, it appears that other receptors or mechanisms are also important (86). Risk factors predisposing patients to increased emesis associated with chemotherapy include female sex, age younger than 30 years, susceptibility to motion sickness, prior chemotherapy with poorly controlled nausea, low alcohol consumption, and the intrinsic emetogenicity of the chemotherapeutic agent (83–87).

Combination antiemetic therapy is now recommended to inhibit multiple receptors involved with nausea and vomiting. Phenothiazines, such as prochlorperazine, chlorpromazine, and thiopropazate have been used as antiemetics for chemotherapy for more than 30 years. They prevent nausea and emesis by blocking dopaminergic D_2 receptors located in the chemoreceptor trigger zone and in the area postrema (84). Metoclopramide, a substituted benzamide, and droperidol, a butyrophenone, are also dopaminergic antagonists. Although effective as single agents at acceptable doses for very mildly emetogenic chemotherapy, the high doses of these agents that would be required to treat moderate- to high-emetogenic chemotherapy can cause the typical extrapyramidal side effects of dystonia or sedation and hypotension (80,84). Combining one of these agents with diphenhydramine, itself a very mild antiemetic, can reduce the extrapyramidal side effects of high-dose dopaminergic antagonists. Short-acting benzodiazepines, such as lorazepam and alprazolam, can also be used as antiemetics. These drugs can also effectively decrease the incidence of extrapyramidal side effects of metoclopromide (83), and their amnesic and anxiolytic properties may contribute to their beneficial effects when given with chemotherapy or for anticipatory nausea. HIV-infected patients taking ritonavir, however, should not be given benzodiazepines because ritonavir potently inhibits the cytochrome P-450 enzyme and can lead to toxic levels of this class of drugs (81).

Corticosteroids, such as dexamethasone, have a minor, but definite antiemetic activity, although the mechanism is unclear (83). When combined with metoclopromide or prochlorperazine, dexamethasone, at intravenous doses of 10–20 mg, has significantly improved the efficacy of either agent alone when used for highly emetogenic chemotherapy (83,86). When combined with the 5-HT_3 antagonists, dexamethasone improves the efficacy of the 5-HT_3 antagonist by 20–30% (83,84,86,87). Dexamethasone, however, can decrease the serum levels of saquinavir, and should be used with caution in patients taking this drug.

An effective antiemetic regimen for moderate- to highly-emetogenic chemotherapy regimens for most HIV-infected patients could consist of a combination of a 5-HT_3 antagonist, a dopaminergic D_2 antagonist, dexamethasone, diphenhydramine and a short-acting benzodiazepine. Smoked marijuana, dronabinol, and other tetrahydrocannabinols have limited efficacy in treating chemotherapy-induced nausea when compared with other antiemetics, but may be tried if a patient is unable to take the first-line drugs (83).

Delayed emesis caused by cisplatin, experienced by about 60% of patients (84), can occur 2–5 days after the chemotherapy is given, and can be severe and difficult to control. Although the mechanism is not well understood, for prevention and treatment of delayed emesis caused by cisplatin, the 5-HT_3 antagonists have not been significantly more effective than placebo (83,84,86). Combination regimens that include metoclopromide and dexamethasone, however, have proved superior to placebo (81% versus 61%) in a double-blind, randomized trial (83). For optimum prevention of delayed nausea, however, these drugs should be taken around-the-clock for 6 or 7 days, starting with a dexamethasone dose of 6 mg four times daily, rapidly tapering to 2 mg twice per day. Physicians should be cautious of the risks of further immunosuppression and greater risk of OIs from extended dexamethasone treatment in an HIV-infected patient.

VII. DIARRHEA

Chemotherapy-induced secretory diarrhea, although not as common as chemo-therapy-associated emesis, can be potentially life-threatening in cancer patients. It can cause electrolyte imbalances, such as hypokalemia, hypercalcemia, hypo-magnesemia, and metabolic acidosis, as well as renal insufficiency and decreased nutrient absorption because of decreased luminal transit time (88). Intractable diarrhea can severely affect the patient's quality of life and ability to function normally in social and professional environments. It is frequently a complication of 5-FU and cisplatin treatment and can also be an unpleasant side effect of metoclopromide. Severe diarrhea is a dose-limiting toxicity of irinotecan (CPT-11), a new topoisomerase-I inhibitor, and mild to moderate diarrhea is a complica-tion of many other chemotherapeutic agents (89). The mechanism of chemother-apy-induced diarrhea is not well understood, but is thought to be associated mainly with mucosal inflammation, increased gastrointestinal secretion, and rapid cell turnover, which results in decreased nutrient absorption. CPT-11 appears to cause a cholinergic syndrome, consisting of abdominal cramps with increased stool frequency, salivation, lacrimation, and diaphoresis (90). The goals of treat-ing chemotherapy-induced diarrhea are to maintain nutrition and fluid and elec-trolyte balance, and to ease patient discomfort, thereby improving overall quality of life.

All cancer patients who receive chemotherapy are susceptible to opportu-nistic infections that can cause diarrhea such as *Escherichia coli, Salmonella* and *Shigella*, as well as *Clostridium difficile*, especially if they are taking antibiotics or have had extensive hospitalization (89). Diarrhea is also very common in pa-tients with AIDS, occurring in up to 80% of patients (80). The reverse tran-scriptase inhibitor, ddI, and all of the currently approved protease inhibitors can cause diarrhea. HIV-infected patients have an enhanced susceptibility to bacterial enteritides as compared to the general population, possibly as a result of achlorhy-dria, found in a large number of these patients (80). In contrast with otherwise immunocompetent cancer patients, these patients are more prone to small bowel invasion by microsporidia, cryptosporidia, and isosporidia, which can cause par-tial villus atrophy and crypt hyperplasia, resulting in malabsorption syndromes. MAC invasion of the small intestine can also cause malabsorption. They are also at a higher risk for CMV enterocolitis, which can cause bowel infarction and perforation (80). HIV-infected patients with lymphoma may have invasion of the gastrointestinal tract as a cause of diarrhea, and KS can also be a rare cause of diarrhea.

A thorough diagnostic workup should be done in all HIV-infected patients with diarrhea who are undergoing chemotherapy. In addition to stool examination for usual enteric pathogens, including *Campylobacter* organisms and *C. difficile* toxin, stool examination or tissue biopsy should be done to look for cryptosporidiosis and isosporidiosis. Spores of microsporidia may be difficult to find in the stool, but in some cases, they can be determined by light microscopic visualization of an intestinal biopsy (80). CMV detection requires an intestinal biopsy, and MAC infection may show acid-fast bacilli in the stool, which should be confirmed by culture. The diagnosis can also be made quickly by biopsy of the intestine.

Fluids and electrolytes should be aggressively replaced and parenteral nutrition should be considered if malabsorption is suspected, or if the patient is unable to take adequate oral nutrition. Empiric antibiotic therapy should be initiated with a fluoroquinolone for suspected bacterial infection while awaiting biopsy, stool culture or toxin results, and the appropriate antibiotic treatment should be given as soon as the infectious agent has been determined.

Antimotility drugs, such as loperamide and diphenoxylate, are commonly used for symptomatic treatment of diarrhea. Loperamide and diphenoxylate act directly on the bowel wall smooth muscle to slow down peristaltic activity by interacting with both cholinergic and noncholinergic receptors. A randomized, double-blind trial of 340 non-HIV patients with acute diarrhea showed both loperamide and diphenoxylate to be safe and effective drugs for treating diarrhea, although patients taking loperamide required fewer doses and experienced a more rapid resolution than did the patients taking diphenoxylate (89,91). Loperamide, when administered every 2 h until 12 h after the last stool event, was able to control diarrhea in patients receiving CPT-11 and allowed higher-dose intensities of this drug (89). Tincture of opium and belladonna have also been used to control severe diarrhea not responsive to loperamide or diphenoxylate.

Octreotide, a stable analogue of somatostatin, prolongs mouth-to-cecum transit time and effectively controls diarrhea in a variety of clinical settings, including diarrhea caused by intestinal tumors, chemotherapy-induced diarrhea, and diarrhea caused by AIDS-associated infections (88,89,92). It inhibits vasoactive intestinal polypeptide (VIP) and serotonin, and directly inhibits the activity of substance P and peptide 5, a peptide fragment of the transmembrane glycoprotein gp41 of HIV (89). The recommended dose for chemotherapy-induced diarrhea is 100 µg subcutaneously every 8 h. Octreotide is generally well tolerated, and this dose can be increased incrementally to an intravenous dose of 2400 µg per day until symptoms are controlled (88). AIDS patients with cryptosporidiosis have been effectively treated with similar doses (92). The most common side effects are injection-site pain and hypoglycemia, although some patients have been noted to develop anorexia, nausea, vomiting, abdominal cramps and bloating, and steatorrhea, as well as cholesterol gallbladder stones and sludge with long-term use (88). HIV-infected patients who are taking ritonavir, which can increase serum cholesterol by 30–40%, should be especially cautious when using octreotide. CMV infection and *C. difficile* toxin are infective agents known to cause toxic megacolon, and if these agents are suspected, drugs that slow the peristaltic activity of the gut should be avoided until these infections are excluded by appropriate tests.

VIII. CONCLUSION

Patients receiving chemotherapy for AIDS-associated tumors may experience all of the same toxicities and side effects from this treatment as do non-HIV-infected persons. These side effects may be potentiated by other diseases, infections, or medications that the patient may have. Preventing and counteracting these side effects and excluding or treating other causes of these symptoms are some of the major tasks of the treating AIDS oncologist. Drug interactions, especially with some of the newer protease inhibitors used to treat HIV infection, must also be considered when treating several of these chemotherapy-induced toxicities. As treatment of HIV and its associated complications improves and patients live longer with HIV infection, the management of the subjective and objective side effects of therapy becomes of greater importance in maintaining a high quality of life for patients.

IX. ACKNOWLEDGMENT

The authors acknowledge the clerical assistance of Ms Nancy Marshello in preparing this manuscript. Supported in part by grants from USPHS, NIH (AI-27660, CA-70080, RR-00865), and a grant from the State of California Universitywide AIDS Research Program (CC96-LA175) to the UCLA AIDS Clinical Research Center.

REFERENCES

1. DW Lyter, J Bryant, R Thackeray, CR Rinaldo, LA Kingsley. Incidence of human immunodeficiency virus-related and nonrelated malignancies in a large cohort of homosexual men. J Clin Oncol 13:2540–2546, 1995.
2. JJ Goedert, J James, TR Cote, ES Jaffe, DW Kingma, RJ Biggar. Additional AIDS-related malignancies. Abstr B.4141. XI Int Conf AIDS, Vancouver, Canada, July 9–11, 1996.
3. U Tirelli, D Errante, M Spina, E Vaccher, D Serraino, M Boiocchi, A Gloghini, A Carbone. Long-term survival of patients with HIV-related systemic non-Hodgkin's lymphomas. Hematol Oncol 14:7–15, 1996.

4. MB Feinberg. Changing the natural history of HIV disease. Lancet 348:239–246, 1996.

5. MA Kosh, PA Volberding, SW Lagakos, DK Booth, C Pettinelli, MW Myers. Toxic effects of zidovudine in asymptomatic human immunodeficiency virus-infected individuals with CD4+ cells counts of 0.50×10^9/L or less: detailed and updated results from protocol 019 of the AIDS Clinical Trials Group. Arch Intern Med 152:2286–2292, 1992.

6. J Hambletoon. Hematologic complications of HIV infection. Oncology 10:671–678, 1996.

7. N Frickhofen, JL Abkowitz, M Safford, JM Berry, J Antunez-de-Mayolo, A Astrow, R Cohen, I Halperin, L King, D Mintzer, B Cohen, NS Young. Persistent B19 parvovirus infection in patients infected with human immunodeficiency virus type 1(HIV-1): a treatable cause of anemia in AIDS. Ann Intern Med 113:926–933, 1990.

8. YS Kim, H Hollander. Polyradiculopathy due to cytomegalovirus: report of two cases in which improvement occurred after prolonged therapy and review of the literature. CID 7:32–37, 1993.

9. AW Harbol, JL Liesveld, PJ Simpson-Haidaris, CN Abboud. Mechanisms of cytopenia in human immunodeficiency virus infection. Blood Review 8:241–251, 1994.

10. RW Price. Neurologic complications of HIV infection. Lancet 348:445–452, 1996.

11. SA Miles. Hematopoietic growth factors as adjuncts to antiretroviral therapy. Acquir Immune Defic Syndr Res Hum Retrovirol 8:1073–1080, 1992.

12. J Janik, L Miller, J Smith. Prechemotherapy granulocyte macrophage colony stimulating factor (GM-CSF) prevents topotecan-induced neutropenia. Proc Am Soc Clin Oncol 12:437, 1993.

13. R de Wit, J Verweij, M Bontenbal, WH Kruit, C Seynaeve, PM Schmitz, G Stoter. Adverse effect on bone marrow protection of prechemotherapy granulocyte colony-stimulating factor support. J Natl Cancer Inst 88:1393–1398, 1996.

14. R Emmanuel, A Holmes, C Blake, PA Pizzo, TJ Walsh. Impairment of neutrophil antifugal activity against hypae of *Aspergillus fumigatus* in children infected with human immunodeficiency virus. J Infec Dis 167:905–911, 1993.

15. RM Rose. The role of colony-stimulating factors in infectious disease: current status, future challenges. Semin Oncol 19:415–421, 1992.

16. KB Gordon, A Tajuddin, J Guitart, et al. Hand-foot syndrome associated with liposome-encapsulated doxorubicin therapy. Cancer 75:2169–2173, 1995.

17. JC Wernz, B Taubes, A Friedberg. Dounoxome-phase II trial for epidemic Kaposi's sarcoma (EKS) [abstr 046B]. Int Conf AIDS 10:18, 1994.

18. T Brown, J Kuhn, M Marshall, et al. A phase I clinical and pharmacokinetic trial of liposomal doxorubicin (NSC-620212). Proc Am Soc Clin Oncol 10:93, 1991.

19. PS Gill, BM Espina, F Muggia, S Cabriales, A Tulpule, JA Esplin, HA Liebman, E Forssen, ME Ross, AM Levine. Phase I/II clinical and pharmacokinetic evaluation of liposomal daunorubicin. J Clin Oncol 13:996–1003, 1995.

20. DW Northfelt, B Dezube, B Miller, et al. Randomized comparative trial of Doxil vs Adrimycin, bleomycin, and vincristine (ABV) in the treatment of severe AIDS-related Kaposi's sarcoma (AIDS-KS) [abstr 1515]. Blood 86:382a, 1995.

21. PS Gill, J Wernz, DT Scadden, P Cohen, GM Mukwaya, JH von Roenn, M Jacobs, S Kempin, I Silverberg, G Gonzales, MU Rarick, AM Myers, F Shepherd, C Sawka, MC Pike, ME Ross. Randomized phase III trial of liposomal daunorubicin versus doxorubicin, bleomycin, and vincristine in AIDS-related Kaposi's sarcoma. J Clin Oncol 14:2353–2364, 1996.

22. M Harrison, D Tomlinson, S Stewart. Liposomal-entrapped doxorubicin: An active agent in AIDS-related Kaposi's sarcoma. J Clin Oncol 13:914–920, 1995.

23. ASCO. American Society of Clinical Oncology recommendations for the use of hematopoietic colony-stimulating factors: evidence-based, clinical practice guidelines. J Clin Oncol 12:2471–2507, 1994.

24. ASCO. Update of recommendations for the use of hematopoietic colony-stimulating factors: Evidence-based clinical practice guidelines. J Clin Oncol 14:1957–1960, 1996.

25. LJ Laubenstein, RL Krigel, CM Odajnyk, KB Hymes, A Friedman-Kien, JC Wernz, FM Muggia. Treatment of epidemic Kaposi's sarcoma with etoposide or a combination of doxorubicin, bleomycin, and vincristine. J Clin Oncol 2:1115–1120, 1984.

26. EP Gelmann, D Longo, HC Lane, AS Fauci, H Masur, M Wesley, OT Preble, J Jacob, R Steis. Combination chemotherapy of disseminated Kaposi's sarcoma in patients with the acquired immune deficiency cyndrome. Am J Med 82:456–462, 1987.

27. PS Gill, M Parick, JA McCutchan, L Slater, B Parker, E Muchmore, M Berstein-Singer, B Akil, BM Espina, M Krailo, A Levine. Systemic treatment of AIDS-related Kaposi's sarcoma: results of a randomized trial. Am J Med 90:427–433, 1991.

28. JR Bonger, U Kronawitter, B Rolinski, K Truebenbach, FD Goebel. Liposomal doxorubicin in the treatment of advanced AIDS-related Kaposi's sarcoma. J AIDS 7: 463–468, 1994.

29. D Sharma, F Muggia, L Lucci, K Chan, E Forseen, PS Gill. Liposomal daunorubicin: tolerance and clinical effects in AIDS-related Kaposi's sarcoma (KS) during a phase I study [abstr]. Proc Am Soc Clin Oncol 9:A9, 1990.

30. MW Saville, J Lietzau, W Wilson, J Pluda, J Bailey, R Cohen, E Feigal, S Broder, R Yarchoan. A trial of paclitaxel (Taxol) in patients with HIV-associated Kaposi's sarcoma (KS) [abstr]. Proc Am Clin Oncol 13:A20, 1994.

31. T Chew, M Jacobs, M Huckabee, M Ross. A phase II clinical trial of DaunoXome (VS103, liposomal daunorubicin) in Kaposi's sarcoma of AIDS patients [abstr WS-B15-3]. Int Conf AIDS 9:58, 1993.

32. PJM Bakker, SA Danner, CHH ten Napel, FP Kroon, HG Sprenger, R van Leusen, PL Meenhorst, A Muusers, CHN Veenhof. Eur J Cancer 31A:188–192, 1995.

33. JC Wernz, B Taubes, A Friedberg. Daunoxome-phase II trial for epidemic Kaposi's sarcoma (EKS) [abstr 046B]. Int Conf AIDS 10:18, 1994.

34. U Tirelli, D Errante, E Oksenhendler, M Spina, E Vaccher, D Serraino, R Gastaldi, L Repetto, G Rizzardini, A Carbone. Prospective study with combined low-dose chemotherapy and zidovudine in 37 patients with poor-prognosis AIDS-related non-Hodgkin's lymphoma. Ann Oncol 3:843–847, 1992.

35. AM Levine, JC Wernz, L Kaplan, N Rodman, P Cohen, C Metroka, JM Bennett, MU Rarick, C Walsh, J Kahn, SA Miles, WC Ehmann, J Feinberg, B Nathawani, PS Gill, RT Mitsuyasu. Low-dose chemotherapy with central nervous system pro-

phylaxis and zidovudine maintenance in AIDS-related lymphoma. JAMA 266:84–
88, 1991.

36. JM Holland, PS Swift. Tolerance of patients with human immunodeficiency virus
     and anal carcinoma to treatment with combined chemotherapy and radiation therapy.
     Radiology 193:251–254, 1994.

37. M Chadha, EA Rosenblatt, S Malamud, J Pisch, A Berson. Squamous-cell carcinoma
     of the anus in HIV-positive patients. Dis Colon Rectum 37:861–865, 1994.

38. JM Timmerman, DW Northfelt, EJ Small. Malignant germ cell tumors in men in-
     fected with the human immunodeficiency virus: natural history and results of ther-
     apy. J Clin Oncol 13:1391–1397, 1995.

39. C-F Perno, DA Cooney, W-Y Gao, Z Hao, DG Johns, A Foli, NR Hartman, R Calio,
     S Broder, R Yarchoan. Effects of bone marrow stimulatory cytokines on human
     immunodeficiency virus replication and the antiviral activity of dideoxynucleosides
     in cultures of monocyte/macrophages. Blood 80:995–1003, 1992.

40. PS Gill, M Berstein-Singer, BM Espina, M Rarick, F Magy, T Montgomery, MS
     Berry, A Levine. Adriamycin, bleomycin and vincristine chemotherapy with recom-
     binant granulocyte-macrophage colony-stimulating factor in the treatment of AIDS-
     related Kaposi's sarcoma. AIDS 6:1477–1481, 1992.

41. P Herman, A Gori, P Franchioly, M Lemone, N Clumeck. Possible role of granulo-
     cyte-macrophage colony stimulating factor (GM-CSF) on the rapid progression of
     AIDS-related Kaposi's sarcoma lesions in vivo. Br J Haematol 87:413–414, 1994.

42. J Ganzalez-Garc'a, A Lorenzo, V Jimenez-Yuste, M De Castro, C Jimenez, MP
     Mart'n, P Herranz, C Fernandez-Capitan, JM Pe-a. Acute myelomonocytic leukemia
     associated with HIV infection and granulocyte colony-stimulating factor therapy
     [abstr B1287]. XI Int Conf AIDS, Vancouver, Canada, July 9–11, 1996.

43. PJM Bakker, SA Danner, CHH ten Napel, et al. Treatment of poor prognosis epi-
     demic Kaposi's sarcoma with doxorubicin, bleomycin, vindesine and recombinant
     human granulocyte-monocyte colony stimulating factor (rhGM-CSF). Eur J Cancer
     31:188–192, 1995.

44. ML Patchen, TJ MacVittie. Granulocyte colony-stimulating factor and amifostine
     (Ethyol) synergize to enhance hematopoietic reconstitution and increase survival in
     irradiated animal. Semin Oncol 21:26–32, 1994.

45. LA Speicher, M Krutzsh, J Wymer, DS Albert, RL Capizzi. Amifostine does not
     inhibit the cytotoxic effects of a broad range of standard anticancer drugs against
     human ovarian and breast cancer cells [abstr]. Proc Annu Meet Am Assoc Cancer
     Res 36:A1727, 1995.

46. D Glover, JH Glick, C Weiler, S Hurowitz, MM Kligerman. WR-2721 against the
     hematologic toxicity of cyclophosphamide: a controlled phase II trial. J Clin Oncol
     4:584–588, 1986.

47. G Kemp, P Rose, J Lurain, M Berman, A Manetta, B Roullet, H Homesley, D Bel-
     pomme, J Glick. Amifostine pretreatment for protection against cyclophosphamide-
     induced and cisplatin-induced toxicities: results of a randomized control trial in pa-
     tients with advanced ovarian cancer. J Clin Oncol 14:2101–2112, 1996.

48. R Dipaola, A Rodriguez, S Riccio, S Goodia, M Orick, J Mollman, S Bird, J Belsh.
     A phase I study of amifostine and paclitaxel in patients with advanced malignancies
     [abstr]. Am Soc Clin Oncol 1996.

49. AF List, R Heaton, B Glinsmann-Gibson, RL Capizzi. Amifostine protects primitive hematopoietic progenitors against chemotherapy cytotoxicity. Semin Oncol 23(4 suppl 8):58–63, 1996.

50. CM Spencer, KL Goa. Amifostine. A review of its pharmacodynamic and pharmacokinetic properties, and therapeutic potential as a radioprotector and cytotoxic chemoprotector. Drugs 50:1001–1031, 1995.

51. GJ Peter, WJF van der Vijgh. Protection of normal tissue from the cytotoxic effects of chemotherapy and radiation by amifostine (WR-2721): Preclinical aspects. Eur J Cancer 31A:S1-S7, 1995.

52. RL Capizzi. Amifostine: the preclinical basis for broad-spectrum selective cytoprotection of normal tissue from cytotoxic therapies. Semin Oncol 23:2–18, 1996.

53. K Matsue, M Harada, S Nakao, M Ueda, K Kondo, K Odaka, T Mori, K Kattori. Controlled study of therapeutic granulocyte transfusions in granulocytopenic patients with severe infections. Jpn J Clin Oncol 14:21–30, 1984.

54. RG Strauss. Current status of granulocyte transfusions to treat neonatal sepsis. J Clin Apheresis 5:25–29, 1989.

55. JE Menitove, RA Abrams. Granulocyte transfusion in neutropenic patients. Crit Rev Oncol Hematol 7:89–113, 1987.

56. CF Whitsett. The role of hematologic growth factor in transfusion medicine. Hematol Oncol Clin North Am 9:23–68, 1995.

57. A Grigg, J Lusk, J Szer. G-CSF stimulated donor granulocyte collections for neutropenic sepsis. Leuk Lymphoma 18:329–334, 1995.

58. LM Williamson, RM Warwick. Transfusion-associated graft-versus-host disease and its prevention. Blood Rev 9:251–261, 1995.

59. HG Klein, RG Strauss, CA Schiffer. Granulocyte transfusion therapy. Semin Hematol 33(4):359–368.

60. J Zaia, P Yam, S Li, H Payne, S Herman, I Sniecinski, B Tegtmeier, S Forman, J Ito. Mobilization of peripheral blood progenitor cells using G-CSF in HIV-1 infected persons [abstr 1985]. Blood 88(suppl 1):499a, 1996.

61. B Rio, A Compagnucci, J Rochemaure, R Zittoun. High dose chemotherapy (CT) and autologous bone marrow transplant (ABMT) for malignant hemophathies in HIV-infected patients [abstr B 1292]. XI Int Conf AIDS 1996.

62. DM Mintzer, FX Real, L Jovino, SE Krown. Treatment of Kaposi's sarcoma and thrombocytopenia with vincristine in patients with the acquired immunodeficiency syndrome. Ann Intern Med 102:200–202, 1985.

63. MW Saville, J Lietzau, JM Pluda, I Feuerstein, J Odom, WH Wilson, RW Humphrey, E Feigal, SM Steinberg, S Broder, R Yarchoan. Treatment of HIV-associated Kaposi's sarcoma with paclitaxel. Lancet 346:26–28, 1995.

64. G van Baelen. Neurologic conditions are difficult to treat. GMHC Treat Iss 9:8–11, 1995.

65. CJ Fichtenbaum, DB Clifford, WG Powderly. Risk factors for dideoxynucleoside-induced toxic neuropathy in patients with human immunodeficiency virus infection. J Acquir Immune Defic Syndr Hum Retrovirol 10:169–174, 1995.

66. M Veilleux, O Paltiel, J Falutz. Sensorimotor neuropathy and abnormal vitamin B12 metabolism in early HIV infection. Can J Neurol Sci 22:43–46, 1995.

67. CA Kemper, A Ganer, G Kent, S Deresinski. Double-blind placebo (P)-controlled

cross-over study fails to show benefit of mexiletine (MX) in painful neuropathy. Natl Conf Hum Retrovirus Relat Infect (2nd) 171, 1995.

68. ST Sonis. Oral complications of cancer therapy. In VT DeVita, S Hellman, SA Rosenberg, eds. Cancer: Principles and Practice of Chemotherapy. Philadelphia: JB Lippincott, 1993, pp 2385–2394.

69. National Institutes of Health Consensus Development Conference Statement. Oral complications of cancer therapies: diagnosis, prevention and treatment. NIH Consensus Statement 7:1–11, 1989.

70. BA Meuller, ET Millheim, EA Farrington, C Brusko, TH Wiser. Mucositis management practices for hospitalized patients: national survey results. 10:310–519, 1995.

71. W Carl. Oral complications of local and systemic cancer treatment. Curr Opin Oncol 10:510–520, 1995.

72. M Weinert, RM Grimes, DP Lynch. Oral manifestations of HIV infection. Ann Intern Med 125:485–496, 1996.

73. JS Greenspan, D Greenspan. Oral complications of HIV infection. IN: MA Sande, PA Volberding, eds. The Medical Management of AIDS, 5th ed. Philadelphia, WB Saunders and Company, 1997, pp 169–180.

74. JR Minor, SC Piscitelli. Thalidomide in diseases associated with human deficiency virus infection. Am J Health-Sys Pharm 53:429–431, 1996.

75. AL Moreira, EP Sampaio, A Zmuidzinas, P Frindt, KS Smith, G Kaplan. Thalidomide exerts its inhibitory action on tumor necrosis factor-α by enhancing mRNA degradation. J Exp Med 177:1675–1680, 1993.

76. JS Greenspan. Proceedings of Clinical Care of the AIDS Patient. San Francisco, 1996.

77. C Porta, M Moroni, G Nastaci. Allopurinol mouthwashes in the treatment of fluorouricil-induced stomatitis. Am J Clin Oncol 17:246–247, 1994.

78. CM Wilcox, DA Schwartz, WS Clark. Esophageal ulceration in human deficiency virus infection. Ann Intern Med 122:143–149, 1995.

79. A Berger, M Henderson, W Nadoolman, V Duffy, D Cooper, L Saberski, L Bartoshuk. Oral capsaicin provides temporary relief for oral mucositis pain secondary to chemotherapy/radiation therapy. J Pain Symptom Manage 10:243–248, 1995.

80. DP Kotler. Gastrointestinal manifestations of human immunodeficiency virus infection. In: T DeVita, S. Hellman, SA Rosenberg, eds. AIDS: Etiology, Diagnosis, Treatment and Prevention. Philadelphia: Lippincott-Raven, 1996, pp 365–391.

81. JG Bartlett. The Johns Hopkins Hospital 1996 Guide to Medical Management of Patients with HIV Infection. 6th ed. Baltimore: Williams and Wilkins, 1996, pp 76–83.

82. MS Saag. Proceedings of Clinical Care of the AIDS Patient. San Francisco, 1996.

83. MK Crow, HM Ghader, R Pazur, G Fraschini. Management of nausea and vomiting. In: R Pazur, ed. Medical Oncology: A Comprehensive Review. New York: PRR, 1996, pp 629–641.

84. SM Grunberg, PJ Hesketh. Control of chemotherapy-induced emesis. N Engl J Med 329:1790–1796, 1993.

85. EA Perez. Review of the preclinical pharmacology and comparative efficacy of 5-hydroxytryptamine-3 receptor antagonists for chemotherapy-induced emesis. J Clin Oncol 13:2417–2426, 1995.

86. J Herrstedt. Development of antiemetic therapy in cancer patients. Acta Oncologica 34:637–640, 1995.

87. The Italian Group for Antiemetic Research. Persistence of efficacy of three antiemetic regimens and prognostic factors in patients undergoing moderately emetogenic chemotherapy. J Clin Oncol 13:2417–2426, 1995.

88. AG Harris, TM O'Dorisio, EA Woltergin, LB Anthony, FR Burton, RB Geller, JH Grendell, B Levin, JS Redfern. Consensus statement: octreotide dose titration in secretory diarrhea. Dig Dis Sci 40:1464–1473, 1995.

89. S Cascinu. Management of diarrhea induced by tumors or cancer therapy. Curr Opin Oncol 7:325–329, 1995.

90. D Gandia, D Abigerges, J-P Armand, G Chabot, L DaCosta, M DeForni. CPT-11-induced cholinergic effects in cancer patients. J Clin Oncol 11:196–197, 1993.

91. JWD Cornett, RL Aspeling, D Mellegol. A double-blind comparative evaluation of loperatmide versus diphenoxylate with atropine in acute diarrhea. Curr Therap Res 21:629–637, 1977.

92. J Romeu, JM Miro, G Sirera, J Mallolas, J Arnal, ME Valls, F Tortosa, B Totet, M Foz. Efficacy of octreotide in the management of chronic diarrhoea in AIDS. AIDS 1495–1499, 1991.

14

Considerations in the Management of HIV Infection in Patients Undergoing Antineoplastic Chemotherapy

Richard F. Little and Robert Yarchoan
National Cancer Institute, National Institutes of Health, Bethesda, Maryland

I. INTRODUCTION

The oncology patient with HIV infection presents unique problems and challenges. When considering antineoplastic chemotherapy, a balance must be struck between the therapeutic effects on the malignancy and the potential for worsening human immunodeficiency virus (HIV)-associated immunosuppression. Ideally, one would like to maximize the antitumor benefit while sparing the immune system from both the detrimental effects of chemotherapy and the progressive immune injury of HIV. However, many questions remain for how best to achieve these goals. In this chapter, we will attempt to review some of what is presently known in this field, to see what conclusions may now be drawn, and to articulate some of the areas for further research.

A particular challenge is posed by the patient whose tumor requires cytotoxic chemotherapy. As a first step, it is worth considering to what extent the patient's prognosis is limited by HIV disease, as opposed to the cancer. If the patient has a tumor that can be reasonably expected to be cured or put into a long-term remission, it is important to consider delivery of adequately dose-intensive chemotherapy to achieve this effect. However, consideration should be given to what extent this may be at the expense of added immune damage, which may increase the likelihood of more rapid mortality from complications of HIV infection (1). In patients with tumor that is not expected to be cured by chemotherapy, palliative approaches are generally used. In such a patient, it may be necessary to give relatively more attention to preventing further immune deterioration and maintaining control of HIV during prolonged palliative therapy. In both instances, it is important to monitor the patient's progress, not only for response to chemotherapy, but also for evidence of unacceptable immune injury. The latter can be relatively difficult in the HIV-infected cancer patient undergoing chemotherapy, as the usual predictive surrogate markers of HIV disease, such as CD4 cell counts and HIV viral load may undergo transient large fluctuations.

An additional challenge in HIV-infected patients with tumor is that such patients are often more intolerant to cytotoxic chemotherapy than HIV-noninfected patients. Factors contributing to this include their underlying immune suppression, decreased bone marrow reserves, poor performance status, or a combination of these factors (2–5). In a sense, strategies to minimize detriment to the immune system from cancer drugs and progressive HIV disease are natural extensions of similar efforts in HIV-noninfected patients. At the same time, the dynamics of HIV infection pose a particular challenge here.

The underlying concerns here are how to balance treatment of the tumor with control of the HIV infection, and how to manage the potential interactions between anti-HIV and antineoplastic therapies. Antiretroviral monotherapy is often reasonably well tolerated when concurrently administered with chemotherapy (6–10). However, more potent combination regimens, including protease inhibitors, have recently been developed for HIV. The combined toxicities of antiretroviral and cancer chemotherapy are not well characterized, and this particularly applies to the HIV protease inhibitors. Certainly, this increases the complexity and cost of treating these patients, and it is not known how the use of various antiretroviral therapy approaches during chemotherapy for various tumors may affect overall survival. For the treating oncologist and his or her patient, the concern of HIV progression during chemotherapy is a compelling factor to include anti-HIV therapy along with chemotherapy. There are fewer data than one would like on the potential usefulness and optimal use of antiretroviral therapy in this setting. Yet, clinicians must make treatment decisions in the face of such incomplete data, and accordingly, it may be worthwhile to summarize the present state of knowledge while at the same time calling attention to the major areas of uncertainty.

II. MONITORING THE STATUS OF HIV INFECTION

It is perhaps worthwhile at the onset to discuss the tools available to monitor the status of HIV disease. The best tools for this purpose currently are the CD4 cell count and the measurement of HIV RNA levels (11). CD4 cell counts are performed by fluorescence-activated cell sorters (FACS), a technique that separates T cells based on fluorescent labeling of lymphocyte surface antigens, particularly the CD4 and CD8 antigens. The CD4 lymphocyte counts are important for assessing the state of the patients immune system and predicting the immediate risk of developing specific opportunistic infections or death. Indeed, most deaths from HIV infection occur only when the CD4 cell count has fallen to fewer than 50/mm^3 (12–16).

There are several techniques employed for the quantification of the HIV viral load in the plasma. The principal ones used today are reverse transcription, followed by the polymerase chain reaction (RT-PCR; 17–20), branched-chain DNA (bDNA) signal amplification (21), and nucleic acid sequence-based amplification (NASBA; 22). Comparable results are obtained with these various methods of RNA quantification (23,24). The techniques all quantify virion-associated cell-free RNA and reflect the amount of circulating virus in the plasma. Most of the assays have a lower detection limit of 400–500 HIV RNA copies per cubic millimeter, and a reported value of undetectable or zero should be considered to represent "fewer than 500 copies per cubic millimeter." More sensitive assays are also available that have a lower limit of detection of 50 HIV RNA copies per cubic millimeter or fewer.

The plasma HIV level is strongly associated with the subsequent pace of HIV disease progression and the time to death (25,26). Additionally, suppression in plasma HIV RNA reduces the hazard of AIDS progression and death (11). At the time of HIV infection, there is an initial burst of viremia followed by steady-state levels of plasma HIV RNA ranging from 10^2 to 10^6 copies per cubic millimeter. This plateau level ("setpoint") of viremia can remain stable for years and has been predictive of the subsequent disease course. Patients with high initial steady-state levels of plasma HIV RNA generally have more rapid disease progression (25–30). Some isolates of HIV readily induce syncytium formation (multinucleated cells that form when cell membranes fuse together) in T cells. Recent studies show that this property is related to the use of CXCR4 as a coreceptor (31). The presence of syncytium-forming viral phenotype is also predictive of subsequent disease progression (30,32).

Patients with low viral burdens (fewer than 5,000–10,000 HIV RNA copies per millimeter of plasma) and near-normal CD4 cell counts may have a particularly prolonged course, sometimes maintaining stable CD4 counts for over 10 years (27,33–36). By contrast, patients with high levels of plasma viremia (more than 30,000–100,000 HIV RNA copies per cubic millimeter) are at a substantially increased risk of rapid clinical progression to AIDS and death, with a median survival of 5.1 years (26,27,29,30,36,37). HIV RNA levels appear to be more predictive of progression than CD4 cell counts, particularly in asymptomatic patients with cell counts of more than 350/mm^3 (25,26). The level of HIV replication, as measured by the viral load, is predictive of the rate of decline in CD4 cells (27). However, the CD4 cell count remains the most important marker for overall disease status and predictor of the immediate hazard of AIDS complications (12,38,39).

Plasma viral RNA levels measure only one compartment of the total body HIV burden. The estimated daily production of HIV virions in infected patients is 10^9–10^{10} virions (20,40), and reducing the plasma viral RNA to levels below the limits of detection by current techniques does not necessarily reflect complete suppression of viral replication. Most viral replication occurs in the lymph nodes, and this is where the bulk of immunological destruction occurs (41). It is still unclear as to what extent suppression of the peripheral viral burden correlates with the dynamics of viral replication in other sites of viral replication (42,43). Although correlations have been found between the level of plasma HIV viremia and proviral DNA in lymph node tissue, the interpretation of this correlation is confounded because there is progressive architectural destruction in the lymph nodes. Architectural integrity in the lymph nodes appears to be better preserved over time in patients with sustained effective antiviral therapy (44).

Decreased HIV DNA burden in the lymphoid tissue associated with decreased peripheral blood mononuclear (PBMC) cell HIV DNA burden in response to reverse transcriptase inhibitor therapy has been reported (45). Yet, there is evidence to suggest that HIV-1 replication can continue in lymphoid tissues following anti-HIV drug-induced reduction in plasma viral RNA by even 2–4 log 10, albeit at a significantly lower rate (46,47). Follicular dendritic cells (FDC) in lymph nodes are another potential reservoir of concern. The concentration of FDC viral RNA can exceed plasma viremia concentrations by factors of 10^2 to more than 10^4 and, perhaps most importantly, some patients receiving reverse transcriptase inhibitors have more than 10^6 copies of viral RNA per gram of lymphoid tissue in the FDC pool at times when the concentration of viral RNA in plasma was below the detection level of the assay (5×10^3 copies per cubic millimeter; 48). More encouraging results have been reported in patients receiving combination therapy, consisting of two nucleoside reverse transcriptase inhibitors and a protease inhibitor: within 6 months, more than 99% of the lymphoid cells actively producing the virus appeared to be eliminated (49). It will be of interest to see how these potent antiretroviral regimens affect this parameter after more prolonged observation.

Even with these uncertainties, the recent findings indicating that HIV-infected patients have an extremely high rate of HIV production, that substantially inhibiting viral replication can reduce the development of resistance, and that early combination therapy can improve survival have caused a shift in our thinking about antiretroviral therapy (50,51). Overall, a consensus is emerging that reducing the viral load (preferably to undetectable levels) is a worthwhile goal of therapy, and initial guidelines have been developed for using plasma HIV RNA levels in individual patient management (52–54). It is now recommended that the plasma HIV RNA level be measured 3–4 weeks after initiating or changing therapy, and then periodically on the same schedule as CD4 cell counts (e.g., every 3–4 months). Given the variability of the RNA PCR assay and fluctuation in the viral load in the absence of therapy, the minimum reduction in HIV RNA titer indicative of antiretroviral activity in a given patient is generally felt to be 0.5 log 10 or more (about threefold) from the pretreatment value (52–54), and it has been suggested that a drop to undetectable levels within 6 months is most desirable (26,28–30,36,54–57). There is evidence that complete suppression of viral replication may prevent or substantially delay the emergence of resistant HIV species, whereas partial suppression may select for resistant mutations (53). At the same time, it is important to remember that HIV-infected cells can persist, even when the plasma HIV RNA cannot be detected with available techniques (49,58).

Surrogate markers other than the viral load and CD4 cell count are generally less helpful. Measurements of p24 antigen (HIV viral core protein) have been used and may be prognostically useful if viral load measurements are unavailable, although it has not been as predictive as RNA PCR. Also changes in levels in response to HIV therapy can not be detected in all patients, further limiting its usefulness (39). β_2-Microglobulin and neopterin have been reported to have prognostic value, as have assessments of IgA, and erythrocyte sedimentation rate (ESR; 39,59–61). However, these surrogate markers have generally not maintained additive predictive value in studies using HIV RNA levels (25,30).

III. ANTIRETROVIRAL THERAPY

A. Introduction

There are, as of this writing, 11 approved antiretroviral drugs for HIV infection. These agents can be categorized into three different drug classes: nucleoside reverse transcriptase inhibitors (NRTIs); nonnucleoside reverse transcriptase inhibitors (NNRTIs); and protease inhibitors (PIs). The NRTIs are 2′,3′-dideoxynucleoside analogues including zidovudine (3′-azidothymidine; AZT), the first drug to be approved for HIV infection (62,63). Other drugs in this class are didanosine (2′,3′-dideoxyinosine; ddI), zalcitabine (2′,3′-dideoxycytidine; ddC) lamivudine (3′-thiacytidine; 3TC), and stavudine (2′,3′-didehydro-2′,3′-dideoxythymidine; D4T). Several nonnucleoside reverse transcriptase inhibitors have been identified, but rapid development of resistance is a problem with this class of drugs. Two drugs of this class, nevirapine and delavirdine, have now been approved. There are four protease inhibitors approved for use in HIV infection: saquinavir, ritonavir, indinavir, and nelfinavir. As will be reviewed in the following, these drugs are most effectively used in combination therapy. The combination regimens are generally designed to incorporate drugs from two or more classes, and to include combination of agents targeted to both resting and dividing cells.

B. Nucleoside Reverse Transcriptase Inhibitors

The NRTIs are not active in themselves, but must be phosphorylated in target cells to their active 3'-triphosphate moieties. In this form they target the reverse transcriptase enzyme (HIV-1 DNA polymerase) of HIV-1, inhibiting its activity and also acting as a chain terminator after being incorporated into the growing proviral DNA chain (62–68). However, the error-prone polymerization of HIV-1 reverse transcriptase produces a myriad of HIV-1 quasispecies, allowing for the eventual emergence of drug-resistant variants against this class of drugs (69–73).

Zidovudine (3'-azidothymidine; AZT), was developed through a collaboration between the National Cancer Institute, Duke University, and the Burroughs Wellcome Company soon after HIV was identified as the etiologic agent of AIDS (62,63). In 1985, a double-blind, placebo-controlled trial of the efficacy of zidovudine in patients with acquired immunodeficiency syndrome (AIDS) or with advanced AIDS-related complex was conducted in 282 patients of whom approximately half received zidovudine and half placebo (66,67). The study was terminated early after 9 months because of striking evidence of a short-term survival advantage in the zidovudine arm; at the time it was terminated 19 placebo recipients, but only 1 zidovudine recipient, had died. As had been observed in the phase I trial of zidovudine (63), a statistically significant, but transient, increase in the number of CD4 cells was noted in subjects receiving zidovudine. The principal toxicities of zidovudine were bone marrow suppression, nausea, and myositis (63,66,67).

Didanosine (2',3'-dideoxyinosine; ddI) and zalcitabine (2',3'-dideoxycytidine; ddC), were subsequently found to be potent inhibitors of HIV replication with clinical activity (68,74–78). Didanosine was the second drug to be approved for HIV infection. AIDS Clinical Trial Group (ACTG) study 175 detected a clinically and statistically significant reduction in the risk of HIV disease progression in patients with 200–500 CD4 cells per cubic millimeter receiving didanosine monotherapy versus those receiving zidovudine monotherapy (50). Also, there is evidence from other studies that patients with more advanced disease who have received at least 8 weeks of zidovudine monotherapy may derive benefit by switching to didanosine (79–81). Didanosine does not cause myelosuppression and is associated with improvement of most hematological parameters in HIV disease (82). The most significant toxicities of didanosine include neuropathy and pancreatitis.

Zalcitabine has modest activity when used alone (74,75). As initial therapy, zalcitabine was inferior to zidovudine in patients with advanced immunosuppression (83). However, in a randomized trial, it was equivalent to didanosine for patients with advanced HIV disease who were intolerant of zidovudine or for whom disease progression occurred despite zidovudine monotherapy (84). Indeed, in this study there was a small, but significant, survival advantage in favor of zalcitabine if a correction was made for the entry CD4 cell count, and this was a basis for its approval. Principal toxicities seen with zalcitabine are neuropathy, oral ulceration, and skin rashes (74,75,84–86). A few patients have been reported to develop esophageal ulceration while receiving zalcitabine (87).

Lamivudine (3′-thiacytidine; 3TC), a cytidine analogue, has only transient activity as monotherapy owing to the rapid development of substantial resistance associated with a mutation in codon 184 of the HIV *pol* gene (88–91). Consequently, the drug has limited use outside of appropriate combination therapy (see later discussion). The drug is extremely well tolerated (91), in part accounting for its widespread interest as a useful component of combination antiretroviral regimens (92).

Stavudine (2′,3′-didehydro-(2′,3′-dideoxythymidine; D4T) is a thymidine analogue that, in initial studies, was well tolerated and showed substantial antiretroviral activity when used as monotherapy or with didanosine (93–96). There are some data that support its continued efficacy in long-term use or following previous prolonged therapy with zidovudine (97,98). The primary toxicity is dose-related peripheral neuropathy (usually reversible) with very little hematotoxicity (93,99,100).

C. Nonnucleoside Reverse Transcriptase Inhibitors

NNRTIs are a chemically diverse group of compounds that are potent and highly specific inhibitors of HIV-1 reverse transcriptase (101–103). There are two NNRTIs, nevirapine and delavirdine, approved by the U.S. Food and Drug Administration (FDA) for use in HIV infection at the time of this writing. Single-amino acid substitutions in the reverse transcriptase that induce high-level resistance to these agents can emerge rapidly, often within weeks, when these drugs are used as monotherapy (102,104,105). Hence, it is recommended that these agents be used in combination with NRTIs (52).

The most clinically significant toxicity of both nevirapine and delavirdine is cutaneous rash, which does not always necessitate stopping therapy (101,103). Slowly escalating the dose over a few weeks can help reduce this toxicity. However, even with this approach, severe life-threatening rash can occur with nevirapine (106). Both drugs can induce the cytochrome P-450 system, leading to increased metabolism and potentially leading to complicated pharmacokinetic interactions with other drugs metabolized by this pathway (103,106).

D. Protease Inhibitors

Protease inhibitors are a class of antiretroviral drugs that inhibit the activity of the HIV-1 protease enzyme. This enzyme is critical for the maturation of infectious virions (107). In the final stages of the HIV-1 life cycle, large nonfunctional HIV-1 polyprotein chains are assembled and packaged at the cell surface, and released into the plasma as immature noninfectious virions. The protease enzyme cleaves these large polyproteins into smaller, functional proteins. Thus, protease inhibitors prevent maturation of these noninfectious virions (108–110). There are now four protease inhibitors licensed by the FDA for use in the United States. The first to be licensed was saquinavir. It is well tolerated, but has relatively poor bioavailability (111,112). It is now approved at a dose of 1800 mg/day. However, a recent study in patients with 200–500 CD4 cells per cubic millimeter suggests that it may be more active at higher doses of up to 7200 mg/day (113). This study compared 3600 mg/day with 7200 mg/day. The lower-dose regimen resulted in a decrease in plasma HIV RNA levels of 1.06 log RNA copies per milliliter of plasma and a mean increase in CD4 cell counts of $72/mm^3$, whereas, the high-dose regimen produced decreases in plasma HIV RNA of 1.34 log RNA copies per cubic millimeter of plasma with a mean CD4 cell increase of $121/mm^3$.

Ritonavir is substantially more potent than saquinavir, partly because of its better oral absorption. Single-agent use has been reported to result in an initial 1.7 log 10 decrease in viremia (114). However, resistance is a problem when it is used as a single agent, and it is best combined with reverse transcriptase inhibitors. The use of ritonavir can be associated with adverse reactions, including gastrointestinal disturbance in approximately 25% of patients, hepatotoxicity, headache, and transient circumoral paresthesia. It is also a strong inhibitor of the hepatic enzyme cytochrome P-450; consequently, it can be complicated to use with other drugs metabolized by this pathway (115). Finally, there is an unproved association of protease inhibitor use and nonketosis-prone hyperglycemia occurring 1–7 months after starting therapy with these agents (116,117), and hemophiliacs using this class of drugs have been reported to have bleeding episodes (118).

Indinavir is very potent, has good bioavailability, and is well tolerated (119–122). It can cause hyperbilirubinemia, mostly indirect and without significant clinical consequence. Also, 3–4% of patients receiving indinavir develop hematuria from nephrolithiasis, composed mainly of precipitated indinavir. In one early study involving heavily pretreated patients with low CD4 cell counts (mean fewer than $100/mm^3$) and high viral loads (mean more than 130,000), the mean increase in CD4 cell counts was $143/mm^3$ and the mean decrease in HIV RNA was more than 1.5 log 10 RNA copies per cubic millimeter (121). Preliminary results from three other studies evaluating indinavir as monotherapy or in combination with nucleoside analogues in nucleoside analogues naive patients resulted in median declines in viral RNA, ranging from -2.0 to more than -2.3 log 10 RNA copies per cubic millimeter and the CD4 T-cell subsets showed increases ranging from 26 to 80/mm^3 (120). At 24 weeks of therapy, 40% of patients receiving indinavir monotherapy had viral RNA levels below the ability of the assay to detect it.

Preliminary data suggest that nelfinavir, the most recently approved protease inhibitor, has high bioavailability, is generally well tolerated, and has potent anti-HIV activity (123–126). The principal toxicity is diarrhea. This drug was rapidly approved by the FDA based on preliminary data that it was well tolerated and effective in lowering the HIV-1 viral RNA and increasing CD4 cell counts in preliminary clinical trials.

E. Combination Antiretroviral Therapy

Even as initial efforts began to develop anti-HIV drugs, researchers envisioned that the disease would probably be most effectively treated with combinations of two or more drugs. As early as 1987, combination regimens of two dideoxynucleosides were explored in the clinic (74), and uncontrolled trials suggested that such regimens may be useful (74,127–131). In 1996, results of two large randomized trials, ACTG 175 and the Delta Trial, demonstrated that zidovudine plus either didanosine or zalcitabine was superior in clinical endpoints compared with zidovudine monotherapy (30,50,51). These results provided clear evidence of the usefulness of combination regimens in HIV infection. More recently, several combination regimens of three drugs (generally two nucleoside analogues and a protease inhibitor) have been reported to reduce the HIV RNA levels to below detectable limits in many patients for prolonged periods and to substantially delay the emergence of resistance (90,132–135). As will be discussed later, such regimens are now considered state-of-the-art therapy for HIV infection for most patients (52–54).

One of the earlier trials of such triple combination therapy used saquinavir as the protease inhibitor (136). In this trial 302 zidovudine-experienced patients were randomly assigned to receive saquinavir (1800 mg/day) plus zidovudine (600 mg/day) and zalcitabine (2.25 mg/day), saquinavir plus zidovudine, or zidovudine plus zalcitabine. In all three treatment groups, CD4 cell counts rose at first and then fell gradually. There were significantly greater reductions in plasma HIV levels with the three-drug combination than with other regimens. There were no major differences in toxic effects among the three treatments (137).

Even greater excitement was generated by preliminary reports in 1996 of the potent and sustained effect of triple combination therapy using zidovudine, lamivudine, and indinavir (138). This double-blinded study randomized 97 HIV-infected zidovudine-experienced patients with between 50 and 400 CD4 cells cubic millimeter, to one of three treatments for up to 52 weeks: 800 mg of indinavir monotherapy every 8 h; combination NRTI therapy with 200 mg of zidovudine every 8 h, and 150 mg of lamivudine twice daily; or all three drugs (133). The decrease in HIV RNA over the first 24 weeks was significantly greater in the three-drug group than in the other groups. In particular, 90% of the triple-drug group had fewer than 500 RNA copies per cubic millimeter at 12 months, compared with less than 30% of the patients in the indinavir monotherapy group, and none of the patients in the NRTI group. Also, approximately 80% of patients on the triple combination had HIV RNA levels below 50 copies per cubic millimeter, compared with none in the other groups. Increases in CD4 cell counts were greater in both groups with indinavir than in the combination NRTI without indinavir group. The triple combination was as well tolerated as monotherapy with indinavir or the NRTI combination.

The clinical efficacy of indinavir in combination with two NRTIs was demonstrated in ACTG 320, a large, randomized, controlled trial of 1156 zidovudine-experienced patients randomly assigned to one of two daily regimens: 600 mg of zidovudine and 300 mg of lamivudine, or that regimen with 2400 mg of indinavir (132). Stavudine could be substituted for zidovudine if patients were zidovudine-intolerant. With a median follow-up of 38 weeks, the proportion of patients whose disease progressed to AIDS or death was significantly lower with the triple combination therapy compared with the double-nucleoside therapy without the protease inhibitor. Moreover, whereas there were substantial increases in the CD4 cell counts among both groups, they were significantly greater for the triple-combination therapy group. In a subset of patients for whom viral RNA PCR measurements were obtained, there were significantly larger drops in viral load for the triple-combination group. At 6 months, the proportion of patients with viral RNA levels of fewer then 500 copies per cubic millimeter was much greater for patients on triple therapy (60%) compared with those without the protease inhibitor (9%). The proportion of adverse events was similar in both groups of patients.

Although saquinavir was the first protease inhibitor approved in the United States, its usefulness, is somewhat limited by its relatively poor oral bioavailability (52). However, there is recent evidence that the area under the time–concentration curve (AUC) of saquinavir as well as certain other protease inhibitors can be increased by its use in combination with ritonavir (139–142). This occurs because of the effect of ritonavir on P-450 (142). There is relatively little cross-resistance between saquinavir and ritonavir, and as such, improved suppression of viral loads may be possible with this combination and in combination with two NRTIs (139,140,143). Preliminary data has indicated that quadruple combination therapy with two nucleoside analogues and two protease inhibitors can be tolerated and yields a substantial anti-HIV effect (139). However, there is still inadequate data to make recommendations.

The use of triple antiretroviral drug therapy with two NRTIs combined with one NNRTI has been evaluated in a randomized, double-blind, placebo-controlled trial of nevirapine added to the combination of zidovudine and didanosine. Three hundred ninety-eight adult patients with CD4 cell counts of 350/mm^3, or fewer, and more than 6 months of previous nucleoside therapy were given either nevirapine or placebo along with open-label zidovudine and didanosine (144). After 48 weeks of study treatment, patients assigned to the triple-combination regimen had an 18% higher mean absolute CD4 cell count, a 0.32 log 10 lower mean infectious HIV-1 titer in PBMC and a 0.25 log 10 lower mean plasma HIV-1 RNA level, compared with zidovudine and didanosine, with the greatest benefit seen in those with CD4 cell counts between 50 and 200/mm^3. Severe rashes were seen in 9% of patients on the triple combination, versus 2% on the double combination. Resistance to NNRTIs can develop in as little as 2 weeks when used as monotherapy, and these drugs should only be used in combination with at least one nucleoside reverse transcriptase inhibitor (52–54).

Preliminary evidence supports the use of delavirdine, the other NNRTI approved for use in HIV infection, for use in combination with two NRTIs (145). In a phase I–II trial of delavirdine, more sustained reductions in branched HIV DNA levels and increases in CD4 counts were seen with the triple-drug combination of delavirdine with zidovudine and didanosine compared with delavirdine monotherapy, combination delavirdine and zidovudine, or combination zidovudine with didanosine.

The recent findings that the viral load (as assessed by HIV RNA PCR) can predict the rate of subsequent immunological deterioration, that the viral load can be suppressed below the level of detection with highly active therapy, and that such suppression can substantially delay the emergence of resistance have dramatically altered our views of anti-HIV therapy. For patients who are treatment-naive, the goal of treatment is now viewed as being to aggressively treat to suppress the viral load below the limit of detection for as long as possible. Such treatment can be associated with substantial immunological improvement, including an increase in CD45 RA-naive CD4 cells (146). There is evidence that such high-level HIV suppression can be sustained for at least 2–3 years in some patients, and one of the important questions now is how long can such virological remission last.

Unfortunately, not all patients achieve undetectable viral loads on triple-combination antiretroviral therapy and others do not sustain such a response. This represents virological failure of the regimen and, as discussed later, is one of the factors used in considering a change of therapy (52,53). Virological failure is more likely to occur in patients who have been previously treated on one- or two-drug regimens with sequential stepwise additions of single antiretroviral agents in the face of apparent virological or clinical failure to the regimen, or for those who have been switched through multiple monotherapy regimens in this setting. Resistance is also likely to develop if plasma drug levels are suboptimal because of drug intolerance or less than excellent compliance (53). Under such conditions, mutations occur, giving rise to HIV quasispecies having relative resistance to various antiretroviral agents (147–150). Although formal data is still incomplete, the experience of many physicians is that it is very difficult to achieve sustained suppression of the HIV viral load once patients have developed resistance to an initial regimen. Even so, the patient's antiretroviral drug history can serve to guide the rational selection of alternative regimens. In general, it is optimal to select second-line regimens, with the goal of again attaining suppression below the limit of detection. For a number of patients who have failed one or more regimens, however, it may be impossible to again attain complete suppression with available agents, and physicians will have to settle for partial suppression. In doing so, they will have to balance the activity of the regimens, their toxicity, and the likely effect of the regimen on other potential regimens in the future. In selecting such regimens, one cannot rely on complete viral suppression to thwart or delay the development of resistance, and it is more important to understand interactions between resistance mutations. Indeed, such patients serve as a reminder that even with 11 approved drugs, the present armamentarium against HIV is insufficient and that additional effective drugs are still urgently needed. Much of the information to guide physicians in such regimens was generated from early trials of combination NRTI therapy.

A mutation at codon 74 of the HIV *pol* gene, which is the most frequent cause of resistance to didanosine, was found by St. Clair et al. to reverse the resistance to zidovudine (73). This provided a strong rationale to test these drugs in combination therapy. In several small studies, the combination didanosine and zidovudine therapy was superior relative to surrogate markers to either monotherapy or to sequential, alternating monotherapy with zidovudine and didanosine (129–131). Some patients on this regimen had prolonged increases in their CD4 cell count, and prolonged survival (129–131,151).

Lamivudine has potent anti-HIV activity and is extremely well tolerated (91), but when it is used as monotherapy, HIV develops a rapid resistance to it that is associated with a mutation at codon 184 of the HIV *pol* gene (88–90). However, this mutation partially reverses HIV resistance to zidovudine associated with a mutation in codon 215 (88), and the combination of lamivudine and zidovudine has been quite effective in both zidovudine-experienced and zidovudine-naive patients (152–156). In 5 multicenter, randomized trials of combination lamivudine and zidovudine, the combination was quite well tolerated and yielded greater and more sustained increases in CD4 cell counts and decreases in viral load than continued zidovudine monotherapy (152–156). As might be predicted by the interaction between the foregoing resistance-conferring mutations, viral mutations associated with zidovudine resistance seem to develop more slowly in patients receiving the combination than in those receiving zidovudine monotherapy (153).

Preliminary studies have shown the safety of stavudine in combination with lamivudine (157–159). A theoretical concern for this combination is that resistance may develop quickly to lamivudine in association with a mutation at codon 184 (88,90), and there does not appear to be any beneficial interaction between this and the mutations causing stavudine resistance. There is some evidence, however, that the combination works somewhat better in practice than one may have predicted; a subset analysis of a large randomized trial comparing two nucleosides (either zidovudine plus lamivudine or stavudine plus lamivudine versus either of these combinations with a protease inhibitor), demonstrated that the combination of stavudine plus lamivudine has prolonged anti-HIV activity, especially when combined with a protease inhibitor (132). It may be that the stavudine–lamivudine combination has its best utility in the setting of complete viral suppression during which the 184 mutation is less likely to appear. Even so, the two-drug combination of stavudine and lamivudine appears to have reasonable activity.

The nucleoside analogue combinations with the most extensively documented clinical benefits to date are zidovudine plus didanosine, zidovudine plus lamivudine, and zidovudine plus zalcitabine (50,74,156,160). The superiority of two of these regimens (zidovudine plus didanosine and zidovudine plus zalcitabine) over zidovudine monotherapy relative to clinical endpoints was recently shown in two large randomized trials. One, ACTG 175, was a double-blinded study of 2467 patients randomly assigned to one of four daily regimens: 600 mg of zidovudine; 600 mg of zidovudine plus 400 mg didanosine; 600 mg of zidovudine plus 2.25 mg of zalcitabine; or 400 mg of didanosine (50). Results of this study showed that progression was significantly less frequent with the combination arms when compared with the zidovudine arm. The combinations resulted in substantially improved outcome, with progression in less than 23% of the patients in each of these arms compared with a progression rate of 32% in the zidovudine monotherapy arm. It is worth noting that the results with the didanosine monotherapy arm were also better than those of the zidovudine monotherapy arm and were overall not significantly different from those of the combination arms. In a subset of the patients studied for virological data, the superior clinical outcomes correlated with greater effects on viral load measurements. A separate study, the European Delta Trial, similarly showed a substantial survival benefit for patients receiving combination therapy with zidovudine plus either didanosine or zalcitabine compared with zidovudine alone among patients who had not received previous zidovudine (51). Patients previously exposed to zidovudine benefited from combination zidovudine and didanosine, but to a smaller extent than did the zidovudine-naive patients. There was no benefit among zidovudine-experienced patients of the zidovudine–zalcitabine combination compared with continued zidovudine monotherapy.

For combination NRTI therapy, physicians should be aware of the phosphorylation patterns of nucleosides. NRTIs are not active against HIV in themselves, but rather, must be phosphorylated by cellular enzymes to the active triphosphate moieties. Thymidine analogues (zidovudine and stavudine) are preferentially activated in replicating cells and are most active in such cells (161,162). By contrast, other NRTIs are relatively more active in resting cells. Regimens that use both a thymidine and nonthymidine NRTIs would thus effectively protect both cell types and, in fact, this helps explain the high activity of such regimens as zidovudine with didanosine or zidovudine with zalcitabine (50,51,128,163). This general principle should be considered as physicians are considering combination regimens.

For patients with more advanced HIV infection, the efficacy of combination nucleoside reverse transcriptase inhibitor therapy may not necessarily be superior to monotherapy, and may, in fact, be less well tolerated (160). For example, in one study of 1102 randomly assigned patients with AIDS or with a CD4 cell count of fewer than 200/mm^3, comparison of zidovudine alone versus zidovudine with either didanosine or zalcitabine showed no differences in the rate of disease progression over a median follow-up of 35 months (160). Most patients had previously received zidovudine. Therapy with zidovudine plus didanosine resulted in more adverse gastrointestinal effects, and treatment with zidovudine plus zalcitabine, resulted in more neuropathy than zidovudine alone. The results of this study are important to consider in thinking about antiretroviral therapy in patients with advanced HIV infection who develop malignancies. However, the ACTG 320 Study Team reported favorable results for patients with advanced immunosuppression receiving combination zidovudine, lamivudine, and indinavir among zidovudine-experienced patients (132).

Certain combinations of nucleosides may have drawbacks that may limit their utility. For example, synergistic toxicity (neuropathy) can be seen with simultaneous zalcitabine and didanosine (74,164,165); cross-reactive resistance of HIV to zalcitabine and lamivudine may decrease the usefulness of this combination (166–168); and there can even be antagonistic activity as in the combination of zidovudine and ribavirin (169), and in the combination of zidovudine with stavudine (170). However, just because two drugs cause a similar toxicity does not mean that they should never be used together. For example, stavudine and didanosine both cause neuropathy, yet there is evidence that they can be used safely together and in combination with protease inhibitors (96,124,171). Such patients should be monitored closely for signs of toxicity.

IV. GENERAL RECOMMENDATIONS FOR ANTIRETROVIRAL THERAPY IN THE NONMALIGNANCY AFFECTED HIV POPULATION

In June 1997, a 13-member panel of the International AIDS Society representing international expertise in antiretroviral research and HIV patient care formulated recommendations for therapy of HIV infection based on CD4 cell count, plasma HIV RNA level, or clinical status (52). At about the same time, an NIH Panel to Define Principles of Therapy of HIV Infection (53) and a panel on Clinical Practices for Treatment of HIV Infection, convened by the Department of Health and Human Services and the Henry J. Kaiser Family Foundation released preliminary guidelines for the use of antiretroviral agents in HIV-infected adults and adolescents (54). Both panels recommended that for treatment-naive patients, the initial regimen should be chosen based on maximum likelihood of suppressing and maintaining the plasma HIV RNA below the level of detection of the most sensitive assays (currently 400–500 copies RNA per milliliter), which can be attained in most antiretroviral-naive patients. The recommended regimen to best achieve these results consists of two nucleoside reverse transcriptase inhibitors with a potent bioavailable protease inhibitor (Tables 1–3). For patients in whom the use of a protease inhibitors is not feasible, an alternative approach is the use of two NRTIs with a nonnucleoside reverse transcriptase inhibitor, but this combination is less reliable in achieving undetectable plasma HIV RNA levels. Two-drug regimens are considered suboptimal, and it is unknown if regimens using two NRTIs would be adequate in patients with a low viral load (i.e., fewer than 10,000 HIV RNA copies per milliliter), and so this strategy was not recom-

Table 1 Initial Recommended Antiretroviral Regimens as Suggested by a Panel of the International AIDS Society in 1997

A   Two nucleoside reverse transcriptase inhibitors with a protease inhibitor

  1. Zidovudine–lamivudine + protease inhibitor
  2. Zidovudine–didanosine + protease inhibitor
  3. Zidovudine–zalcitabine + protease inhibitor
  4. Stavudine–lamivudine + protease inhibitor
  5. Stavudine–didanosine + protease inhibitor

B   Combination nucleosides with nonnucleoside reverse transcriptase inhibitor
      Any of the above nucleoside combinations can also be administered with a NNRTI

Source: Ref. 52.

Table 2 Possible Alternative Regimens if Changing Antiretroviral Therapy is Needed Owing to Drug Failure of Three-Drug Regimens

Current regimen	Alternative regimen
Zidovudine–lamivudine–protease inhibitor	Stavudine–didanosine–new protease inhibitor
	Stavudine–didanosine–NNRTI
	Ritonavir–saquinavir–NRTI
Stavudine–lamivudine–protease inhibitor	Zidovudine–didanosine–new protease inhibitor
	Zidovudine–didanosine–NNRTI
	Ritonavir–saquinavir–NRTI
Zidovudine–didanosine–protease inhibitor	Stavudine–lamivudine–new protease inhibitor
	Stavudine–lamivudine–NNRTI
	Ritonavir–saquinavir–NRTI
Stavudine–didanosine–protease inhibitor	Zidovudine–lamivudine–new protease inhibitor
	Zidovudine–lamivudine–NNRTI
	Ritonavir–saquinavir–NRTI
Zidovudine–didanosine–NNRTI	Stavudine–lamivudine–protease inhibitor
	Zidovudine–lamivudine–protease inhibitor

Source: Ref. 52.

Table 3 Possible Alternative Regimens for Treatment Failure on a Selected Double-NRTI Combinations

Current regimen	Alternative regimen
Zidovudine–didanosine	Zidovudine–lamivudine–protease inhibitor
	Stavudine–lamivudine–protease inhibitor
	Ritonavir–saquinavir–NRTI
Zidovudine–zalcitabine	Zidovudine–lamivudine–protease inhibitor
	Stavudine–lamivudine–protease inhibitor
	Stavudine–didanosine–protease inhibitor
	Ritonavir–saquinavir–NRTI
Zidovudine–lamivudine	Stavudine–didanosine–protease inhibitor
	Ritonavir–saquinavir–NRTI
Stavudine–didanosine	Zidovudine–lamivudine–protease inhibitor
	Ritonavir–saquinavir–NRTI
Stavudine–lamivudine	Zidovudine–didanosine–protease inhibitor
	Ritonavir–saquinavir–NRTI

Source: Ref. 52.

mended for most circumstances. Monotherapy was considered substandard by the panels. The recommendations reflected the panels' agreement that plasma HIV RNA measurements are important for predicting risk of clinical progression and that recent clinical trials of combination therapies demonstrated that reductions in plasma HIV RNA levels are associated with increased survival and decreased progression to AIDS (132,160,172,173).

These panels noted that there is evidence to suggest that the selection of appropriate early therapeutic intervention may be instrumental in delaying the evolution of drug-resistant mutants (53,54,57). Although patients may initially be infected with a single virion, viral genomic variation occurs during the course of HIV infection (even during the first cycles of replication) and, even in the absence of selective pressure, this process yields a number of HIV quasispecies, some of which are spontaneously resistant to antiretroviral drugs (147,148,174). The prevalence of such mutants in the population of virus before the initiation of antiretroviral therapy is believed to be a function of the number of prior rounds of viral replication, the mutation rate, and the selective advantage (fitness) possessed by wild-type virus over variants that have incorporated mutations conferring drug resistance (147). An extension of this concept is that early intervention and effective suppression of viral replication may delay the emergence of mutant resistant clones. A more durable response would thus be expected with earlier intervention, as opposed to the later stages of HIV disease when a broader pattern of drug-resistant quasispecies would be expected to have previously evolved. Another driving force in the recommendations was evidence that reductions in plasma viremia correlate with increased CD4 cell numbers and AIDS-free survival (11,25,27,30,175). Treatments that achieve a greater and more durable suppression of HIV replication were thus assumed to be of greater clinical benefit. Finally, the panels noted that there is recent evidence that relatively complete suppression of the viral load can delay the emergence of resistance (52–54, 90,176,177).

The viral load and CD4 cell count were recommended by these panels as useful tools for assessing when to initiate antiretroviral therapy (52–54,57). The panels noted that for patients who are asymptomatic and have CD4 cell counts of more than 500/mm^3, there is no clear clinical trial data to define the optimal treatment strategy. However, given that there appears to be no threshold of HIV replication below which immune destruction does not occur, aggressive treatment can be considered for any patient if HIV RNA is detected in the plasma. Treatment is strongly recommended in those patients with CD4 cell counts of fewer than 500/mm^3, patients with rapidly declining CD4 cell counts (i.e., a greater than 300/mm^3 loss over 12–18 months), or for asymptomatic patients who have high viral load (i.e. more than 20,000 RNA copies per cubic millimeter). The panels recommended including a protease inhibitor in the initial regimen for any patient in whom therapy is indicated, particularly for patients at higher risk for

progression. In particular, a protease inhibitor could be considered for symptomatic patients, patients with lower or rapidly falling CD4 cell counts, and asymptomatic patients with high plasma HIV RNA levels, regardless of the CD4 count
(52–54,57). However, the panels noted that there is no firm clinical trial data to
address this point (especially in patients with a CD4 cell count of more than 500/
mm^3), and that the recommendations to consider therapy in this population is
based on recent advances in understanding viral dynamics and resistance. Of
certain importance is that patients understand the required commitment of adher-
ence to stringent drug schedules and dosing, and the potential consequences
(emergence of drug-resistant HIV) of less than excellent compliance. Moreover,
there are potential problems related to long-term toxicity, tolerance, and possible
induction of drug-resistant virus. Several other groups are currently formulating
recommendations for using antiretroviral therapy and clinical trial data are emerging rapidly. As such, clinicians should be alert for changes in these recommendations as scientific advances occur and new clinical trial results become available.

An important principle for managing antiretroviral therapy is that in the
setting of drug failure in a three-drug regimen, all three drugs should ideally be
changed when possible to drugs that the patient has not failed. At a minimum,
two drugs that the patient has not failed should be substituted in a three-drug
regimen (Table 2; 52–54). The choice of new drugs should be guided by past
drug history, and the new agents should be selected to minimize cross-resistance
with the likely mutations conferring resistance to the previous regimens. Specifically, stepwise and sequential addition of one adjunct agent to a failing regimen
should be avoided, as this is likely to result in the development of resistance to
the newly added agent in short order (53). Drug failure is a complex issue, but
there are some salient points that suggest virological failure of the regimen: a
less than tenfold (1.0 log) reduction in plasma HIV RNA by 4 weeks following
initiation of therapy; failure to suppress plasma HIV RNA to undetectable levels
within 4–6 months of initiating therapy; reemergence of detectable viral RNA
on repeated determinations after an initial complete suppression, or reproducible
threefold or greater increase from the nadir RNA level on a regimen (54). However, the overall clinical picture including quality of life, immunological standing
as reflected by the CD4 counts, and remaining therapeutic options for control of
HIV must be considered before defining treatment failure and prompting a change
in therapy.

V. ANTIRETROVIRAL THERAPY DURING CANCER CHEMOTHERAPY

As we can see from the foregoing discussion, the physician treating the HIV-
infected patient now has a wide number of therapeutic options. The complexity

of treatment is increased considerably in patients who also have tumors. The treatment plan must balance tumor treatment and HIV therapy and, moreover, complex interactions among the treatments and disease process may occur. One concern is the potential for overlapping drug toxicities and for interactions that, for example, may change the pharmacokinetics of a given agent, resulting in unexpected and potentially deleterious toxicities or changes in activity. The treatment of tumors in patients with low CD4 cell counts who are also receiving drugs to prevent or treat opportunistic infections poses further challenges. One underlying question in all such patients is how to treat the HIV infection while cancer chemotherapy is administered. Unfortunately, there has been relatively little research directed toward this question.

It is fair to say that, although the general principles of antiviral therapy can apply to the patients with tumors, the complexity of interactions in therapy may be such that the current specific recommendations for anti-HIV therapy may not necessarily apply in patients receiving chemotherapy. Even in patients with advanced HIV infection, for whom anti-HIV therapy is clearly recommended, this issue may have to be reconsidered in the setting of active chemotherapy. The criteria for stopping or changing antiviral therapy are likewise not entirely appropriate during chemotherapy. For example, the International Panel stated three general reasons for changing or stopping antiretroviral therapy (57). The first is treatment failure as inferred by increased viral replication, indicated by increases in viral load (e.g., a return toward or within 0.3–0.5 log 10 of pretreatment plasma HIV RNA levels), decreases in CD4 cell counts (or percentages), or clinical progression. Chemotherapy-induced lymphopenia invalidates the CD4 count as a marker of HIV disease progression, and it is not yet completely clear what effect chemotherapy has on viral load. Opportunistic infections may also occur during chemotherapy independently of HIV disease. The second reason to stop or change antiretroviral therapy is toxicity, intolerance, or nonadherence. Patients with more advanced or complicated disease are more likely to experience overlapping toxicity with other drugs, to have fewer therapeutic options and, consequently, a potentially impaired ability to adhere to a given antiretroviral regimen. Yet, they may be able to resume the antiviral drugs after the chemotherapy. The third reason for stopping or altering antiretroviral therapy is if the current regimen represents substandard practice, such as in zidovudine monotherapy (57), yet even this recommendation might need further consideration for the unique case of the patient receiving active cancer chemotherapy.

An important fundamental issue that has not been adequately addressed is the risk of AIDS progression in patients during active chemotherapy in various patient groups. A relevant issue is the effect of the chemotherapy on HIV replication. The killing of lymphocytes during chemotherapy may destroy the target cells for HIV replication, and even eliminate a reservoir of infected cells. Preliminary findings in eight patients with AIDS-related non–Hodgkin's lymphoma (NHL) treated at the National Cancer Institute with EPOCH (infusional etoposide, vincristine, and doxorubicin, with bolus cyclophosphamide and oral prednisone) chemotherapy would support this view (178). In such patients, there was a trend toward decreased HIV RNA levels during the actual 96-h chemotherapy infusions. These transient dips not withstanding, the viral load remained relatively stable during the course of therapy after an initial small rebound following cessation of antiretroviral therapy. In another small study of six patients receiving CHOP (cyclophosphamide, doxorubicin, vincristine, and prednisone) for AIDS-related NHL, plasma viremia measured by PCR only transiently increased toward the completion of all the chemotherapy cycles, then return to baseline in four of six patients (179). In the other two patients, however, viral loads remained high. In a separate study of CHOP in patients with AIDS-related lymphomas, chemotherapy was associated with a decrease in p24 antigen (180). More data will be needed, however, to formulate an assessment of the effects of chemotherapy on HIV viral burden, and there is a need for additional investigation in this area.

One also has to consider the potential interactions between HIV-induced and chemotherapy-induced immunosuppression. Chemotherapy can induce profound immune suppression independent of HIV. Recovery of lymphocytes following chemotherapy is delayed relative to that of other cell types, and a relative lymphocytopenia can last for years (181–183). This may be important in patients who also have HIV infection. One can hypothesize that because HIV replication is greater in dividing cells, suppression of viral replication may be most important during lymphocyte recovery. Another concern is that HIV-infected patients have thymic damage (35,184,185) and may thus have an impaired ability to produce new thymic-derived (naive) T cells. However, this may not pose an insurmountable problem, as T cell expression after chemotherapy in adults without HIV infection largely involves postthymus expansion of peripheral T cells (186,187). Additionally, some expansion of the RA+ (naive) CD4 pool has been observed in adults receiving highly active antiretroviral therapy (HAART; 146).

Also, remember that there may be substantial differences between the immunosuppression induced by HIV and that by chemotherapy. There are, for example, distinctive differences in functional characteristics of natural killer cells (NK) and lymphokine-activated killer cells (LAK) in chemotherapy versus HIV-induced immune dysfunction (2,5). Findings indicate that cytotoxic NK pool size is increased in breast cancer patients, but is diminished consequent to administration of cytotoxic chemotherapy. However, the functional capacity of individual NK and LAK cells remains intact in this setting. By contrast, in HIV-1 seropositive individuals, derangements of NK and LAK cells have been observed, with marked reductions in cytolytic functions in addition to reductions of NK and LAK pool sizes (2). This may partly account for some of the differences in the clinical expression of immune compromise relative to cell number in the setting of cytotoxic chemotherapy versus HIV disease.

Even in the absence of HIV infection, chemotherapy regimens have been associated with varying rates of complicating opportunistic infections. For example, aggressive chemotherapy regimens such as ProMACE-CytaBOM (prednisone, methotrexate with leucovorin, doxorubicin, cyclophosphamide, etoposide, cytarabine, bleomycin, vincristine, methotrexate with leucovorin) for lymphoma (188), or a recently described combined modality regimen using low-dose paclitaxel and radiation therapy for small cell lung cancer (189) have been associated with opportunistic infections, including *Pneumocystis carinii* pneumonia. HIV has a deleterious immune influence beyond lymphocytopenia (190–194), and may thus exacerbate chemotherapy-induced immunosuppression. However, HIV infection is also associated with overstimulation of certain immune functions (such as IL-6 production), and may have complex interactions with the immune effects of cytotoxic therapy.

It is important to consider what influence chemotherapy has on viral load and what the implications of observed changes are. Ideally, one would like to administer aggressive anti-HIV therapy during antineoplastic chemotherapy. However, it is important to consider whether this is possible, or whether it may adversely affect the delivery of the chemotherapy to a greater extent than it provides benefit to the patients. It is important to determine whether pharmacokinetic interactions among the various agents exert a consequential influence. It is important to consider how combined toxicities may affect the ability to administer adequate doses of chemotherapy. In addition, it is important to determine whether inclusion of antiretroviral therapy during chemotherapy influences the development of mutant viral strains that are resistant to therapy, particularly if doses of the antiviral drugs are reduced because of toxicities. These issues are likely to be disease- and regimen-specific.

Monitoring viral load in HIV-infected cancer patients undergoing active cancer chemotherapy may not be entirely straightforward. Patients undergoing chemotherapy may have periods of lymphocyte killing interspersed with periods of regeneration fueled by endogenous cytokines and growth factors. Additionally, antigenic or cytokine-mediated stimuli (for example, from sepsis) can induce transient increases in HIV replication (20,40,56,195–199). Moreover, administered exogenous growth factors can lead to changes in HIV disease activity. For example, granulocyte–macrophage colony-stimulating factor (GM-CSF) increases HIV replication in monocytes and macrophages in vitro and in vivo (161,200–202), including patients undergoing lymphoma therapy with CHOP (180). On the other hand, filgrastim (granulocyte colony-stimulating factor; G-CSF) has no apparent effect on HIV replication (200,201,203). Also, growth factors may influence the effects of dideoxynucleoside reverse transcriptase inhibitors on HIV replication through an effect on dideoxynucleoside phosphorylation. For example, in vitro GM-CSF can increase the antiviral effect of zidovudine in monocytes, but it slightly decreases the antiviral activity of zalcitabine and didanosine (201,204).

Another consideration is that, during chemotherapy, other surrogate markers, such as viral load and CD4 cell count measurements, may be affected and thus may not be reliable indicators of long-term HIV progression. Standard doses of some cancer chemotherapeutic drugs can result in transient losses of 50% or more of circulating lymphocytes (2). Given these confounding variables, a determination that a given antiretroviral drug or drug combination has failed during chemotherapy may not be straightforward, and one may have to proceed relatively blindly. Incorporating the measurement of viral loads and CD4 cell counts into chemotherapy protocols in an attempt to understand the dynamics of HIV disease as modified by chemotherapy, with or without antiretroviral therapy, may provide important information on these issues. In this way, we can begin to develop a rational approach to the use or omission of antiretroviral therapy during chemotherapy.

It is perhaps worthwhile to consider some of the information that is currently available to address this point. The use of the antiretroviral didanosine was investigated in a pilot study of infusional CDE (cyclophosphamide, doxorubicin, and etoposide), along with filgrastim in 25 patients with HIV-related NHL (9). The overall CR rate in this study was 58% (50% for patients with CD4 fewer than 100, and 67% for patients with CD4 more than 100). Patients were assigned to one of two groups with differing schedules of didanosine inclusion or exclusion by cycle. Didanosine usage was associated with relatively less leukopenia, neutropenia, and thrombocytopenia. Fewer red blood cell and platelet transfusions were required on the cycles in which patients received didanosine. Overall, however, CDE resulted in a significant decrease in CD4 and CD8 cell counts, and this was not affected by coadministration of didanosine. The CD4 cell counts returned to baseline 3 months following chemotherapy, but the study design did not allow a determination of didanosine's effect on CD4 cell recovery. Also, serum p24 antigen did not change substantially when comparing the pre-CDE value with those obtained during CDE therapy, regardless of whether didanosine was included in the cycle. There were no clinical or biochemical episodes of pancreatitis, only one episode of mild peripheral neuropathy that resolved after discontinuation of didanosine, and no other toxicities that appeared to be due to the didanosine.

In this study the mean steady-state plasma etoposide concentrations were 11–38% lower during cycles in which didanosine was administered (9). Indeed, the lower etoposide concentrations likely accounted for the favorable myelotolerance observed with the didanosine inclusive cycles. Although this study seems to provide evidence that combining an effective monotherapeutic antiretroviral agent with chemotherapy in patients with HIV-associated lymphoma does not necessarily cause substantial increased toxicity in such a regimen, it did not answer the question of whether there was any added benefit from its inclusion in the treatment plan. This study also highlighted the potential for complex interactions between antiretroviral and cancer chemotherapeutic agents.

The complexity of interactions with chemotherapy and other agents was again underscored in a trial of CHOP chemotherapy, with or without GM-CSF, for HIV-related non–Hodgkin's lymphoma (180). In that study, GM-CSF administration was associated with improved quality of life in that patients randomized to the GM-CSF arm had fewer episodes of neutropenic fever, shorter periods of neutropenia, and shorter hospitalizations. The GM-CSF cycles had fewer dose reductions and fewer cycle delays compared with the non–GM-CSF cycles, but complete response rates were similar in the groups receiving GM-CSF and those not. CHOP chemotherapy was associated with a slight decrease in p24 antigen among patients who did not receive the GM-CSF. However, p24 levels were increased over 200% in patients also receiving the GM-CSF. The long-term consequence of these increases in p24 antigen are not clear. The effects of GM-CSF on HIV replication were further examined by Scadden et al. (205). This group studied a group of patients with CD4 cell counts of $200/mm^3$ or fewer, who were given GM-CSF along with zidovudine. In this setting, addition of GM-CSF was not associated with changes in viral load by PCR measurements, changes in p24 antigen, or zidovudine levels, either intracellular or in the plasma (205). It is quite possible that no net effect in HIV replication was observed in these patients because the increase in HIV replication induced by GM-CSF was counterbalanced by the GM-CSF-induced increase in zidovudine phosphorylation and effectiveness.

An important issue that is not completely understood is the effect of various chemotherapeutic regimens on HIV viral dynamics. Some cytotoxic drugs may themselves have antiretroviral activity. For example, doxorubicin inhibits HIV replication by a variety of mechanisms, including inhibition of the HIV-1 long terminal repeat, and possibly direct inhibition of HIV-1 reverse transcriptase (206–211). The clinical effect of various chemotherapeutic regimens on the HIV viral load was studied in a very small pilot study of AIDS-related KS and AIDS-related lymphoma in which five patients were followed prospectively (212). The four KS patients were treated with combination bleomycin, methotrexate, and vincristine, and the lymphoma patient received vincristine, etoposide, mitozanthrone, and prednisone. Various effects in plasma HIV viremia were seen, with little change for the Kaposi's sarcoma patients and, in the lymphoma patient, the viral load actually decreased (212).

In a study by Levine et al. (213), HIV RNA levels were measured in ten patients with relapsed or refractory AIDS-related lymphoma who were being treated with mitoguazone (MGBG). In this study, five patients experienced an increase in HIV RNA copies per cubic millimeter of plasma, whereas five experienced a decrease. There was no relation between baseline HIV RNA levels and either the response to therapy or survival. Another study examined patients receiving low-dose methotrexate, bleomycin, doxorubicin, cyclophosphamide, vincristine, and dexamethasone (m-BACOD) chemotherapy with zalcitabine (10).

In this study, 64% of patients had HIV p24 antigen levels, which either fell or remained consistently negative, whereas 36% experienced an increase. Interestingly, no patient developed peripheral neuropathy, even though vincristine and zalcitabine can both cause it. Finally, in a case report of a patient with HIV infection and ovarian cancer in whom antiretroviral (monotherapy with zidovudine) was stopped before chemotherapy with combination cyclophosphamide and cisplatin, HIV-1 p24 antigen, neopterin, β_2-microglobulin, and CD4 values remained stable (214). Overall, these studies do provide some information on the effects of cancer therapies on the parameters of HIV infection. However, many questions remain, and there is still a need for investigators to develop these data in future protocols.

It is also important to consider the potential for overlapping toxicity and pharmacokinetic interactions in patients receiving chemotherapy along with antiretroviral therapy. Several such interactions have already been identified (Tables 4 and 5), and the therapeutic plan should take into account overlapping toxicities or the potential for changes in toxicity and alterations in effective dose intensity of antineoplastic drugs because of pharmacokinetic interactions. This issue is complex, and physicians are encouraged to carefully examine the package labels for the various drugs and other pharmacological reference works such as the American Society of Health-System Pharmacists Drug Information manual for detailed information on such potential interactions (215). In overlapping toxicity, a particular concern is myelosuppression, as this is so commonly caused by cytotoxic chemotherapy. The myelotoxicity of antineoplastic drugs may be enhanced when used with HIV drugs or opportunistic infection-related drugs, such as zidovudine and trimethoprim–sulfamethoxazole. In such a case, it can be difficult to determine which agent is the predominant contributor to toxicity. Physicians can elect to discontinue or substitute the antiretroviral drug(s), or alternatively, modify the dose of the antineoplastic agent in the face of overlapping toxicity. Choosing antiretroviral therapy in a way that minimizes potential adverse interactions (or even omitting it) may be preferable in certain circumstances. This issue highlights the need for physicians with training in both oncology and treatment of HIV infection or, alternatively, close coordination between those with expertise in these two fields.

How does one choose the optimal anti-HIV regimen in a patient receiving chemotherapy? This decision can be quite complex and there are still no firm guidelines. The physician's decision of what to use should be made with an understanding of the overlapping toxicities and of the interactions among the agents (see Tables 4 and 5; 215,216). Ideally, one would like to use aggressive three-drug therapy. However, concern for multiple drug interactions and combined toxicities, in certain instances, may prompt consideration for alternative regimens or even completely withholding anti-HIV treatment for a patient who is actively receiving cancer chemotherapy. Antiretroviral regimens that are less

Table 4 Potential Overlapping Toxicities of Some HIV Antiretroviral Drugs and Antineoplastic Drugs

	Zidovudine	Didanosine	Zalcitabine	Stavudine	Lamivudine
Bleomycin	—	—	Oral ulcers/mucositis	—	—
Doxorubicin	Myelotoxicity	—	Oral ulcers/mucositis	—	—
Interferon	—	—	—	—	—
Cyclophosphamide	Myelotoxicity	—	—	—	—
Paclitaxel	Myelotoxicity	Neuropathy	Neuropathy (oral ulcers/mucositis)	Neuropathy	Neuropathy
Carboplatin	Myelotoxicity	?Neuropathy	—	—	—
Cisplatin	—	Neuropathy	Neuropathy	Neuropathy	Neuropathy
Cytarabine	Myelotoxicity	—	—	—	—
Daunorubicin	Myelotoxicity	Neuropathy	Oral ulcers/mucositis	—	—
Etoposide	Myelotoxicity	—	—	—	—
Mechlorethamine	Myelotoxicity	—	—	—	—
Methotrexate	Myelotoxicity	Neuropathy	Oral ulcers/mucositis	—	—
Procarbazine	Myelotoxicity	Neuropathy	Oral ulcers/mucositis	—	—
Vincristine	—	Neuropathy	Neuropathy	Neuropathy	Neuropathy
Vinblastine	Myelotoxicity	Neuropathy	Oral ulcers/mucositis	Neuropathy	Neuropathy
Fluorouracil	Myelotoxicity	—	Oral ulcers/mucositis	—	—
Ifosfamide	Myelotoxicity	?Pancreatitis	—	—	—
Dacarbazine	Myelotoxicity	—	—	—	—

Source: Ref. 215, 216, 227.

Table 5 Potential Pharmacokinetic Interactions of Combined Antiretroviral and Antineoplastic Drugs

	Saquinavir (SQV)	Ritonavir (RTV)	Indinavir (IDV)	Nelfinavir (NFV)	Nucleoside analogue reverse transcriptase inhibitors
Interferon (IFN)	Increased SQV levels owing to P-450 depression by IFN	Increased RTV levels owing to P-450 depression by IFN	Increased IDV levels owing to P-450 depression by IFN	Increased NFV levels owing to P-450 depression by IFN	Possible synergy
Bleomycin	Possible	Possible	Possible	Possible	—
Cyclophosphamide (CTX)	Possible increase in CTX owing to P-450 interaction	Possible increase in CTX owing to P-450 interaction	Possible increase in CTX owing to P-450 interaction	Possible increase in CTX owing to P-450 interaction	—
Paclitaxel	Possible	Large increases in paclitaxel levels	Possible	Possible	—
Carboplatin	Possible	Possible	Possible	Possible	—
Cisplatin	Possible	Possible	Possible	Possible	—
Cytarabine	Possible	Possible	Possible	Possible	—
Doxorubicin	Possible	Possible increase in doxorubicin owing to P-450 interaction	Possible	Possible	—
Daunorubicin	Possible	Possible increase in daunorubicin owing to P-450 interaction	Possible	Possible	—
Etoposide	Possible	Large increases in etoposide levels	Possible	Possible	ddI decreases plasma concentration of etoposide

Mechlorethamine	Possible	Possible	Possible	Possible	—
Methotrexate	Possible	Possible	Possible	Possible	—
Procarbazine	Possible increase in procarbazine owing to P-450 interaction	Possible increase in procarbazine owing to P-450 interaction	Possible increase in procarbazine owing to P-450 interaction	Possible increase in procarbazine owing to P-450 interaction	—
Vinblastine	Possible increase in vinblastine owing to P-450 interaction	Possible increase in vinblastine owing to P-450 interaction	Possible increase in vinblastine owing to P-450 interaction	Possible increase in vinblastine owing to P-450 interaction	—
Vincristine	Possible increase in vincristine owing to P-450 interaction	Possible increase in vincristine owing to P-450 interaction	Possible increase in vincristine owing to P-450 interaction	Possible increase in vincristine owing to P-450 interaction	—
Fluorouracil	Possible	Possible	Possible	Possible	—
Ifosfamide	Possible increase in ifosfamide owing to P-450 interaction	Possible increase in ifosfamide owing to P-450 interaction	Possible increase in ifosfamide owing to P-450 interaction	Possible increase in ifosfamide owing to P-450 interaction	—
Dacarbazine	Possible	Possible but possibly decreased metabolism to active form	Possible	Possible	—
Tamoxifen	Increased SQV levels owing to P-450 depression by tamoxifen	Increased RTV levels owing to P-450 depression by tamoxifen	Increased IDV levels owing to P-450 depression by tamoxifen	Increased NFV levels owing to P-450 depression by tamoxifen	—

Source: Refs. 9, 215, 216, 227.

than completely suppressive increase the likelihood that resistant HIV quasispecies will develop, thereby limiting future therapeutic options for the control of
HIV (53), and the best suppressive regimens now comprise two NRTIs and a
potent protease inhibitor (52,54). However, for carefully selected patients, physicians may want to consider the combinations of zidovudine with didanosine,
zidovudine with zalcitabine, or zidovudine with lamivudine. Combined stavudine
and didanosine has antiretroviral potency that appears comparable with other two-
drug combinations (96), but both are neurotoxic and should be given cautiously
with neurotoxic agents such as vincristine or paclitaxel. Combined stavudine and
lamivudine is well tolerated, particularly for patients with limited bone marrow
reserve who are poor candidates for zidovudine-containing regimens. However,
the contribution of lamivudine in this combination is unclear once lamivudine-
resistant HIV with a 184 codon mutation is selected (and this can occur within
4–8 weeks; 88). The choice of whether to add a protease inhibitor should be
made on the basis of the possibility of achieving complete viral suppression with
the protease inhibitor during the period of chemotherapy, the assessed risk of
HIV progression during this period, and the potential for adverse drug interactions. The combinations of cytotoxic agents used in effective lymphoma regimens
may, by themselves, have myriad potential drug interactions, and the potential
for substantial pharmacokinetic changes in the presence of protease inhibitors
(see Table 5) may result in profound anticipated and unanticipated interactions
(9,215,216). In this setting, it may be particularly difficult to employ protease
inhibitors.

A related question in this context is whether it is best to omit antiretroviral
therapy altogether in certain patients receiving cancer chemotherapy. Control of
HIV infection is overall highly desirable, and one should strive for this. However,
optimal antiviral therapy can cause problems in patients receiving chemotherapy.
There are few specific clinical trials addressing this issue and one needs to make
the best decision possible with incomplete data. During more prolonged palliative
treatment regimens, such as for Kaposi's sarcoma, aggressive antiretroviral therapy is almost always indicated. In this setting, the control of HIV infection can
be crucial to the overall prognosis, and one may do well to focus on monitoring
toxicity from both the antiviral drugs and chemotherapy while ensuring that the
tumor remains under control and antiretroviral drug levels remain therapeutic.
Single-agent cytotoxic chemotherapy regimens are often effective in KS, and as
such, combinations of nucleoside reverse transcriptase inhibitors and inclusion
of protease inhibitors may be considered. On the other hand, in lymphoma regimens that involve multiple drugs over a relatively short period (6 months or less)
and in which cure of the lymphoma may be possible, consideration might be
given to not using anti-HIV therapy in certain instances, especially in patients
with low viral loads. Indeed there are only limited data on the feasibility of combining highly active three-drug antiretroviral regimens with cytotoxic lymphoma

therapy: Nadler et al. are now conducting a trial testing the feasibility of combining such therapy with CHOP for AIDS-related lymphoma. Further clinical trials will surely be needed to clarify these issues.

It is important to stress that dose-reduction of antiretroviral drugs should be avoided if possible because resistance can be hastened with subtherapeutic levels of antiviral drugs. This is especially important with protease inhibitors (217). Consequently, it may be better to withhold antiretroviral therapy during periods of actual or anticipated chemotherapy-induced toxicity, and restart the agents when deemed safe to do so (e.g., during the second half of chemotherapy cycles), rather than to attempt dose attenuation.

It is not possible to make specific recommendations to guide the use of antiretroviral therapy simultaneously with antineoplastic chemotherapy because adequate data to formulate such recommendations are not available. There are many considerations to be made, and a variety of options to take. One can consider four basic approaches: (1) continuing aggressive three-drug anti-HIV treatment during chemotherapy; (2) using "attenuated" anti-HIV treatment with combination NRTIs and omitting protease inhibitors; (3) withholding the antiretroviral drugs during chemotherapy infusions; and (4) temporarily suspending antiretroviral therapy during the full course of chemotherapy. Each scenario has advantages and disadvantages. Continued aggressive antiretroviral therapy may offer the best control of HIV and would, under usual circumstances, be the optimal therapy. However, pharmacokinetic interactions may result in suboptimal drug levels, leading to poor control of HIV and emergence of resistant HIV, thereby limiting future therapeutic options for control of HIV. Also, such interactions may similarly affect the antineoplastic drugs, resulting in poor tumor control. Pharmacokinetic interactions may lead to toxic levels of various agents, or overlapping toxicities may require dose reductions of both classes of drugs, or delays in administration of antineoplastic drugs. These factors may be associated with reduced ability to eradicate potentially curable malignancy, such as lymphoma. Opting for fewer drugs in the anti-HIV combination may decrease the likelihood of adverse pharmacokinetic interactions, but as reviewed in the foregoing, does not eliminate it. Furthermore, poorer suppression of HIV replication may lead to resistant HIV quasispecies. Holding the antiretroviral drugs during the chemotherapy infusions may eliminate problems with pharmacokinetic interactions, but does not address the problems with overlapping toxicities of the various agents. Furthermore, with repeated cessation and reinstitution of antiretroviral drugs, there is greater exposure to suboptimal drug levels, which could promote development of resistant HIV quasispecies and greater HIV-induced immunological deterioration may occur. It is clear that the simplest approach is to suspend the antiretroviral temporarily during finite-course chemotherapy, but the relative safety of this approach is unknown and is likely to be limited to a distinct minority of patients with low-baseline HIV replication and no antecedent history of AIDS or low CD4 cell counts. Clearly, we need to learn more about the feasibility and the potential problems associated with administering aggressive multidrug anti-HIV therapy during complex lymphoma therapy and the optimal strategy for addressing these problems.

VI. CONCLUSIONS

The results of recent studies on combination nucleoside analogues and protease inhibitors for HIV infection have created an environment of optimism for the long-term control and prevention of HIV disease and even consideration of the eradication of the virus from certain infected persons (55,218–220). Combinations of reverse transcriptase inhibitors with protease inhibitors can, in some patients, result in decreases in circulating virus below the levels of our ability to detect virus in plasma using the most sensitive PCR techniques available. And yet, many challenges remain, particularly for the patient with both HIV infection and tumors.

There has been relatively little research to address the best ways to manage HIV therapy during chemotherapy. Combinations of antineoplastic and antiretroviral drugs have potentially deleterious interactions of which physicians should be aware. The effect of chemotherapy on HIV dynamics is still unknown, and well-planned clinical trials are needed to evaluate the optimal role of antiretroviral drugs in patients receiving chemotherapy. Such trials should ideally include a period of follow-up after the chemotherapy is concluded to assess the long-term effects of such regimens. At the same time, we must begin to use the present knowledge base to develop the best treatment strategies. For patients with low-baseline viral load and no history of advanced immunosuppression, who are receiving short-term, potentially curative chemotherapy regimens, as for lymphomas, it may be reasonable to consider an emphasis toward optimizing the treatment of the tumor. This may include avoiding unwanted toxic effects from multiple drug interactions and eliminating antiretroviral drugs that complicate the cancer therapy while, at the same time, preserving future options for HIV control. For patients, receiving longer-term palliative cancer therapy, as in Kaposi's sarcoma, or patients with advanced immunosuppression and high-baseline viral load, one should consider an emphasis on maintaining effective antiretroviral therapy and striking a balance to best achieve control of the malignancy, minimize toxicity, and ensure effective dosing of the antiretroviral agents to minimize the development of resistant HIV.

Future directions in HIV therapy with aggressive attempts to control the virus could conceivably involve the oncologist in curative intent. Interestingly, the field of medical oncology has already pioneered efforts toward HIV eradica-

tion, and bone marrow transplantation has been entertained as a means to recon-
stitute the immune system, especially if there were an approach to prevent the
infused donor marrow from being infected by HIV. In one patient who received
an allogeneic bone marrow transplant following high-dose cyclophosphamide
and total-body irradiation with concurrent zidovudine for HIV-related non–Hodgkin's lymphoma, HIV was not found at necroscopy by culture or by PCR (221).
However, this result has not been confirmed. The use of animal marrow not susceptible to infection by HIV has been attempted (222). The first patient was given
a low inoculum of a baboon zenograft following preparative radiation. Although
long-term engraftment was not achieved, this patient had improved health and a
reduced viral load, suggesting that this therapy (including the preparative regimen
and xenostimulation) may have somehow reduced the burden of HIV-infected
cells (223–225). A modified version of this approach may be contemplated based
on the recent finding that CKR5 is a second receptor for monocytotropic stains
of HIV, and that persons homozygous for a human structural gene mutation giving rise to a defective receptor are naturally resistant to infection by HIV (226).
It may be possible to replace the damaged immune system in an HIV-infected
patient with a marrow from a donor homozygous for the altered CKR5 receptor,
thus rendering the patient relatively resistant to HIV infection. The recent discoveries concerning the accessory receptors for HIV highlight the possibility that
advances in our basic understanding may lead to new therapeutic advances in
the treatment of AIDS. At the same time, substantial advances in the treatment
of HIV-related tumors, particularly involving pathogenesis-based strategies, may
avoid some of the marrow-suppressive and immunosuppressive toxicities associated with most available cytotoxic chemotherapeutic agents. It is also likely that
progress in the treatment of patients with HIV and tumors will require substantial
clinical involvement to optimize the best way of combining complex therapies.
Through advances in both basic and applied research, it is reasonable to contem-
plate making substantial advances in the treatment of such patients.

REFERENCES

1. AM Levine. Acquired immunodeficiency syndrome-related lymphoma. Blood 80:
   8–20, 1992.
2. BG Brenner, C Vo, MA Wainberg. Different effects of breast cancer, HIV-1 infection and chemotherapy on inducible natural immunity. Leukemia 8(suppl 1):S183–
   185, 1994.
3. DD Von Hoff. MGBG: teaching an old drug new tricks. Ann Oncol 5:487–493,
   1994.
4. MA Conant. Management of human immunodeficiency virus-associated malignancies. Recent Results Cancer Res 139:423–432, 1995.

5. M Wainberg, B Brenner, G Margolese. Immune responsiveness and the effects of adjuvant chemotherapy. In: G. Margolese, ed. Breast Cancer. New York, Churchill Livingstone 1983:223–248.
6. D Errante, U Tirelli, R Gastaldi, D Milo, AM Nosari, G Rossi, G Fiorentini, A Carbone, E Vaccher, S Monfardini. Combined antineoplastic and antiretroviral therapy for patients with Hodgkin's disease and human immunodeficiency virus infection. A prospective study of 17 patients. The Italian Cooperative Group on AIDS and Tumors (GICAT). Cancer 73:437–444, 1994.
7. CF von Gunten, JH Von Roenn. Clinical aspects of human immunodeficiency virus-related lymphoma. Curr Opin Oncol 4:894–899, 1992.
8. PS Gill, AM Levine, M Krailo, MU Rarick, C Loureiro, L Deyton, P Meyer, S Rasheed. AIDS-related malignant lymphoma: results of prospective treatment trials. J Clin Oncol 5:1322–1328, 1987.
9. J Sparano, P Wiernik, X Hu, C Sarta, E Schwartz. Pilot trial of infusional cyclophosphamide, doxorubicin, and etoposide plus didanosine and filgrastim in patients with human immunodeficiency virus-associated non–Hodgkin's lymphoma. J Clin Oncol 14:3026–3035, 1996.
10. AM Levine, A Tulpule, B Espina, W Boswell, J Buckley, S Rasheed, S Stain, J Parker, B Nathwani, PS Gill. Low dose methotrexate, bleomycin, doxorubicin, cyclophosphamide, vincristine, and dexamethasone with zalcitabine in patients with acquired immunodeficiency syndrome-related lymphoma. Effect on human immunodeficiency virus and serum interleukin-6 levels over time. Cancer 78:517–526, 1996.
11. MD Hughes, VA Johnson, MS Hirsch, JW Bremer, T Elbeik, A Erice, DR Kuritzkes, WA Scott, SA Spector, N Basgoz, MA Fischl, RT D'Aquilla. Monitoring plasma HIV-1 RNA levels in addition to CD4+ lymphocyte count improves assessment of antiretroviral therapeutic response. ACTG 241 Protocol Virology Substudy Team. Ann Intern Med 126:929–938, 1997.
12. R Yarchoan, DJ Venzon, JM Pluda, J Lietzau, KM Wyvill, AA Tsiatis, SM Steinberg, S Broder. CD4 count and the risk for death in patients infected with HIV receiving antiretroviral therapy. Ann Intern Med 115:184–189, 1991.
13. AN Phillips, CA Lee, J Elford, A Webster, G Janossy, PD Griffiths, PBA Kernoff p24 Antigenaemia, CD4 lymphocyte counts and the development of AIDS. AIDS 5:1217–1222, 1991.
14. AN Phillips, CA Lee, J Elford, G Janossy, A Timms, M Bofill, PBA Kernoff. Serial CD4 lymphocyte counts and the development of AIDS. Lancet 337:389–392, 1991.
15. AN Phillips, J Elford, C Sabin, M Bofill, G Janossy, CA Lee. Immunodeficiency and risk of death in HIV infection. JAMA 268:2662–2666, 1992.
16. V De Gruttola, M Wulfsohn, MA Fischl, A Tsiatis. Modeling the relationship between survival and CD4 lymphocytes in patients with AIDS and AIDS-related complex. J Acquir Immune Defic Syndr 6:359–365, 1993.
17. M Piatak Jr, MS Saag, LC Yang, SJ Clark, JC Kappes, KC Luk, BH Hahn, GM Shaw, JD Lifson. Determination of plasma viral load in HIV-1 infection by quantitative competitive polymerase chain reaction. AIDS 7(suppl 2):S65–71, 1993.
18. M Piatak Jr, MS Saag, LC Yang, SJ Clark, JC Kappes, KC Luk, BH Hahn, GM

Shaw, JD Lifson. High levels of HIV-1 in plasma during all stages of infection determined by competitive PCR. Science 259:1749–1754, 1993.

19. DD Ho, AU Neumann, AS Perelson, W Chen, JM Leonard, M Markowitz. Rapid turnover of plasma virions and CD4 lymphocytes in HIV-1 infection. Nature 373: 123–126, 1995.

20. X Wei, SK Ghosh, ME Taylor, VA Johnson, EA Emini, P Deutsch, JD Lifson, S Bonhoeffer, MA Nowak, BH Hahn, MS Saag, GM Shaw. Viral dynamics in human immunodeficiency virus type 1 infection. Nature 373:117–122, 1995.

21. MS Urdea, JC Wilber, T Yeghiazarian, JA Todd, DG Kern, SJ Fong, D Besemer, B Hoo, PJ Sheridan, R Kokka, P Neuwald, CA Pachl. Direct and quantitative detection of HIV-1 RNA in human plasma with a branched DNA signal amplification assay. AIDS 7(suppl 2):S11–14, 1993.

22. S Bruisten, B van Gemen, M Koppelman, M Rasch, D van Strijp, R Schukkink, R Beyer, H Weigel, P Lens, H Huisman. Detection of HIV-1 distribution in different blood fractions by two nucleic acid amplification assays. AIDS Res Hum Retroviruses 9:259–265, 1993.

23. H Revets, D Marissens, S de Wit, P Lacor, N Clumeck, S Lauwers, G Zissis. Comparative evaluation of NASBA HIV-1 RNA QT, AMPLICOR-HIV monitor, and QUANTIPLEX HIV RNA assay, three methods for quantification of human immunodeficiency virus type 1 RNA in plasma. J Clin Microbiol 34:1058–1064, 1996.

24. AM Vandamme, JC Schmit, S Van Dooren, K Van Laethem, E Gobbers, W Kok, P Goubau, M Witvrouw, W Peetermans, E De Clercq, J Desmyter. Quantification of HIV-1 RNA in plasma: comparable results with the NASBA HIV-1 RNA QT and the AMPLICOR HIV monitor test. J Acquir Immune Defic Syndr Hum Retrovirol 13:127–139, 1996.

25. W O'Brien, PM Hartigan, D Martin, J Esinhart, A Hill, S Benoit, M Rubin, MS Simberkoff, JD Hamilton. Changes in plasma HIV-1 RNA and CD4+ lymphocyte counts and the risk of progression to AIDS. Veterans Affairs Cooperative Study Group on AIDS. N Engl J Med 334:426–431, 1996.

26. JW Mellors, CR Rinaldo Jr, P Gupta, RM White, JA Todd, LA Kingsley. Prognosis in HIV-1 infection predicted by the quantity of virus in plasma. Science 272:1167–1170, 1996.

27. JW Mellors, A Munoz, JV Giorgi, JB Margolick, CJ Tassoni, P Gupta, LA Kingsley, JA Todd, AJ Saah, R Detels, JP Phair, CR Rinaldo Jr. Plasma viral load and CD4+ lymphocytes as prognostic markers of HIV-1 infection. Ann Intern Med 126:946–954, 1997.

28. JW Mellors, LA Kingsley, CR Rinaldo Jr, JA Todd, BS Hoo, RP Kokka, P Gupta. Quantitation of HIV-1 RNA in plasma predicts outcome after seroconversion. Ann Intern Med 122:573–579, 1995.

29. A Galetto-Lacour, S Yerly, TV Perneger, C Baumberger, B Hirschel, L Perrin. Prognostic value of viremia in patients with long-standing human immunodeficiency virus infection. Swiss HIV Cohort Study Group. J Infect Dis 173:1388–1393, 1996.

30. DA Katzenstein, SM Hammer, MD Hughes, H Gundacker, JB Jackson, S Fiscus, S Rasheed, T Elbeik, R Reichman, A Japour, TC Merigan, MS Hirsch. The relation of virologic and immunologic markers to clinical outcomes after nucleoside therapy

in HIV-infected adults with 200 to 500 CD4 cells per cubic millimeter. AIDS Clinical Trials Group Study 175 Virology Study Team. N Engl J Med 335:1091–1098, 1996.

31. RI Connor, KE Sheridan, D Ceradini, S Choe, NR Landau. Change in coreceptor use correlates with disease progression in HIV-1–infected individuals. J Exp Med 185:621–628, 1997.

32. R D'Aquila, VA Johnson, SL Welles, AJ Japour, DR Kuritzkes, V DeGruttola, PS Reichelderfer, RW Coombs, CS Crumpacker, JO Kahn, DD Richman. Zidovudine resistance and HIV-1 disease progression during antiretroviral therapy. AIDS Clinical Trials Group Protocol 116B/117 Team and the Virology Committee Resistance Working Group. Ann Intern Med 122:401–408, 1995.

33. J Ferbas, AH Kaplan, MA Hausner, LE Hultin, JL Matud, Z Liu, DL Panicali, H Nerng-Ho, R Detels, JV Giorgi. Virus burden in long-term survivors of human immunodeficiency virus (HIV) infection is a determinant of anti-HIV CD8+ lymphocyte activity. J Infect Dis 172:329–339, 1995.

34. A Ruffault, C Michelet, C Jacquelinet, O Guist'hau, N Genetet, C Bariou, R Colimon, F Cartier. The prognostic value of plasma viremia in HIV-infected patients under AZT treatment: a two-year follow-up study. J Acquir Immune Defic Syndr Hum Retrovirol 9:243–248, 1995.

35. AS Fauci, G Pantaleo, S Stanley, D Weissman. Immunopathogenic mechanisms of HIV infection. Ann Intern Med 124:654–663, 1996.

36. G Pantaleo, S Menzo, M Vaccarezza, C Graziosi, OJ Cohen, JF Demarest, D Montefiori, JM Orenstein, C Fox, LK Schrager, JB Margolick, S Buchbinder, JV Giorgi, AS Fauci. Studies in subjects with long-term nonprogressive human immunodeficiency virus infection. N Engl J Med 332:209–216, 1995.

37. NL Michael, M Vahey, DS Burke, RR Redfield. Viral DNA and mRNA expression correlate with the stage of human immunodeficiency virus (HIV) type 1 infection in humans: evidence for viral replication in all stages of HIV disease. J Virol 66:310–316, 1992.

38. MD Hughes, DS Stein, HM Gundacker, FT Valentine, JP Phair, PA Volberding. Within-subject variation in CD4 lymphocyte count in asymptomatic human immunodeficiency virus infection: implications for patient monitoring. J Infect Dis 169:28–36, 1994.

39. JL Fahey, JM Taylor, R Detels, B Hofmann, R Melmed, P Nishanian, JV Giorgi. The prognostic value of cellular and serologic markers in infection with human immunodeficiency virus type 1. N Engl J Med 322:166–172, 1990.

40. AS Perelson, AU Neumann, M Markowitz, JM Leonard, DD Ho. HIV-1 dynamics in vivo: virion clearance rate, infected cell life-span, and viral generation time. Science 271:1582–1586, 1996.

41. G Pantaleo, AS Fauci. New concepts in the immunopathogenesis of HIV infection. Annu Rev Immunol 13:487–512, 1995.

42. S Sei, H Akiyoshi, J Bernard, DJ Venzon, CH Fox, DJ Schwartzentruber, BD Anderson, JB Kopp, BU Mueller, PA Pizzo. Dynamics of virus versus host interaction in children with human immunodeficiency virus type 1 infection. J Infect Dis 173:1485–1490, 1996.

43. BU Mueller, S Sei, B Anderson, K Luzuriaga, M Farley, DJ Venzon, G Tudor-

Williams, DJ Schwartzentruber, C Fox, JL Sullivan, PA Pizzo. Comparison of virus burden in blood and sequential lymph node biopsy specimens from children infected with human immunodeficiency virus. J Pediatr 129:410–418, 1996.

44. JM Schapiro, OW Kamel, MA Winters, M Vierra, B Efron, TC Merigan. Lymph Node histopathology in HIV-infected patients correlates with duration of response to antiretroviral therapy. 4th Conference on Retroviruses and Opportunistic Infections. Washington, DC, 1997.

45. OJ Cohen, G Pantaleo, M Holodniy, S Schnittman, M Niu, C Graziosi, GN Pavlakis, J Lalezari, JA Bartlett, RT Steigbigel, J Cohn, R Novak, M Deborah, AS Fauci. Decreased human immunodeficiency virus type 1 plasma viremia during antiretroviral therapy reflects downregulation of viral replication in lymphoid tissue. Proc Natl Acad Sci USA 92:6017–6021, 1995.

46. J Wong, H Gunthard, D Havlir, A Haase, Z Zhang, S Kwok, C Ignacio, N Keating, J Chodakewitz, E Emini, A Meibohm, L Jonas, D Richman. Reduction of HIV in blood and lymph nodes after potent antiretroviral therapy. 4th Conference on Retroviruses and Opportunistic Infections. Washington, DC, 1997.

47. D Kotler, T Shimada, F Clayton. Effect of Combination antiretroviral therapy upon mucosal viral RNA burden and apoptosis. 4th Conference on Retroviruses and Opportunistic Infections. Washington, DC, 1997.

48. AT Haase, K Henry, M Zupancic, G Sedgewick, RA Faust, H Melroe, W Cavert, K Gebhard, K Staskus, Z-Q Zhang, PJ Dailey HH Balfour Jr, A Erice, AS Perelson. Quantitative image analysis of HIV-1 infection in lymphoid tissue. Science 274: 985–989, 1996.

49. W Cavert, DW Notermans, K Staskus, SW Wietgrefe, M Zupancic, K Gebhard, K Henry, ZQ Zhang, R Mills, H McDade, J Goudsmit, SA Danner, AT Haase. Kinetics of response in lymphoid tissues to antiretroviral therapy of HIV-1 infection. Science 276:960–964, 1997.

50. SM Hammer, DA Katzenstein, MD Hughes, H Gundacker, RT Schooley, RH Haubrich, WK Henry, MM Lederman, JP Phair, M Niu, MS Hirsch, TC Merigan. A trial comparing nucleoside monotherapy with combination therapy in HIV-infected adults with CD4 cell counts from 200 to 500 per cubic millimeter. AIDS Clinical Trials Group Study 175 Study Team. N Engl J Med 335:1081–1090, 1996.

51. Delta: a randomised double-blind controlled trial comparing combinations of zidovudine plus didanosine or zalcitabine with zidovudine alone in HIV-infected individuals. Delta Coordinating Committee. Lancet 348:283–291, 1996.

52. CC Carpenter, MA Fischl, SM Hammer, MS Hirsch, DM Jacobsen, DA Katzenstein, JS Montaner, DD Richman, MS Saag, RT Schooley, MA Thompson, S Vella, PG Yeni, PA Volberding. Antiretroviral therapy for HIV infection in 1997. Updated recommendations of the International AIDS Society–USA panel. JAMA 277:1962–1969, 1997.

53. Report of the NIH panel to define principles of therapy of HIV infection. National Institutes of Health: Bethesda, MD, 1997.

54. Guidelines for the Use of Antiretroviral Agents in HIV-Infected Adults and Adolescents. Department of Health and Human Services: Washington, DC, 1997.

55. DD Ho. Viral counts count in HIV infection. Science 272:1124–1125, 1996.

56. MA Nowak. AIDS pathogenesis: from models to viral dynamics in patients. J Acquir Immune Defic Syndr Hum Retrovirol 10(suppl 1):S1–S5, 1995.

57. CC Carpenter, MA Fischl, SM Hammer, MS Hirsch, DM Jacobsen, DA Katzenstein, JS Montaner, DD Richman, MS Saag, RT Schooley, MA Thompson, S Vella, PG Yeni, PA Volberding. Antiretroviral therapy for HIV infection in 1996. Recommendations of an international panel. International AIDS Society–USA. JAMA 276:146–154, 1996.

58. TW Chun, L Carruth, D Finzi, X Shen, JA DiGiuseppe, H Taylor, M Hermankova, K Chadwick, J Margolick, TC Quinn, YH Kuo, R Brookmeyer, MA Zeiger, P Barditch-Crovo, RF Siliciano. Quantification of latent tissue reservoirs and total body viral load in HIV-1 infection. Nature 387:183–188, 1997.

59. SE Krown, D Niedzwiecki, RB Bhalla, N Flomenberg, D Bundow, D Chapman. Relationship and prognostic value of endogenous interferon-alpha, beta$_2$-microglobulin, and neopterin serum levels in patients with Kaposi sarcoma and AIDS. J Acquir Immune Defic Syndr 4:871–880, 1991.

60. MJ Morfeldt, I Julander, LV von Stedingk, J Wasserman, B Nilsson. Elevated serum beta-2-microglobulin—a prognostic marker for development of AIDS among patients with persistent generalized lymphadenopathy. Infection 16:109–110, 1988.

61. B Schwartlander, B Bek, H Skarabis, J Koch, J Burkowitz, MA Koch. Improvement of the predictive value of CD4+ lymphocyte count by beta$_2$-microglobulin, immunoglobulin A and erythrocyte sedimentation rate. The Multicentre Cohort Study Group. AIDS 7:813–821, 1993.

62. H Mitsuya, KJ Weinhold, PA Furman, MH St Clair, S Nusinoff Lehrman, RC Gallo, D Bolognesi, DW Barry, S Broder. 3′-Azido-3′-deoxythymidine (BW A509U): an antiviral agent that inhibits the infectivity and cytopathic effect of human T-lymphotropic virus type III/lymphadenopathy-associated virus in vitro. Proc Natl Acad Sci USA 82:7096–7100, 1985.

63. R Yarchoan, RW Klecker, KJ Weinhold, PD Markham, HK Lyerly, DT Durack, E Gelmann, SN Lehrman, RM Blum, DW Barry, GM Shearer, MA Fischl, H Mitsuya, RC Gallo, JM Collins, DP Bolognesi, CE Myers, S Broder. Administration of 3′-azido-3′-deoxythymidine, an inhibitor of HTLV-III/LAV replication, to patients with AIDS or AIDS-related complex. Lancet 1:575–580, 1986.

64. H Mitsuya, R Yarchoan, S Broder. Molecular targets for AIDS therapy. Science 249:1533–1544, 1990.

65. R Yarchoan, H Mitsuya, CE Myers, S Broder. Clinical pharmacology of 3′-azido-2′,3′-dideoxythymidine (zidovudine) and related dideoxynucleosides. N Engl J Med 321:726–738, 1989.

66. MA Fischl, DD Richman, MH Grieco, MS Gottlieb, PA Volberding, OL Laskin, JM Leedom, JE Groopman, D Mildvan, RT Schooley, GG Jackson, DT Durack, D King, TACW Group. The efficacy of azidothymidine (AZT) in the treatment of patients with AIDS and AIDS-related complex. A double-blind, placebo-controlled trial. N Engl J Med 317:185–191, 1987.

67. DD Richman, MA Fischl, MH Grieco, MS Gottlieb, PA Volberding, OL Laskin, JM Leedom, JE Groopman, D Mildvan, MS Hirsch, GG Jackson, DT Durack, S Nusinoff-Lehrman, the AZT Collaborative Working Group. The toxicity of azido-

thymidine (AZT) in the treatment of patients with AIDS and AIDS-related complex. A double-blind, placebo-controlled trial. N Engl J Med 317:192–197, 1987.

68. H Mitsuya, S Broder. Inhibition of the in vitro infectivity and cytopathic effect of human T-lymphotropic virus type III/lymphadenopathy virus-associated virus (HTLV-III/LAV) by 2′,3′-dideoxynucleosides. Proc Natl Acad Sci USA 83:1911–1915, 1986.

69. R Rooke, M Tremblay, H Soundeyns, L DeStephano, X-J Yao, M Fanning, JSG Montaner, M O'Shaughnessy, K Gelmon, C Tsoukas, J Gill, J Ruedy, MA Wainberg, the Canadian Zidovudine Multi-Center Study Group. Isolation of drug-resistant variants of HIV-1 from patients on long-term zidovudine therapy. AIDS 3: 411–415, 1989.

70. BA Larder, SD Kemp. Multiple mutations in HIV-1 reverse transcriptase confer high-level resistance to zidovudine (AZT). Science 246:1155–1158, 1989.

71. BA Larder, SD Kemp, PR Harrigan. Potential mechanism for sustained antiretroviral efficacy of AZT–3TC combination therapy. Science 269:696–699, 1995.

72. YK Chow, MS Hirsch, DP Merrill, LJ Bechtel, JJ Eron, JC Kaplan, RT D'Aquilla. Use of evolutionary limitations of HIV-1 multidrug resistance to optimize therapy [published erratum appears in Nature 1993 Aug 19;364:679, 737]. Nature 361:650–654, 1993.

73. MH St Clair, JL Martin, G Tudor-Williams, MC Bach, CL Vavro, DM King, P Kellam, SD Kemp, BA Larder. Resistance to ddI and sensitivity to AZT induced by a mutation in HIV-1 reverse transcriptase. Science 253:1557–1559, 1991.

74. R Yarchoan, CF Perno, RV Thomas, RW Klecker, J-P Allain, RJ Wills, N McAtee, MA Fischl, R Dubinsky, MC McNeely, H Mitsuya, JM Pluda, TJ Lawley, M Leuther, B Safai, JM Collins, CE Myers, S Broder. Phase I studies of 2′,3′-dideoxycytidine in severe human immunodeficiency virus infection as a single agent and alternating with zidovudine (AZT). Lancet 1:76–81, 1988.

75. TC Merigan, G Skowron, SA Bozzette, D Richman, R Uttamchandani, M Fischl, R Schooley, M Hirsch, W Soo, C Pettinelli, H Schaumburg, the ddC Study Group of the AIDS Clinical Trials Group. Circulating p24 antigen levels and responses to dideoxycytidine in human immunodeficiency virus (HIV) infections. Ann Intern Med 110:189–194, 1989.

76. R Yarchoan, H Mitsuya, RV Thomas, JM Pluda, NR Hartman, C-F Perno, KS Marczyk, J-P Allain, DG Johns, S Broder. In vivo activity against HIV and favorable toxicity profile of 2′,3′-dideoxyinosine. Science 245:412–415, 1989.

77. TP Cooley, LM Kunches, CA Saunders, JK Ritter, CJ Perkins, M Colin, RP McCaffrey, HA Liebman. Once-daily administration of 2′,3′-dideoxyinosine (ddI) in patients with the acquired immunodeficiency syndrome or AIDS-related complex. N Engl J Med 322:1340–1345, 1990.

78. JS Lambert, M Seidlin, RC Reichman, CS Plank, M Laverty, GD Morse, C Knupp, C McLaren, C Pettinelli, FT Valentine, R Dolin. 2′,3′-Dideoxyinosine (ddI) in patients with the acquired immunodeficiency syndrome or the AIDS-related complex. A phase I trial. N Engl J Med 322:1333–1340, 1990.

79. JO Kahn, SW Lagakos, DD Richman, A Cross, C Pettinetti, S-H Liou, M Brown, PA Volberding, CS Crumpacker, G Beall, HS Sacks, TC Merigan, M Beltangady, L Smaldone, R Dolin, the NIAID AIDS Clinical Trials Group. A controlled trial

comparing continued zidovudine with didanosine in human immunodeficiency virus infection. N Engl J Med 327:581–587, 1992.

80. SL Spruance, AT Pavia, D Peterson, A Berry, R Pollard, TF Patterson, I Frank, SC Remick, M Thompson, RD MacArthur, GE Morey Jr, CH Ramirez-Ronda, BM Bernstein, DE Sweet, L Crane, EA Peterson, CT Pachucki, SL Green, J Brand, A Rios, LM Dunkle, A Cross, MJ Brown, P Ingraham, R Gugliotti, AH Schindzielorz, L Smaldone, and tB-MSA-S Group. Didanosine compared with continuation of zidovudine in HIV-infected patients with signs of clinical deterioration while receiving zidovudine. A randomized, double-blind clinical trial. Ann Intern Med 120: 360–368, 1994.

81. JS Montagner, A Rachlis, J Gill, R Beaulieu, C Tsoukas, M Fanning, W Cameron, R Lalonde, M Bergeron, W Schlech, L Dunkle, A Schindzielorz, L Smaldone, M Wainberg, M O'Schaughnessy, J Singer, P Phillips, J Ruedy, MT Schecter. A double blind study of ddI vs. continued AZT among HIV+ individuals with CD4 counts 200 to 500/mm^3 treated with AZT for at least six months. VIII International Conference on AIDS/III STD World Congress. Amsterdam, 1992.

82. LP Schacter, M Rozencweig, M Beltangady, JD Allan, R Canetta, TP Cooley, R Dolin, S Kelley, J Lambert, HA Liebman, M Messina, C Nicaise, M Seidlin, FT Valentine, R Yarchoan, LF Smaldone. Effects of therapy with didanosine on hematologic parameters in patients with advanced human immunodeficiency virus disease. Blood 80:2969–2976, 1992.

83. SA Bozzette, DE Kanouse, S Berry, N Duan. Health status and function with zidovudine or zalcitabine as initial therapy for AIDS. A randomized controlled trial. Roche 3300/ACTG 114 Study Group. JAMA 273:295–301, 1995.

84. DI Abrams, AI Goldman, C Launer, JA Korvick, JD Neaton, LR Crane, M Grodesky, S Wakefield, K Muth, S Kornegay, DL Cohn, A Hallen, R Luskin-Hawk, N Markowitz, JH Sampton, M Thompson, L Deyton, tTBCPfCRo AIDS. A comparative trial of didanosine or zalcitabine after treatment with zidovudine in patients with human immunodeficiency virus infection. N Engl J Med 330:657–662, 1994.

85. RM Dubinsky, R Yarchoan, M Dalakas, S Broder. Reversible axonal neuropathy from the treatment of AIDS and related disorders with 2',3'-dideoxycytidine (ddC). Muscle Nerve 12:856–860, 1989.

86. MC McNeely, R Yarchoan, S Broder, TJ Lawley. Dermatologic complications associated with administration of 2',3'-dideoxycytidine in patients with human immunodeficiency virus infection. J Am Acad Dermatol 21:1213–1217, 1989.

87. AS Indorf, PS Pegram. Esophageal ulceration related to zalcitabine (ddC). Ann Intern Med 117:133–134, 1992.

88. MF Kavlick, T Shirasaka, E Kojima, JM Pluda, F Hui Jr, R Yarchoan, H Mitsuya. Genotypic and phenotypic characterization of HIV-1 isolated from patients receiving (−)-2',3'-dideoxy-3'-thiacytidine. Antiviral Res 28:133–146, 1995.

89. R Schuurman, M Nijhuis, R van Leeuwen, P Schipper, D de Jong, P Collis, SA Danner, J Mulder, C Loveday, C Christopherson, S Kwok, J Sninsky, CAB Boucher. Rapid changes in human immunodeficiency virus type 1 RNA load and appearance of drug-resistant virus populations in persons treated with lamivudine (3TC). J Infect Dis 171:1441–1449, 1995.

90. BA Larder. Viral resistance and the selection of antiretroviral combinations. J Acquir Immune Defic Syndr Hum Retrovirol 10(suppl):S28–S33, 1995.

91. JM Pluda, TP Cooley, JS Montaner, LE Shay, NE Reinhalter, SN Warthan, J Ruedy, HM Hirst, CA Vicary, JB Quinn, GJ Yuen, MR Wainberg, M Rubin, R Yarchoan. A phase I/II study of 2′-deoxy-3′-thiacytidine (lamivudine) in patients with advanced human immunodificiency virus infection. J Infect Dis 171:1438–1447, 1995.

92. C Cohen, P Shalit, M Conant, R Scott, T Wong, K Campbell, J Smith, K Frost, NY The AmFAR Community-Based Clinical Trials Network. American Foundation for AIDS Research, NY. Lamivudine (3TC) and stavudine (d4T) combination therapy: HIV viral load and CD4 changes in a retrospective study of 330 patients. 4th Conference on Retroviruses and Opportunistic Infections. Washington, DC, 1997.

93. HW Murray, KE Squires, W Weiss, S Sledz, HS Sacks, J Hassett, A Cross, RE Anderson, LM Dunkle. Stavudine in patients with AIDS and AIDS-related complex: AIDS clinical trials group 089. J Infect Dis 171(suppl 2):S123–130, 1995.

94. MJ Browne, KH Mayer, SBD Chafee, MN Dudley, MR Posner, SM Steinberg, KK Graham, SM Geletko, SH Zinner, SL Denman, LM Dunkle, S Kaul, C McLaren, G Skowron, NM Kouttab, TA Kennedy, AB Weitberg, G Curt. 2′,3′-Didehydro-3′-deoxythymidine (d4T) in patients with AIDS or AIDS-related complex: a phase I trial. J Infect Dis 167:21–29, 1993.

95. BP Griffith, H Brett-Smith, G Kim, JW Mellors, TM Chacko, RB Garner, YC Cheng, P Alcabes, G Friedland. Effect of stavudine on human immunodeficiency virus type 1 virus load as measured by quantitative mononuclear cell culture, plasma RNA, and immune complex-dissociated antigenemia. J Infect Dis 173: 1252–1255, 1996.

96. R Pollard, D Peterson, D Hardy, L Pedneault, V Rutkiewicz, J Pottage, R Murphy, J Gathe, G Beall, J Skovronski, A Cross, L Dunkle. Antiviral effect and safety of stavudine (d4T) and didanosine (ddI) combination therapy in HIV-infected subjects in an ongoing pilot randomized double-blind trial. 2nd National Conference on Human Retroviruses and Related Infections. Washington, DC, 1996.

97. C Deminie, C Bechtold, K Riccardi, P-F Lin, R Colonno. HIV-1 isolates from subjects on prolonged stavudine therapy remain sensitive to stavudine. XI International Conference on AIDS. Vancouver, BC, 1996.

98. S Mauss, O Adams, R Willers, D Haussinger, H Jablonowski. Stavudine (d4T)—HIV 1 viral load and CD4 positive cell count in HIV+ individuals pretreated with zidovudine. XI International Conference on AIDS. Vancouver, BC, 1996.

99. EA Petersen, CH Ramirez-Ronda, WD Hardy, R Schwartz, HS Sacks, S Follansbee, DM Peterson, A Cross, RE Anderson, LM Dunkle. Dose-related activity of stavudine in patients infected with human immunodeficiency virus. J Infect Dis 171(suppl 2):S131–139, 1995.

100. G Skowron. Biologic effects and safety of stavudine: overview of phase I and II clinical trials. J Infect Dis 171(suppl 2):S113–117, 1995.

101. D Havlir, SH Cheeseman, M McLaughlin, R Murphy, A Erice, SA Spector, TC Greenough, JL Sullivan, D Hall, M Myers, M Lamson, DD Richman. High-dose nevirapine: safety, pharmacokinetics, and antiviral effect in patients with human immunodeficiency virus infection. J Infect Dis 171:537–545, 1995.

102. SH Cheeseman, D Havlir, MM McLaughlin, TC Greenough, JL Sullivan, D Hall, SE Hattox, SA Spector, DS Stein, M Myers, DD Richman. Phase I/II evaluation of nevirapine alone and in combination with zidovudine for infection with human immunodeficiency virus. J Acquir Immune Defic Syndr Hum Retrovirol 8:141–151, 1995.

103. WW Freimuth. Delavirdine mesylate, a potent non-nucleoside HIV-1 reverse transcriptase inhibitor. Adv Exp Med Biol 394:279–289, 1996.

104. DD Richman, D Havlir, J Corbeil, D Looney, C Ignacio, SA Spector, J Sullivan, S Cheeseman, K Barringer, D Pauletti, C-K Shih, M Myers, J Griffin. Nevirapine resistance mutations of human immunodeficiency virus type 1 selected during therapy. J Virol 68:1660–1666, 1994.

105. MD de Jong, S Vella, A Carr, CA Boucher, A Imrie, M French, J Hoy, S Sorice, S Pauluzzi, F Chiodo, GJ Weverling, ME van der Ende, PJ Frissen, HM Weigel, RH Kauffmann, JM Lange, R Yoon, M Moroni, E Hoenderdos, G Leitz, DA Cooper, D Hall, P Reiss. High-dose nevirapine in previously untreated human immunodeficiency virus type 1-infected persons does not result in sustained suppression of viral replication. J Infect Dis 175:966–970, 1997.

106. Viramune (nevirapine) Tablets package insert, Roxane Laboratories, Inc., A Boehringer Ingelheim Company.

107. NE Kohl, EA Emini, WA Schleif, LJ Davis, JC Heimbach, RA Dixon, EM Scolnick, IS Sigal. Active human immunodeficiency virus protease is required for viral infectivity. Proc Natl Acad Sci USA 85:4686–4690, 1988.

108. TJ McQuade, AG Tomasselli, L Liu, V Karacostas, B Moss, TK Sawyer, RL Heinrikson, WG Tarpley. A synthetic HIV-1 protease inhibitor with antiviral activity arrests HIV-like particle maturation. Science 247:454–456, 1990.

109. PY Lam, PK Jadhav, CJ Eyermann, CN Hodge, Y Ru, LT Bacheler, JL Meek, MJ Otto, MM Rayner, YN Wong, C-H Chang, PC Weber, DA Jackson, TR Sharpe, S Erickson-Viitanen. Rational design of potent, bioavailable, nonpeptide cyclic ureas as HIV protease inhibitors. Science 263:380–384, 1994.

110. RW Humphrey, DA Davis, H Mitsuya, R Yarchoan. HIV virions produced by cells treated with the HIV-1 protease inhibitor KNI-272 do not acquire infectivity after viral budding. J Invest Med 44:252A, 1996.

111. VS Kitchen, C Skinner, K Ariyoshi, EA Lane, IB Duncan, J Burckhardt, HU Burger, K Bragman, AJ Pinching, JN Weber. Safety and activity of saquinavir in HIV infection. Lancet 345:952–955, 1995.

112. V Kitchen, F Stewart, K Bragman, J Weber. Emerging proteinase inhibitors. Lancet 345:1512, 1995.

113. JM Schapiro, MA Winters, F Stewart, B Efron, J Norris, MJ Kozal, TC Merigan. The effect of high-dose saquinavir on viral load and CD4+ T-cell counts in HIV-infected patients. Ann Intern Med 124:1039–1050, 1996.

114. M Markowitz, M Saag, WG Powderly, AM Hurley, A Hsu, JM Valdes, D Henry, F Sattler, A La Marca, JM Leonard, DD Ho. A preliminary study of ritonavir, an inhibitor of HIV-1 protease, to treat HIV-1 infection. N Engl J Med 333:1534–1539, 1995.

115. SA Danner, A Carr, JM Leonard, LM Lehman, F Gudiol, J Gonzales, A Raventos, R Rubio, E Bouza, V Pintado, AG Aguado, J Gacia de Lomas, R Delgado, JCC

Borleffs, A Hsu, JM Valdes, CAB Boucher, DA Cooper, tE-ACRS Group. A short-term study of the safety, pharmacokinetics, and efficacy of ritonavir, an inhibitor of HIV-1 protease. European-Australian Collaborative Ritonavir Study Group. N Engl J Med 333:1528–1533, 1995.

116. MP Dube, DL Johnson, JS Currier, JM Leedom. Protease inhibitor-associated hyperglycaemia. Lancet 350:713–714, 1997.

117. A Ault. FDA warns of potential protease-inhibitor link to hyperglycaemia. Lancet 349:1819, 1997.

118. Monitoring but no drug-regimen changes advised for hemophilia patients taking protease inhibitors. Am J Health Syst Pharm 53:1999, 1996.

119. EA Emini, J Condra, W Schleif, F Massari, R Leavitt, P Deutsch, J Chodakewitz. Maintenance of long-term virus suppression in patients treated with the HIV-1 protease inhibitor Crixivan (indinavir). XI International Conference on AIDS. Vancouver, BC, 1996.

120. JA Chodakewitz, R Leavitt, F Massari, C Hildebrand, K Arcuri, L Gilde, M Nessly, A Meibohm, K Ghosh, R Radkowski, A Getson, F Rockhold. Crixivan: summary of 24-week experience with Crixivan at 2.4 g/d in phase II trials. XI International Conference on AIDS. Vancouver, BC, 1996.

121. DS Stein, DG Fish, JA Bilello, SL Preston, GL Martineau, GL Drusano. A 24-week open-label phase I/II evaluation of the HIV protease inhibitor MK-639 (indinavir). AIDS 10:485–492, 1996.

122. D Stein, G Drusano, R Steigbigel, P Berry, J Mellors, D McMahon, H Teppler, C Hildebrand, M Nessly, J Chodakewitz. Two year follow-up of patients treated with indinavir 800 mg q8h. 4th Conference on Retroviruses and Opportunistic Infections. Washington, DC, 1997.

123. Viracept (nelfinavir mesylate) package insert, Agouron Pharmaceuticals, Inc.

124. L Pendeault, R Elion, M Adler, R Anderson, T Kelleher, C Knupp, S Kaul, B Kerr, A Cross, L Dunkle, CCC Bristol-Myers Squibb Pharmaceutical Research Institute, Washington, DC, Agouron Pharmaceuticals. Stavudine (d4T), didanosine (ddI), and nelfinavir combination therapy in HIV-infected subjects: antiviral effect and safety in an ongoing pilot study. 4th Conference on Retroviruses and Opportunistic Infections. Washington, DC, 1997.

125. K Henry, A Lamarca, R Myers, S Chapman, ftVCSGA Pharmaceuticals. The safety of Viracept (nelfinavir mesylate, NFV) in pivotal phase II/III double-blind randomized controlled trials as monotherapy and in combination with either d4T or AZT/3TC. 4th Conference on Retroviruses and Opportunistic Infections. Washington, DC, 1997.

126. W Powderly, M Sension, M Conant, A Stein, N Clendeninn, ftVCSGA Pharmaceuticals. The Efficacy of Viracept (nelfinavir mesylate, NFV) in pivotal Phase II/III double-blind randomized controlled trials as monotherapy and in combination with d4T or AZT/3TC. 4th Conference on Retroviruses and Opportunistic Infections. Washington, DC, 1977.

127. G Skowron, SA Bozzette, L Lim, CB Pettinelli, HH Schaumberg, J Arezzo, MA Fischl, WG Powderly, DJ Gocke, DD Richman, JC Pottage, D Antoniskis, GF McKinley, NE Hyslop, G Ray, G Simon, N Reed, ML LoFaro, RB Uttamchandani, LD Gelb, SJ Sperber, RL Murphy, JM Leedom, MH Grieco, J Zachary, MS Hirsch,

SA Spector, J Bigley, W Soo, TC Merigan. Alternating and intermittent regimens of zidovudine and dideoxycytidine in patients with AIDS or AIDS-related complex. Ann Intern Med 118:321–330, 1993.

128. T-C Meng, MA Fischl, AM Boota, SA Spector, D Bennett, Y Bassiakos, S Lai, B Wright, DD Richman. A phase I/II study of combination therapy with zidovudine and dideoxycytidine in subjects with advanced human immunodeficiency virus (HIV) disease. Ann Intern Med 116:13–20, 1992.

129. AC Collier, RW Coombs, MA Fischl, PR Skolnik, D Northfelt, P Boutin, CJ Hooper, LD Kaplan, PA Volberding, LG Davis, DR Henrard, S Weller, L Corey. Combination therapy with zidovudine and didanosine compared with zidovudine alone in HIV-1 infection. Ann Intern Med 119:786–793, 1993.

130. R Yarchoan, JA Lietzau, BY Nguyen, OW Brawley, JM Pluda, MW Saville, KM Wyvill, SM Steinberg, R Agbaria, H Mitsuya, S Broder. A randomized pilot study of alternating or simultaneous zidovudine and didanosine therapy in patients with symptomatic human immunodeficiency virus infection. J Infect Dis 169:9–17, 1994.

131. MV Ragni, DA Amato, ML LoFaro, V DeGruttola, C Van Der Horst, ME Eyster, CM Kessler, GF Gjerset, M Ho, DM Parenti, U Dafni, R Suraiya, JA Korvick, TC Merigan, TACT Group. Randomized study of didanosine monotherapy and combination therapy with zidovudine in hemophilic and nonhemophilic subjects with asymptomatic human immunodeficiency virus-1 infection. AIDS Clinical Trial Groups. Blood 85:2337–2346, 1995.

132. SM Hammer, KE Squires, MD Hughes, JM Grimes, LM Demeter, JS Currier, JJ Eron Jr, JE Feinberg, HH Balfour Jr, LR Deyton, JA Chodakewitz, MA Fischl. A controlled trial of two nucleoside analogues plus indinavir in persons with human immunodeficiency virus infection and CD4 cell counts of 200 per cubic millimeter or less. AIDS Clinical Trials Group 320 Study Team. N Engl J Med 337:725–733, 1997.

133. RM Gulick, JW Mellors, D Havlir, JJ Eron, C Gonzalez, D McMahon, DD Richman, FT Valentine, L Jonas, A Meibohm, EA Emini, JA Chodakewitz. Treatment with indinavir, zidovudine, and lamivudine in adults with human immunodeficiency virus infection and prior antiretroviral therapy. N Engl J Med 337:734–739, 1997.

134. D Kempf, A Molla, E Sun, S Danner, C Boucher, J Leonard. The duration of viral suppression is predicted by viral load during protease inhibitor therapy. 4th Conference on Retroviruses and Opportunistic Infections. Washington, DC, 1997.

135. RW Shafer, AK Iversen, MA Winters, E Aguiniga, DA Katzenstein, TC Merigan. Drug resistance and heterogeneous long-term virologic responses of human immunodeficiency virus type 1-infected subjects to zidovudine and didanosine combination therapy. The AIDS Clinical Trials Group 143 Virology Team. J Infect Dis 172:70–78, 1995.

136. AC Collier, RW Coombs, DA Schoenfeld, RL Bassett, J Timpone, A Baruch, M Jones, K Facey, C Whitacre, VJ McAuliffe, HM Friedman, TC Merigan, RC Reichman, C Hooper, L Corey. Treatment of human immunodeficiency virus infection with saquinavir, zidovudine, and zalcitabine. AIDS Clinical Trials Group. N Engl J Med 334:1011–1017, 1996.

137. AC Collier, RW Coombs, DA Schoenfeld, R Bassett, A Baruch, L Corey. Combination therapy with zidovudine, didanosine and saquinavir. Antiviral Res 29:99, 1996.
138. R Gulick, J Mellors, D Havlir, et al. Potent and sustained antiretroviral activity of indinavir (IDV) in combination with zidovudine (ZDV) and lamivudine (3TC). 3rd Conference on Retroviruses and Opportunistic Infections. Washington, DC, 1996.
139. I Barbour, O Clayton. Efficacy and safety of quadruple combination therapy in treatment experienced HIV/AIDS patient. 4th Conference on Retroviruses and Opportunistic Infections. Washington, DC, 1997.
140. C Steinhart, S George, R Mann. "Salvage therapy" using the combination of ritonavir and saquinavir in patients with advanced HIV infection. 4th Conference on Retroviruses and Opportunistic Infections. Washington, DC, 1997.
141. DJ Kempf, KC Marsh, G Kumar, AD Rodrigues, JF Denissen, E McDonald, MJ Kukulka, A Hsu, GR Granneman, PA Baroldi, E Sun, D Pizzuti, JJ Plattner, DW Norbeck, JM Leonard. Pharmacokinetic enhancement of inhibitors of the human immunodeficiency virus protease by coadministration with ritonavir. Antimicrob Agents Chemother 41:654–660, 1997.
142. G Granneman, A Hsu, E Sun, J Leonard, Y Xu, R Rode, tr-ss group. Pharmacokinetics pharmacodynamics of ritonavir—saquinavir combination therapy. 4th Conference on Retroviruses and Opportunistic Infections. Washington, DC, 1997.
143. DS Berger, G Bucher, K Delaney, H Wittert, P Gomatos. Further reduction in plasma HIV load in patients with advanced AIDS when a second protease inhibitor was added to triple drug combination therapy. 4th Conference on Retroviruses and Opportunistic Infections. Washington, DC, 1997.
144. RD Aquila, MD Hughes, VA Johnson, MA Fischl, JP Sommadossi, SH Liou, J Timpone, M Myers, N Basgoz, M Niu, MS Hirsch. Nevirapine, zidovudine, and didanosine compared with zidovudine and didanosine in patients with HIV-1 infection. A randomized, double-blind, placebo-controlled trial. National Institute of Allergy and Infectious Diseases AIDS Clinical Trials Group Protocol 241 Investigators. Ann Intern Med 124:1019–1030, 1996.
145. RT Davey Jr, DG Chaitt, GF Reed, WW Freimuth, BR Herpin, JA Metcalf, PS Eastman, J Falloon, JA Kovacs, MA Polis, RE Walker, H Masur, J Boyle, S Coleman, SR Cox, L Wathen, CL Daenzer, HC Lane. Randomized, controlled phase I/II, trial of combination therapy with delavirdine (U-90152S) and conventional nucleosides in human immunodeficiency virus type 1-infected patients. Antimicrob Agents Chemother 40:1657–1664, 1996.
146. B Autran, G Carcelain, TS Li, C Blanc, D Mathez, R Tubiana, C Katlama, P Debre, J Leibowitch. Positive effects of combined antiretroviral therapy on CD4+ T cell homeostasis and function in advanced HIV disease. Science 277:112–116, 1997.
147. JM Coffin. HIV population dynamics in vivo: implications for genetic variation, pathogenesis, and therapy. Science 267:483–489, 1995.
148. SD Frost, AR McLean. Quasispecies dynamics and the emergence of drug resistance during zidovudine therapy of HIV infection. AIDS 8:323–332, 1994.
149. P Kellam, CA Boucher, JM Tijnagel, BA Larder. Zidovudine treatment results in the selection of human immunodeficiency virus type 1 variants whose genotypes confer increasing levels of drug resistance. J Gen Virol 75:341–351, 1994.
150. M Holodniy, L Mole, D Margolis, J Moss, H Dong, E Boyer, M Urdea, J Kolberg,

S Eastman. Determination of human immunodeficiency virus RNA in plasma and cellular viral DNA genotypic zidovudine resistance and viral load during zidovudine–didanosine combination therapy. J Virol 69:3510–3516, 1995.

151. BY Nguyen, R Yarchoan, KM Wyvill, DJ Venzon, JM Pluda, H Mitsuya, S Broder. Five-year follow-up of a phase I study of didanosine in patients with advanced human immunodeficiency virus infection. J Infect Dis 171:1180–1189, 1995.

152. S Staszewski. Zidovudine and lamivudine: results of phase III studies. J Acquir Immune Defic Syndr Hum Retrovirol 10(suppl 1):S57, 1995.

153. C Katlama, D Ingrand, C Loveday, N Clumeck, J Mallolas, S Staszewski, M Johnson, AM Hill, G Pearce, H McDade. Safety and efficacy of lamivudine–zidovudine combination therapy in antiretroviral-naive patients. A randomized controlled comparison with zidovudine monotherapy. Lamivudine European HIV Working Group. JAMA 276:118–125, 1996.

154. S Staszewski, C Loveday, JJ Picazo, P Dellarnonica, P Skinhoj, MA Johnson, SA Danner, PR Harrigan, AM Hill, L Verity, H McDade. Safety and efficacy of lamivudine–zidovudine combination therapy in zidovudine-experienced patients. A randomized controlled comparison with zidovudine monotherapy. Lamivudine European HIV Working Group. JAMA 276:111–117, 1996.

155. JJ Eron, SL Benoit, J Jemsek, RD MacArthur, J Santana, JB Quinn, DR Kuritzkes, MA Fallon, M Rubin, the North American HIV Working Party. Treatment with lamivudine, zidovudine, or both in HIV-positive patients with 200 to 500 CD4+ cells per cubic millimeter. N Engl J Med 333:1662–1669, 1996.

156. JA Bartlett, SL Benoit, VA Johnson, JB Quinn, GE Sepulveda, WC Ehmann, C Tsoukas, MA Fallon, PL Self, M Rubin. Lamivudine plus zidovudine compared with zalcitabine plus zidovudine in patients with HIV infection. A randomized, double-blind, placebo-controlled trial. North American HIV Working Party. Ann Intern Med 125:161–172, 1996.

157. D Rouleau, B Conway, J Raboud, P Patenaude, MT Schechter, M O'Shaughnessy, JSG Montaner. A pilot, open label study of the antiviral effect of stavudine (d4T) and lamivudine (3TC) in advanced HIV disease. XI International Conference on AIDS. Vancouver, BC, 1996.

158. CR Steinhart, D Jacobsen, S George. Combination antiretroviral therapy with stavudine (D4T) and lamivudine (3TC): a retrospective analysis. XI International Conference on AIDS. Vancouver, BC, 1996.

159. RM Novak, J Colombo, M Linares-Diaz, L Moreira. Comparison of AZT/3TC vs. d4T/3TC for the treatment of HIV in persons with CD4 counts < 300 and prior AZT experience. XI International Conference on AIDS. Vancouver, BC, 1996.

160. LD Saravolatz, DL Winslow, G Collins, JS Hodges, C Pettinelli, DS Stein, N Markowitz, R Reves, MO Loveless, L Crane, M Thompson, D Abrams. Zidovudine alone or in combination with didanosine or zalcitabine in HIV-infected patients with the acquired immunodeficiency syndrome or fewer than 200 CD4 cells per cubic millimeter. Investigators for the Terry Beirn Community Programs for Clinical Research on AIDS. N Engl J Med 335:1099–1106, 1996.

161. C-F Perno, R Yarchoan, DA Cooney, NR Hartman, DSA Webb, Z Hao, H Mitsuya, DG Johns, S Broder. Replication of human immunodeficiency virus in monocytes. Granulocyte/macrophage colony-stimulating factor (GM-CSF) potentiates viral

production yet enhances the antiviral effect mediated by 3′-azido-2′3′-dideoxy-thymidine (AZT) and other dideoxynucleoside congeners of thymidine. J Exp Med 169:933–951, 1989.

162. W-Y Gao, T Shirasaka, DG Johns, S Broder, H Mitsuya. Differential phosphorylation of azidothymidine, dideoxycytidine, and dideoxyinosine in resting and activated peripheral blood mononuclear cells. J Clin Invest 91:2326–2333, 1993.

163. E Kojima, T Shirasaka, BD Anderson, S Chokekijchai, SM Steinberg, S Broder, R Yarchoan, H Mitsuya. Human immunodeficiency virus type-1 (HIV-1) viremia changes and development of drug-related mutations in patients with symptomatic HIV-1 infection receiving alternating or simultaneous zidovudine and didanosine therapy. J Infect Dis 171:1152–1159, 1995.

164. TC Merigan, G Skowron, SA Bozzette, D Richman, R Uttamchandani, M Fischl, R Schooley, M Hirsch, W Soo, C Pettinelli, H Schaumburg, and the ddc Study Group of the AIDS Clinical Trials Group. Circulating p24 antigen levels and responses to dideoxycytidine in human immunodeficiency virus (HIV) infections. A phase I and II study. Ann Intern Med 110:189–194, 1989.

165. R Yarchoan, H Mitsuya, J Pluda, KS Marczyk, RV Thomas, NR Hartman, P Brouwers, C-F Perno, J-P Allain, DG Johns, S Broder. The National Cancer Institute phase I study of ddI administration in adults with AIDS or AIDS-related complex: analysis of activity and toxicity profiles. Rev Infect Dis 12(suppl 5):S522–S533, 1990.

166. Z Gu, RS Fletcher, EJ Arts, MA Wainberg, MA Parniak. The K65R mutant reverse transcriptase of HIV-1 cross-resistant to 2′, 3′-dideoxycytidine, 2′,3′-dideoxy-3′-thiacytidine, and 2′,3′-dideoxyinosine shows reduced sensitivity to specific dideoxynucleoside triphosphate inhibitors in vitro. J Biol Chem 269:28118–28122, 1994.

167. Q Gao, Z Gu, J Hiscott, G Dionne, MA Wainberg. Generation of drug-resistant variants of human immunodeficiency virus type 1 by in vitro passage in increasing concentrations of 2′, 3′-dideoxycytidine and 2′, 3′-dideoxy-3′-thiacytidine. Antimicrob Agents Chemo 37:130–133, 1993.

168. Z Gu, H Salomon, JM Cherrington, AS Mulato, MS Chen, R Yarchoan, A Foli, KM Sogocio, MA Wainberg. K65R mutation of HIV-1 reverse transcriptase encodes cross-resistance to 9-(2-phosphonylmethoxyethyl)adenine. Antimicrob Agents Chemother 39:1888–1891, 1995.

169. MW Vogt, KL Hartshorn, PA Furman, T-C Chou, JA Fyfe, LA Coleman, C Crumpacker, RT Schooley, MS Hirsch. Ribavirin antagonizes the effect of azidothymidine on HIV replication. Science 235:1376–1379, 1987.

170. QY Zhu, A Scarborough, B Polsky, TC Chou. Drug combinations and effect parameters of zidovudine, stavudine, and nevirapine in standardized drug-sensitive and resistant HIV type 1 strains. AIDS Res Hum Retroviruses 12:507–517, 1996.

171. R Pollard, D Peterson, D Hardy, L Pedneault, V Rutkiewicz, J Pottage, R Murphy, J Gathe, G Beall, J Skovronski, A Cross, L Dunkle. Stavudine (d4T) and didanosine (ddI) combination therapy in HIV-infected subjects: antiviral effect and safety in an on-going pilot randomized double-blinded trial. XI International Conference on AIDS. Vancouver, BC, 1996.

172. NM Graham, DR Hoover, LP Park, DS Stein, JP Phair, JW Mellors, R Detels, AJ

Saah. Survival in HIV-infected patients who have received zidovudine: comparison of combination therapy with sequential monotherapy and continued zidovudine monotherapy. Multicenter AIDS Cohort Study Group. Ann Intern Med 124:1031–1038, 1996.

173. MA Fischl, K Stanley, AC Collier, JM Arduino, DS Stein, JE Feinberg, JD Allan, JC Goldsmith, WG Powderly. Combination and monotherapy with zidovudine and zalcitabine in patients with advanced HIV disease. The NIAID AIDS Clinical Trials Group. Ann Intern Med 122:24–32, 1995.

174. SM Wolinsky, BT Korber, AU Neumann, M Daniels, KJ Kunstman, AJ Whetsell, MR Furtado, Y Cao, DD Ho, JT Safrit, RA Koup. Adaptive evolution of human immunodeficiency virus-type 1 during the natural course of infection. Science 272: 537–542, 1996.

175. W O'Brien, PM Hartigan, ES Daar, MS Simberkoff, JD Hamilton. Changes in plasma HIV RNA levels and CD4+ lymphocyte counts predict both response to antiretroviral therapy and therapeutic failure. VA Cooperative Study Group on AIDS. Ann Intern Med 126:939–945, 1997.

176. DA Katzenstein, M Holodniy. HIV viral load quantification, HIV resistance, and antiretroviral therapy. AIDS Clin Rev 277–303, 1995–1996.

177. MD de Jong, J Veenstra, NI Stilianakis, R Schuurman, JM Lange, RJ de Boer, CA Boucher. Host-parasite dynamics and outgrowth of virus containing a single K70R amino acid change in reverse transcriptase are responsible for the loss of human immunodeficiency virus type 1 RNA load suppression by zidovudine. Proc Natl Acad Sci USA 93:5501–5506, 1996.

178. R Little, G Franchini, D Pearson, P Ellwood, R Yarchoan, W Wilson. HIV-1 viral burden (VB) during EPOCH chemotherapy (CT) for HIV-related lymphomas. 1st National AIDS Malignancy Conference. Bethesda, MD, Philidelphia: Lippincott–Raven, 1997.

179. S Zanussi, C Simonelli, M D'Andrea, M Comar, E Bidoli, M Giacca, U Tirelli, E Vaccher, PD Paoli. The effects of antineoplastic chemotherapy on HIV disease. AIDS Res Hum Retroviruses 12:1703–1707, 1996.

180. LD Kaplan, JO Kahn, S Crowe, D Northfelt, P Neville, H Grossberg, DI Abrams, J Tracey, J Mills, PA Volberding. Clinical and virologic effects of recombinant human granulocyte–macrophage colony-stimulating factor in patients receiving chemotherapy for human immunodeficiency virus-associated non–Hodgkin's lymphoma: results of a randomized trial. J Clin Oncol 9:929–940, 1991.

181. GR Weiss, JG Kuhn, J Rizzo, LS Smith, GI Rodriguez, JR Eckardt, HA Burris 3rd, S Fields, K VanDenBerg, DD von Hoff. A phase I and pharmacokinetics study of 2-chlorodeoxyadenosine in patients with solid tumors. Cancer Chemother Pharmacol 35:397–402, 1995.

182. DC Betticher, MF Fey, A von Rohr, A Tobler, H Jenzer, A Gratwohl, A Lohri, P Pugin, U Hess, O Pagani, G Zulian, T Cerny. High incidence of infections after 2-chlorodeoxyadenosine (2-CDA) therapy in patients with malignant lymphomas and chronic and acute leukaemias. Ann Oncol 5:57–64, 1994.

183. CL Mackall, TA Fleisher, MR Brown, IT Magrath, AT Shad, ME Horowitz, LH Wexler, MA Adde, LL McClure, RE Gress. Lymphocyte depletion during treatment with intensive chemotherapy for cancer. Blood 84:2221–2228, 1994.

184. AE Davis Jr. The histopathological changes in the thymus gland in the acquired immunodeficiency syndrome. Ann NY Acad Sci 437:493–502, 1984.

185. HJ Schuurman, WJ Krone, R Broekhuizen, J van Baarlen, P van Veen, AL Goldstein, J Huber, J Goudsmit. The thymus in acquired immunodeficiency syndrome. Comparison with other types of immunodeficiency diseases, and presence of components of human immunodeficiency virus type 1. Am J Pathol 134:1329–1338, 1989.

186. CL Mackall, L Granger, MA Sheard, R Capeda, RE Gress. T-cell regeneration after bone-marrow transplantation: differential CD45 isoform expression on thymic-derived versus thymic-independent progeny. Blood 82:2585–2594, 1993.

187. CL Mackall, TA Fleisher, MR Brown, MP Andrich, CC Chen, IM Feuerstein, ME Horowitz, IT Magrath, AT Shad, SM Steinberg, LH Wexler, RE Gress, Age, thymopoiesis, and CD4+ T-lymphocyte regeneration after intensive chemotherapy. N Engl J Med 332:143–149, 1995.

188. MJ Browne, SM Hubbard, DL Longo, R Fisher, R Wesley, DC Ihde, RC Young, PA Pizzo. Excess prevalence of *Pneumocystis carinii* pneumonia in patients treated for lymphoma with combination chemotherapy. Ann Intern Med 104:338–344, 1986.

189. B Reckzeh, H Merte, KH Pfluger, R Pfab, M Wolf, K Havemann. Severe lymphocytopenia and interstitial pneumonia in patients treated with paclitaxel and simultaneous radiotherapy for non–small-cell lung cancer. J Clin Oncol 14:1071–1076, 1996.

190. GM Shearer, M Clerici. Abnormalities of immune regulation in human immunodeficiency virus infection. Pediatr Res 33:S71–S74; [discussion S74–S75], 1993.

191. A Kinter, AS Fauci. Interleukin-2 and human immunodeficiency virus infection: pathogenic mechanisms and potential for immunologic enhancement. Immunol Res 15:1–15, 1996.

192. C Graziosi, KR Gantt, M Vaccarezza, JF Demarest, M Daucher, MS Saag, GM Shaw, TC Quinn, OJ Cohen, CC Welbon, G Pantaleo, AS Fauci. Kinetics of cytokine expression during primary human immunodeficiency virus type 1 infection. Proc Natl Acad Sci USA 93:4386–4391, 1996.

193. AS Fauci. AIDS: newer concepts in the immunopathogenic mechanisms of human immunodeficiency virus disease. Proc Assoc Am Physicians 107:1–7, 1995.

194. D Goletti, AL Kinter, EC Hardy, G Poli, AS Fauci. Modulation of endogenous IL-1 beta and IL-1 receptor antagonist results in opposing effects on HIV expression in chronically infected monocytic cells. J Immunol 156:3501–3508, 1996.

195. B Rosok, P Voltersvik, R Bjerknes, M Axelsson, LR Haaheim, B Asjo. Dynamics of HIV-1 replication following influenza vaccination of HIV+ individuals. Clin Exp Immunol 104:203–207, 1996.

196. SI Staprans, BL Hamilton, SE Follansbee, T Elbeik, P Barbosa, RM Grant, MB Feinberg. Activation of virus replication after vaccination of HIV-1-infected individuals. J Exp Med 182:1727–1737, 1995.

197. DV Havlir, DD Richman. Viral dynamics of HIV: implications for drug development and therapeutic strategies. Ann Intern Med 124:984–994, 1996.

198. AV Herz, S Bonhoeffer, RM Anderson, RM May, MA Nowak. Viral dynamics in

vivo: limitations on estimates of intracellular delay and virus decay. Proc Natl Acad Sci USA 93:7247–7251, 1996.

199. S Stanley, MA Ostrowski, JS Justement, K Gantt, S Hedayati, M Mannix, K Roche, DJ Schwartzentruber, CH Fox, AS Fauci. Effect of immunization with a common recall antigen on viral expression in patients infected with human immunodeficiency virus type 1. N Engl J Med 334:1222–1230, 1996.

200. Y Koyanagi, WA O'Brien, JQ Zhao, DW Golde, JC Gasson, ISY Chen. Cytokines alter production of HIV-1 from primary mononuclear phagocytes. Science 241: 1673–1675, 1988.

201. CF Perno, DA Cooney, WY Gao, Z Hao, DG Johns, A Foli, NR Hartman, R Calio, S Broder, R Yarchoan. Effects of bone marrow stimulatory cytokines on human immunodeficiency virus replication and the antiviral activity of dideoxynucleosides in cultures of monocyte/macrophages. Blood 80:995–1003, 1992.

202. JM Pluda, R Yarchoan, PD Smith, N McAtee, LE Shay, D Oette, M Maha, SM Wahl, CE Myers, S Broder. Subcutaneous recombinant granulocyte–macrophage colony-stimulating factor used as a single agent and in an alternating regimen with azidothymidine in leukopenic patients with severe human immunodeficiency virus infection. Blood 76:463–472, 1990.

203. S Miles, J Glaspy, Y Chung, K Lee, L Souza, G Baldwin. Recombinant granulocyte colony stimulating factor (r-metHuG-CSF) increases neutrophil number and function, but does not alter HIV expression in patients with AIDS. V International Conference on AIDS. Montreal, 1989.

204. CF Perno, DA Cooney, MJ Currens, G Rocchi, DG Johns, S Broder, R Yarchoan. Ability of anti-HIV agents to inhibit HIV replication in monocyte/macrophages or U937 monocytoid cells under conditions of enhancement by GM-CSF or anti-HIV antibody. AIDS Res Hum Retroviruses 6:1051–1055, 1990.

205. DT Scadden, O Pickus, SM Hammer, B Stretcher, J Bresnahan, J Gere, J McGrath, JM Agosti. Lack of in vivo effect of granulocyte–macrophage colony-stimulating factor on human immunodeficiency virus type 1. AIDS Res Hum Retroviruses 12: 1151–1159, 1996.

206. R Jeyaseelan, M Kurabayashi, L Kedes. Doxorubicin inhibits Tat-dependent transactivation of HIV type 1 LTR. AIDS Res Hum Retroviruses 12:569–576, 1996.

207. CF Perno, R Yarchoan, J Balzarini, A Bergamini, G Milanese, R Pauwels, E De Clercq, G Rocchi, R Calio. Different pattern of activity of inhibitors of the human immunodeficiency virus in lymphocytes and monocyte/macrophages. Antiviral Res 17:289–304, 1992.

208. A Bergamini, CF Perno, J Balzarini, M Capozzi, L Marinelli, G Milanese, CD Pesce, R Calio, G Rocchi. Selective inhibition of HIV replication by Adriamycin in macrophages but not in lymphocytes. AIDS Res Hum Retroviruses 8:1239–1247, 1992.

209. Y Tomita, T Kuwata. Effects of Adriamycin on the reverse transcriptase and the production of murine leukemia virus. Cancer Res 36:3016–3019, 1976.

210. L Bogdany, E Csanyi. Inhibition of RNA dependent DNA polymerases by anthracycline antibiotics. Neoplasma 29:37–42, 1982.

211. KV Dhananjaya, A Antony. Inhibition of avian myeloblastosis virus reverse transcriptase and its associated activities by daunomycin and Adriamycin. Indian J Biochem Biophys 24:265–270, 1987.
212. OT Rutschmann, P Lorenzi, M Pechere, J Krischer, A Rosay, S Hulliger, S Yerly, L Perrin, B Hirschel. HIV viremia during antitumoral chemotherapy. XI International Conference on AIDS. Vancouver, BC, 1996.
213. A Levine, A Tulpule, J Rochat, B Espina, R McPhee, D Tessman, D VonHoff. Short term impact of mitoguazone (MGBG) chemotherapy on HIV viral load in patients with relapsed/refractory AIDS-lymphoma. American Society of Hematology Thirty-Eighth Annual Meeting. 1996. Orlando, FL. Philadelphia: WB Saunders, 1996.
214. DA Fishman, RR Viscarello, I Cass, PE Schwartz. Effect of combination chemotherapy with cisplatin and cyclophosphamide on human immunodeficiency virus type-1 surrogate markers in a patient with advanced epithelial ovarian cancer. Gynecol Oncol 57:105–108, 1995.
215. GK McEvoy, ed. American Hospital Formulatory Service. 1996 ed. AHFS 96 Drug Information. K Litvak, J Olin, H Welsh, eds. Bethesda, MD: American Society of Health-System Pharmacists, 1996:2813.
216. SG Deeks, M Smith, M Holodniy, JO Kahn. HIV-1 protease inhibitors. A review for clinicians. JAMA 277:145–153, 1997.
217. L Moutouh, J Corbeil, DD Richman. Recombination leads to the rapid emergence of HIV-1 dually resistant mutants under selective drug pressure. Proc Natl Acad Sci USA 93:6106–6111, 1996.
218. DD Ho. How long should treatment be given if we had an antiretroviral regimen that completely blocks HIV replication? XI International Conference on AIDS. Vancouver, BC 1996.
219. K Luzuriaga, Y Bryson, P Krogstad,J Robinson, B Stechenberg, M Lamson, P Gagnier, JL Sullivan. Triple combination therapy in early vertical HIV-1 infection: potential for eradication of infection. 4th Conference on Retroviruses and Opportunistic Infections. Washington, DC, 1997.
220. T-W Chun, L Carruth, D Finzi, X Shen, J Digiuseppi, H Taylor, K Chadwick, J Margolick, M Zeiger, P Barditch-Crovo, RF Siliciano. Quantitative analysis of latent integrated and unintegrated HIV-1 provirus in lymph nodes and peripheral blood: implications for virus eradication. 4th Conference on Retroviruses and Opportunistic Infections. Washington, DC, 1997.
221. HK Holland, R Saral, JJ Rossi, AD Donnenberg, WH Burns, WE Beschorner, H Farzadegan, RJ Jones, GV Quinnan, GB Vogelsang, HM Vriesendorp, JR Wingard, JA Zaia, GW Santos. Allogeneic bone marrow transplantation, zidovudine, and human immunodeficiency virus type 1 (HIV-1) infection. Studies in a patient with non–Hodgkin lymphoma. Ann Intern Med 111:973–981, 1989.
222. C Ricordi, AG Tzakis, WB Rybka, P Fontes, ED Ball, M Trucco, M Kocova, D Triulzi, J McMichael, H Doyle, P Gupta, JJ Fung, TE Starzl. Xenotransplantation of hematopoietic cells resistant to HIV as a potential treatment for patients with AIDS. Transplant Proc 26:1302–1303, 1994.
223. ST Ildstad. Xenotransplantation for AIDS. Lancet 347:761, 1996.

224. B Thorne, J Getty, M Sharp, V Parks, D Mahon. Patient initiated research; Jeff
      Getty, Project Inform and the baboon bone marrow transplant. XI International
      Conference on AIDS. Vancouver, BC, 1996.
225. R Taylor. Baboon graft fails, but patient thrives. Nat Med 2:259, 1996.
226. M Dean, M Carrington, C Winkler, GA Huttley, MW Smith, R Allikmets, JJ Goed-
      ert, SP Buchbinder, E Vittinghoff, E Gomperts, S Donfield, D Vlahov, R Kaslow,
      A Saah, C Rinaldo, R Detels, OB SJ. Genetic restriction of HIV-1 infection and
      progression to AIDS by a deletion allele of the CKR5 structural gene. Hemophilia
      Growth and Development Study, Multicenter AIDS Cohort Study, Multicenter He-
      mophilia Cohort Study, San Francisco City Cohort, ALIVE Study. Science 273:
      1856–1862, 1996.
227. BA Chabner, JM Collins, eds. Cancer Chemotherapy: Principles and Practice. Phil-
      adelphia: JB Lippincott, 1990:545.

15
Management of Opportunistic Infections

Kirk D. Miller
Georgetown University School of Medicine, Washington, D.C., and National Institutes of Health, Bethesda, Maryland

Henry Masur
George Washington University School of Medicine, Washington, D.C., and National Institutes of Health, Bethesda, Maryland

I. INTRODUCTION

Although the clinical course of human immunodeficiency virus type 1 (HIV-1) infection varies greatly from patient to patient, the hallmark of the disease is progressive immunosuppression, primarily owing to destruction of CD4+ T lymphocytes. This results in impaired cell-mediated immunity and, ultimately, in wide-ranging immune dysfunction (1,2). Eventually patients develop certain opportunistic infections or malignancies, or experience a decline in CD4+ lymphocyte cell counts to levels of fewer than 200/mm^3, thereby fulfilling the case-definition for the acquired immunodeficiency syndrome (AIDS; 3)

The number of ''AIDS-defining'' and ''AIDS-associated'' infections is vast—the present discussion, therefore, will focus on general principles of management and on individual opportunistic infections (OIs) that are most common, serious, treatable, and preventable. For the most part these are new or reactivated latent infections of the central nervous system (CNS) and eye, the respiratory system, and the gastrointestinal tracts. Others typically present as systemic febrile illnesses without organ-specific localizing signs or symptoms. Infectious agents that are manifest primarily through their role in the pathogenesis of HIV-associated malignancies (e.g., human herpesvirus-8 [HHV-8] and Epstein–Barr virus [EBV]) are presented in detail in Chapters 4 and 5.

II. THE RISK OF OPPORTUNISTIC INFECTION

Although the level of immunosuppression is without question the most important risk factor for developing an opportunistic process following infection with HIV, other influences on risk also warrant consideration.

A. Level of Immunosuppression: CD4+ Lymphocyte Count

Studies of the natural history of HIV infection in adults have shown that 90% of AIDS-defining illnesses in adults occur in individuals with CD4+ lymphocyte counts of fewer than 200/mm^3, and certain of these rarely occur in individuals with CD4+ lymphocytes counts of 50/mm^3, or more (Table 1; 4,5). Moreover, there appears to be an ongoing trend for OIs to occur at ever lower CD4+ counts, probably reflecting expanded use of prophylaxis and generally improved clinical care of these patients. (6).

Ideally, one will have several relatively recent CD4+ values (i.e., values determined before the onset of the patient's current acute process) at one's disposal for use in evaluating a patient's risk of given opportunistic infection. Numerous factors have the effect of transiently lowering CD4+ lymphocyte counts, including acute (especially viral) infections, brief corticosteroid therapy, and major surgery. In addition, there is significant diurnal and even seasonal variability,

Table 1 Development of Opportunistic Infection by Level of Immunosuppression (CD4+ Lymphocyte Count)

Infections associated with mild immunosuppression (CD4+ 200–500 range)
    Tuberculosis
    Herpes simplex (severe or frequently recurring mucocutaneous infections)
    Herpes zoster (localized cutaneous infections/shingles)
    Candidiasis (oral thrush and recurrent or severe vaginal infections)
    Pyogenic infections (e.g., bacterial "community-acquired" pneumonia)
    Oral hairy leukoplakia (presumed due to Ebstein–Barr virus infection)
Infections seen with moderate immunosuppression (CD4+ < 100–200 range)
    Pneumocystis carinii pneumonia
    Cryptococcal meningitis
Infections seen with profound immunosuppression (CD4+ < 50–100 range)
    Mycobacterium avium complex bacteremia
    Cytomegalovirus (retinal and enteral infections)
    Progressive multifocal leukencephalopathy (caused by JC virus infection)
    Cryptosporidial enteritis
    Toxoplasma gondii encephalitis

---

as well as considerable laboratory-to-laboratory variability. In general there seems to be less variation in the CD4+ percentage value than in the absolute value (7).

With the initiation of highly active antiretroviral therapy (HAART) and with immunomodulator therapy with interleukin-2 (IL-2), patients often experience increases in CD4+ lymphocyte counts to levels higher than key thresholds for developing opportunistic infections. Whether these augmented CD4+ lymphocyte counts provide a level of protection equivalent to that present in patients with similar CD4+ lymphocyte counts who have never dropped below key thresholds is not well studied. However, recent modifications to guidelines for opportunistic infection prevention acknowledge that discontinuation of certain types of prophylaxis may be reasonable (8).

B. Viral Load

The level of circulating HIV RNA (as measured by reverse transcriptase–polymerase chain reaction [RT–PCR] and bDNA assays) is an independent risk factor for development of opportunistic infection, as well as being the most important predictor or overall prognosis. However, how to incorporate viral load information into prophylactic strategies is not yet clear.

C. Previous and Concomitant OIs

A history of a previous AIDS-defining opportunistic infection places the patient in a high-risk category for a new opportunistic process, or a new episode of a previously diagnosed and treated process. Similarly, the presence or a history of other less serious HIV-associated infections should increase the level of suspicion of a new serious opportunistic process—for example, the presence of oral thrush is an independent risk factor for developing *Pneumocystis carinii* pneumonia (PCP; 9)

D. Antimicrobial Use

A detailed history of the patient's current use of prophylactic and therapeutic antimicrobial medications is important in assessing the risk for various opportunistic infections. Trimethoprim–sulfamethoxazole (TMP–SMZ) is probably the antimicrobial agent most widely used by patients, primarily for prophylaxis against *P. carinii*. However, this agent also provides prophylaxis against a wide range of pathogens, including *Toxoplasma gondii*, *Isospora belli*, and respiratory pathogens, such as *Streptococcus pneumoniae* and *Haemophilus influenzae* (10). Conversely, treatment or ongoing prolonged suppression of CNS toxoplasmosis with dapsone will provide some level of prophylaxis against PCP (11,12). There

Table 2 Examples of Antimicrobial Agents Widely Used in the Prevention and Treatment of AIDS-Related Infections That May Influence the Likelihood of Other Infections

Typical clinical setting	Agent(s)	Other potential influences
Prevention of PCP	TMP–SMX	Decreased incidence of toxoplasmosis, isosporiasis, and infection with susceptible bacteria
Treatment of toxoplasmosis	Dapsone, clindamycin	Decreased incidence of PCP (with dapsone) and decreased incidence of infection with susceptible bacteria (clindamycin)
Prevention of MAC	Clarithromycin, azithromycin	Decreased incidence of infection with susceptible bacteria
Treatment of MAC	Ethambutol, rifabutin	Decreased incidence of infection with other susceptible mycobacteria
Treatment or prevention candidiasis or cryptococcal disease	Fluconazole, itraconazole	Decreased incidence of infection of with other susceptible fungi
Treatment or prevention of CMV disease	Ganciclovir, foscarnet, cidofovir	Decreased incidence of herpes simplex and zoster infections

are several examples of antimicrobials used in the prevention and treatment of AIDS-related opportunistic infections that may influence the incidence of other infections (Table 2). The level of such influence in most of these situations, however, has yet to be quantified (13).

E. Chemotherapy

The effect of chemotherapy on the development of opportunistic infection is also less than adequately quantified in the setting of HIV disease. In the absence of data to the contrary, it would seem reasonable to assume that the immunosuppressive effects of chemotherapeutic agents are at least additive to those of the underlying HIV infection. Indeed, early studies of intensive therapy for HIV-associated lymphoma demonstrated rates of opportunistic infection as high as 78%, whereas more recent studies of less-intensive regimens suggest more acceptable rates (see

Chapter 9; 14–17). Corticosteroids appear to enhance the risk for opportunistic infection when administered for long periods (>21 days).

Several principles concerning opportunistic infection in HIV-infected patients undergoing chemotherapy are generally accepted: (1) Patients receiving antimicrobials for the prevention and treatment of opportunistic infections should continue to receive these agents during chemotherapy unless otherwise contraindicated; (2) patients receiving intensive combination chemotherapy regimens generally should receive PCP prophylaxis, regardless of CD4+ lymphocyte count; and (3) HIV-infected patients undergoing chemotherapy are subject to profound and prolonged myelosuppression that can be lessened by the prophylactic use of G-CSF (see Chapter 9). Agents commonly used in HIV-infected patients that are likely to contribute to chemotherapy-induced neutropenia include zidovudine (AZT), TMP–SMZ, dapsone, foscarnet, ganciclovir, pentamidine, pyrimethamine, flucytosine, interferon alfa, and trimetrexate (18).

F. Geographic Location

The incidence of many opportunistic process varies markedly by geographic location. A prime example is PCP, which is much less common in developing countries, notably in Africa, than in the United States and Europe. Differences have also been noted within Europe, with a higher incidence noted in southern European countries. The converse is true for tuberculosis (19,20). Another is toxoplasmosis, the incidence of which varies with the seroprevalence rate of *T. gondii* infection in the population. Thus, toxoplasmosis is much more common in Europe, particularly France and Germany, than it is in the United States and in the United States, toxoplasmosis is more common among Hispanics than among whites (21).

Other notable examples of the influence of geography on the incidence of opportunistic infection include histoplasmosis and coccidioidomycosis, which are hyperendemic and much more common in HIV-infected patients in central and south-central and southwestern United States, respectively (22,24). Gastrointestinal infections with opportunistic pathogens are especially locale-specific. The high incidence of infection with *Isospora* and *Cyclospora* in Haiti and Central America are two among many such examples (25,26).

G. Asplenia

Although less common now than earlier in the AIDS epidemic, splenectomy remains one of the therapies for HIV-associated idiopathic thrombocytopenia (ITP). Splenectomized patients have artificially elevated absolute CD4+ lymphocyte counts (owing to augmention of total white blood cell [WBC] counts, rather than increased CD4+ lymphocyte percentage); therefore, following splenectomy, greater reliance should be placed in the percentage of CD4+ lymphocytes when assessing the likelihood of a given opportunistic infection or the need for prophylaxis (27). It can also be assumed that HIV-infected patients are subject to increased risk of infection with encapsulated organisms such as *H. influenzae* and *Streptococcus pneumoniae*. As in other settings, HIV-infected patients should be immunized with the polyvalent pneumococcal vaccine and conjugate *H. influenzae* b vaccine before elective splenectomy, even though patients with HIV infection are less likely to respond to immunization, especially if their CD4+ lymphocyte cell count is fewer than 200/mm^3 (8).

H. Animal Exposures

Several opportunistic infections have been associated with exposure to pets and farm animals. Most important among these is the association of exposure to cats with infections caused by *Bartonella henselae*, the etiologic agent of cat-scratch disease and bacillary angiomatosis (28). Cats also expose patients to the risk of primary toxoplasmosis. Cats and dogs can transmit *Cryptosporidium*, *Campylobacter*, and *Salmonella*. Birds can carry *Cryptococcus neoformans*, *Mycobacterium avium*, and *Histoplasma capsulatum* (29).

III. PRINCIPLES OF MANAGEMENT

Survival among HIV-infected patients has improved steadily since the mid-1980s (30). Although the relative contribution of newer antiretroviral therapies to this welcome trend cannot easily be separated from that provided by improved management of infectious complications, it is clear that AIDS patients have benefitted considerably from numerous new diagnostic techniques and therapies for OIs, many of which were developed in response to the needs of these patients (31).

A. Opportunistic Pathogens in the Setting of HIV Infection

Patients with AIDS have also benefitted from an increased appreciation for the natural history of infection with opportunistic agents peculiar to this setting. Cytomegalovirus (CMV), *P. carinii*, *T. gondii*, and *C. neoformans* are notable examples of pathogens that cause disease with distinguishing, if not unique, features in the setting of HIV infection (32–36).

One can divide HIV-associated opportunistic infections into two broad groups: those for which there is effective therapy, and those for which there is not. Fortunately, the former far outnumber the latter. Also, investigational therapies of varying promise exist for most of the relatively few OIs in the ''untreatable'' category, such as progressive multifocal leukoencephalopathy (PML), crypt-osporidiosis, and *Enterocytozoan bieneusi* (one of the causitive agents of mi-crosporidiosis).

After specific therapy for an OI is begun, it may take longer to appreciate a clinical response in HIV-infected patients than in other settings. Prolonged re-sponses are the rule in HIV-infected patients with PCP and cryptococcal meningi-tis (37,38). When reassessing patients with poor therapeutic responses, two other possibilities merit consideration. First is that an additional undiagnosed and un-treated pathogen might be contributing to the clinical picture. In one series of patients with PCP, 14% of patients had a second "copathogen" identified at the time of bronchoscopy (39). The other possibility is drug resistance, as might contribute to poor clinical response in CMV and herpes simplex virus (HSV) infections, tuberculosis, and candidiasis, among others (40–43).

Some patients, for example, those with presumed CMV retinitis and CNS toxoplasmosis, are usually treated without confirmatory microbiological or histo-logical studies, because of the risk associated with obtaining clinical specimens (21,44). Others, for example, those with fever and meningeal signs or symptoms and normal imaging studies, should never be treated empirically. Less clear, is the case for empiric therapy for PCP. Proponents argue that bronchoscopy is invasive, uncomfortable, costly, and time-consuming in patients with a high like-lihood of PCP (Table 3; 45) Opponents argue that up to 25% of these patients will have a diagnosis other than PCP, a figure too high to support the concept of empiric therapy for PCP, given that misdiagnosed patients will have been denied timely definitive therapy, will have been exposed unnecessarily to the

Table 3　Factors Mitigating for and Against the Diagnosis of PCP

Mitigating for the diagnosis of PCP	Mitigating against the diagnosis of PCP
Gradual onset	Sudden onset
Oral thrush	Prophylaxis with TMP–SMX or dapsone
Significant hypoxemia	Shaking chills
Elevated LDH	Pleuritic chest pain
Diffuse infiltrate	Purulent or copious sputum production
Pneumothorax	Hemoptysis
Prior episode of PCP	CD4+ cell count > $200/mm^3$
	Leukocytosis
	Focal infiltrate with consolidation
	Pleural effusion
	Intrathoracic adenopathy

toxicities of anti-PCP therapy, and will have been allowed to expose contacts to *M. tuberculosis* should tuberculosis be the correct diagnosis (46). Obviously, an accurate diagnosis is preferable and should be pursued whenever feasible.

B. Use of Antimicrobials in the Setting of HIV Infection

Agents used to prevent and treat OIs may have unusual properties in HIV-infected patients, particularly for safety. The level of intolerance to sulfonamides in these patients—fully 30% experience some form of toxicity to TMP–SMZ—is perhaps the most notable example of an altered safety profile (47). Another is the frequency with which antimicrobial agents (e.g., TMP—SMZ, dapsone, cidofovir, flucytosine, ganciclovir, and pyrimethamine) produce drug-induced neutropenia, ostensibly owing to the myelosuppressive effect of drugs combined with the effect of HIV itself on the bone marrow (48). Occasional differences in efficacy have also been noted. Although acyclovir provides bone marrow and renal transplant patients with protection from CMV infection, studies have not shown a similar effect in AIDS patients (49).

AIDS is also unparalleled as a setting for potential drug interactions (Table 4). Many interactions with clinically important consequences have been described, as have serious interactions between antimicrobials and antiretrovirals, especially the protease inhibitors (18). The addition of chemotherapeutic agents to regimens combining antimicrobials and antiretrovirals obviously only compounds this complexity (17).

Several antimicrobials commonly used by AIDS patients can cause fever mimicking OIs. Although TMP–SMZ and dapsone should be particularly suspect, fever can be a side effect, however rare, of most antimicrobials. Identifying a specific drug as the cause of fever in these patients can provide a not-inconsiderable clinical challenge (50).

C. Diagnostic Evaluation of the Febrile Patient

The scope of the diagnostic evaluation of the febrile patient will depend on his or her presenting signs and symptoms and level of immunosuppression. Evaluation of early-stage patients will generally be similar to that undertaken for an immunocompetent patient. Patients with significant evidence of immunosuppression (particularly those with a CD4+ cell count of fewer than 200/mm^3 or a history of OIs) require special consideration, especially in the absence of an obvious focus of infection (50). When examining such patients, particular attention should be given to the skin (including intravenous catheter sites), mucous membranes, sinuses, lymph nodes, abdomen, chest, and to the neurological examination. An expert ophthalmological examination is required for febrile patients with fewer than 50/mm^3 CD4+ cells and no obvious source of infection (32).

Table 4 Toxicities and Drug Interactions of Commonly Used Medications in the Treatment of Opportunistic Infections in HIV-Infected Patients

Agent	Side effects	Drug interactions
Acyclovir (Zovirax)	Infrequent with oral administration Renal toxicity has been associated with IV use	The potential for renal toxicity may be increased by concurrent use of other nephrotoxic drugs.
Amphotericin (Fungizone)	Fever, chills, renal toxicity, anemia, low serum calcium and magnesium levels	The potential for renal toxicity may be increased by concurrent use of other nephrotoxic drugs
Atovaquone (Mepron)	Rash, GI intolerance, diarrhea	No known significant interactions.
Azithromycin (Zithromax)	GI intolerance, diarrhea	Antacids reduce absorption.
Cidofovir (Vistide)	Renal toxicity, neutropenia	Requires administration with probenecid to minimize renal effects.
Ciprofloxacin (Cipro)	GI intolerance, CNS toxicity (drowsiness, headache, insomnia)	Absorption is decreased with antacids and ddI. Levels of theophylline are increased.
Clarithromycin (Biaxin)	GI intolerance	Levels of terfenadine (Seldane and astemizole (Hismanal) are increased and may cause life-threatening arrhythmias. Theophylline and carbamazepine levels are increased
Clindamycin (Cleocin)	Pseudomembranous (*C. difficile*) colitis, rash	Activity of neuromuscular blocking agents may be enhanced.
Dapsone	Rash, fever, neutropenia, severe hemolytic anemia in G6PD-deficient patients	Absorption is decreased with ddI, antacids, and H_2 blockers. Dapsone levels are decreased with rifampin and rifabutin, and increased with trimethoprim.
Ethambutol (Myambutol)	Ocular toxicity (dose-related)	No known significant interactions.

Table 4 Continued

Agent	Side effects	Drug interactions
Fluconazole (Diflucan)	GI intolerance, rash, elevated liver enzymes	P-450 enzyme inhibition in liver causes decreased metabolism of many drugs (e.g., rifampin, rifabutin, phenytoin, coumadin). Increased levels of ternfenadine (Seldane) may cause life-threatening arrhythmia. Rifampin decreases fluconazole levels.
Flucytosine (Ancabon)	Leukopenia, thrombocytopenia, rash, GI intolerance	Concurrent use of other agents with bone marrow toxicity may enhance toxic effects.
Foscarnet (Foscavir)	Renal toxicity, low serum calcium, magnesium, potassium levels; electrolyte imbalances may cause seizures	Concurrent pentamidine may cause severe hypocalcemia. Other nephrotoxic drugs should be avoided.
Ganciclovir (Cytovene)	Neutropenia, thrombocytopenia, CNS toxicity (headache, seizure, confusion)	Severe, life-threatening bone marrow suppression has occurred in patients receiving simultaneous AZT and ganciclovir. Concurrent use of other agents with bone marrow toxicity may also enhance toxicity.
Isoniazid (INH)	Hepatitis (age-related), peripheral neuropathy (patients on INH should receive pyridoxine)	Alcohol increases incidence of hepatitis. INH increases the effects of many drugs (e.g., coumadin, benzodiazepines, carbamazipine, cycloserine, ethionamide, phenytoin, theophylline). Antacids may decrease absorption.

Table 4 Continued

Agent	Side effects	Drug interactions
Itraconazole (Sporanox)	GI intolerance, rash, hepatitis (rare)	Increased levels of certain drugs (e.g., cyclosporine, oral hypoglycemics, digoxin). Increased levels of ternfenadine (Seldane) may cause life-threatening arrhythmia.
Ketoconazole (Nizoral)	GI intolerance, hepatitis, adrenal suppression, gynecomastia	Levels markedly reduced when administered with antacids or H_2 blockers. Levels of cyclosporine are increased. Rifampin causes marked decrease in ketoconazole levels.
Paromomycin (Humatin)	GI intolerance	No known significant interactions.
Pentamidine (NebuPent)	IV: renal toxicity, pancreatitis, hypotension, hypoglycemia, thrombocytopenia, hypocalcemia; aerosol: cough, wheezing	Concurrent use of other (Pentam), nephrotoxic drugs may increase.
Primaquine	Severe hemolytic anemia in G6PD-deficient patients, methemoglobinemia	No known significant interactions.
Pyrazinamide	Hepatitis, hyperuricemia	No known significant interactions.
Pyrimethamine (Daraprim)	Bone marrow toxicity and megaloblastic anemia caused by folate deficiency	Other antifolate drugs (e.g., dapsone, TMP–SMX) may increase potential for bone marrow toxicity. Hepatotoxicity has been reported when used concurrently with lorazepam.

Table 4 Continued

Agent	Side effects	Drug interactions
Rifabutin (Mycobutin)	Orange discoloration of secretions, rash, GI intolerance, neutropenia, uveitis	Levels of numerous drugs are decreased (e.g., coumadin, barbiturates, benzodiazepines, beta-blockers, oral contraceptives, corticosteroids, dapsone, ketoconazole, phenytoin, methadone, trimethoprim) by rifabutin. Clarithromycin and fluconazole increase rifabutin levels and may increase the incidence of uvetis. Rifabutin should not be used in patients taking ritonavir, saquinavir soft gel capsules, or delaviradine, due to decrease in levels of these antiretroviral drugs. Rifabutin dosage should be reduced by one-half in patients on indinavir, nelfinavir, or amprenavir. Rifabutin dosage should be increased in patients taking efavirenz.
Rifampin (Rifadin; Rimactane)	Orange discoloration of secretions rash, GI intolerance, jaundice, hepatitis, thrombocytopenia, leukopenia, dyspnea, wheezing	Levels of numerous drugs are decreased (see listing for rifabutin) by rifampin. Rifampin should not be used in patients taking protease inhibitors (indinavir, saquinavir, ritonavir, nelfinavir, amprenavir) or non-nucleoside reverse transcriptase inhibitors (delaviradine, nevirapine, efavirenz).

Table 4 Continued

Agent	Side effects	Drug interactions
Trimethoprim–sulfamethoxazole (Bactrim; Septra)	Rash, pruritis, neutropenia, hepatic enzyme elevations, fever, GI intolerance, hyperkalemia	Levels of coumadin, phenytoin, and procainamide are increased by TMP–SMX.
Trimetrexate (Neutrexin)	Must be used with leucovorin to minimize serious antifolate-type toxicities including severe bone marrow suppression and hepatic, GI, and renal toxicities.	Concurrent use of other agents with bone marrow, hepatic, or renal (rarely) toxicity may increase toxicity. Numerous drugs may increase trimetrexate levels (e.g., erythromycin, rifampin, rifabutin, ketoconazole, fluconazole).

All newly febrile patients should have a chest x-ray film. In the absence of another likely source of infection, patients with normal chest x-ray films should undergo sputum induction and bronchoscopy for bronchoalveolar lavage (BAL)—especially in the presence of factors suggesting the diagnosis of PCP (see Table 3). Although PCP is the primary consideration in this situation, aliquots of sputum and BAL specimens should also be examined and cultured for mycobacteria and fungi (39,51). Cultures of sputum or BAL fluid for *Candida*, HSV, and CMV are of no use in determining the pathogenesis of pulmonary dysfunction.

In addition to standard laboratory tests (e.g., CBC, hepatic enzymes, and renal function tests and electrolytes), late-stage febrile patients should have blood cultures drawn for mycobacterial, fungal, and bacterial pathogens (52). Blood cultures and urine cultures for CMV are not useful in this setting (33). Cryptococcal antigen is highly useful, as are serological studies for histoplasmosis and coccidioidomycosis in endemic areas (23–25,35,37).

Ulcerative lesions of skin and mucous membranes should be cultured for HSV. Newly enlarged, hard, fixed, or matted lymph nodes require aspiration for culture and cytological examination, or biopsy for culture and histological examination. Liver biopsy (particularly in the presence of an elevated alkaline phosphatase) and bone marrow biopsy (particularly in the presence of new or unexplained cytopenias) have reasonable diagnostic yields, but their role in the diagnostic workup is debated (53,55). Although MAC is commonly isolated from both sites, mycobacterial blood cultures will be positive in nearly all of these patients, thus diminishing the diagnostic usefulness of these biopsies (56).

At some point in the diagnostic workup, computed tomography (CT) scans of the chest and abdomen are often undertaken to find an occult focus of infection or evidence of malignancy. Plain films or CT scans of the sinuses may identify asymptomatic sinusitis, a not uncommon source of fever in these patients (57). Fever, drenching night sweats, or weight loss in excess of 10% normal body weight are each considered systemic "B" symptoms, which are seen in approximately 80–90% of patients with AIDS-related lymphoma at presentation. Furthermore, Kaposi's sarcoma may also be associated with fever.

D. Intensive Care for Critically Ill Patients

Seriously ill HIV-infected patients who develop acute respiratory failure requiring endotracheal intubation and mechanical ventilation do not have prognoses as dismal as once believed. Reports in the early 1980s suggested that such patients had 10% chance of survival, but studies from the mid- to late-1980s demonstrated survival rates of 40% (58,59–61). Patients with HIV infection need to be assessed similarly to other patients in terms of the appropriateness of intensive care. Functional status before the current acute event, the time elapsed before intensive care during which the efficacy of therapy could be assessed, the certainty of the diagnosis, and the patient's wishes, all are factors that must be considered.

IV. NEUROLOGICAL AND OPHTHALMOLOGICAL INFECTIONS

Most HIV-infected individuals will develop a symptomatic neurological condition at some time during their illness (62). Of these, opportunistic infections of the CNS are of greatest concern. The initial workup of these patients requires a CT or magnetic resonance imaging (MRI) scan to divide conditions that typically present as mass lesions from those that typically do not, such as meningitis and encephalitis. MRI is preferable because of its greater sensitivity in identifying small lesions. Patients who have normal CT scans in the presence of signs and symptoms of focal CNS disease should have a contrast-enhanced MRI scan (63).

A. Mass Lesions of the CNS

Patients with mass lesions usually present with any combination of the expected signs and symptoms, such as altered mental status, focal neurological deficits, and seizures; headache is less common. The presence of fever can be helpful in differentiating infectious from noninfectious causes. Three entities account for more than 80% of CNS mass lesions in late-stage HIV infection—non-Hodgkin's lymphoma (see Chapter 5), toxoplasmosis, and progressive multifocal leuko-

Table 5 HIV-Associated Infections of the CNS and Eye

Common causes of infectious CNS mass lesions:
  Toxoplasma gondii, progressive multifocal leukoencephalopathy
Less common causes of infectious CNS mass lesions:
  Cryptococcus neoformans ("cryptococcoma"), cytomegalovirus, *Histoplasma capsulatum*.
  Coccidiodes immitis, herpes simplex, mycobacteria ("tuberculoma"), brain abscess
Common causes of meningitis/encephalitis:
  C. neoformans, cytomegalovirus
Less common causes of meningitis or encephalitis:
  H. capsulatum and *Coccidioides immitis* (more common in highly endemic areas)
  Listeria monocytogenes, Mycobacterium tuberculosis, Nocardia asteroides, Streptococcus pneumoniae, Haemophilus influenzae, Neisseria meningitides, Treponema pallidum
  Group B streptococcus (children)
  Herpes simplex, varicella–zoster virus
Common cause of retinitis:
  Cytomegalovirus
Less common causes of retinitis:
  Toxoplasma gondii, Candida albicans, Treponema pallidum, herpes zoster virus, *Pneumocystis carinii*

---

encephalopathy (PML; 64). Other infectious agents cause mass lesions in these patients much less commonly (Table 5).

1. Toxoplasmosis

Toxoplasmosis of the CNS is caused by reactivation of latent infection with the protozoan *T. gondii* (21,36). Primary infection occurs through ingestion of undercooked meat (beef, lamb, or pork) or ingestion of cat feces. It characteristically causes multiple ring-enhancing lesions on CT and MRI scans. The lesions of toxoplasmosis are so characteristic that patients are usually begun on therapy presumptively and followed closely for response (65). Serum antitoxoplasma IgG titers, which are positive in almost all patients with proven disease, provide corroborative evidence for the diagnosis (i.e., a negative serological result makes a diagnosis of toxoplasmosis very unlikely). Brain biopsy is usually reserved for patients who have not responded to presumptive therapy for toxoplasmosis. Unless there is a contraindication based on physical examination, such as papilledema or on neuroradiologic abnormality, this latter group of patients should also have a lumbar puncture.

The treatment regimen of choice for toxoplasmosis is sulfadiazine and pyrimethamine (Table 6). Patients unable to tolerate sulfadiazine can be treated with clindamycin and pyrimethamine. Other regimens include atovaquone and pyrimethamine, and dapsone and pyrimethamine. In the absence of clear clinical and radiographic improvement within 14–21 days, the diagnosis should be questioned and a biopsy of the lesions should be performed.

Patients with toxoplasmosis may require steroids (e.g., an initial dose of dexamethasone 10 mg IV, followed by dexamethasone 4 mg IV or PO every 6 h) to control edema and increased intracranial pressure. However, their use should be reserved for clear neurological indications and should be limited to the shortest possible course to avoid additional immunosuppression. Steroid administration obfuscates the assessment of both clinical and radiographic improvement—patients can show early improvement from steroids alone. Seizures require standard anticonvulsant therapy. Prophylactic medication for seizures is not generally recommended.

Infections with *T. gondii.* outside of the CNS (e.g., pulmonary and eye infections) are relatively rare (66,67).

2. Progressive Multifocal Leukoencephalopathy

The JC virus, one of the human papovaviruses, causes PML. It causes diffuse lesions, that are often multiple and are limited to the white matter. They do not enhance with contrast. Although rare cases of spontaneous remission have been reported, the general rule is inexorable (but painless) progressive neurological dysfunction that is not relieved by known therapies (68–70). Trials of cytarabine (ara-C) have failed to demonstrate efficacy (71). Formal investigation of cidofovir will be required to corroborate anecdotal successes (72). Optimization of antiretroviral therapy is generally recommended (73).

B. Meningitis

In contrast with patients with parenchymal mass lesions, as described in the foregoing, patients with disease primarily involving the leptomeninges have fewer focal neurological deficits, although cranial nerve palsies do occur. Fever and headache tend to predominate (acute sinusitis is a common cause of headache and fever in HIV-infected individuals and must be differentiated from the more serious intracranial processes; 57). Nuchal rigidity, photophobia, and altered sensorium may also be present. Because of the high incidence of CNS mass lesions in HIV-infected patients, lumbar puncture is often delayed until the individual has been evaluated for CNS mass lesions by a CT or MRI scan, although this is unnecessary in the absence of focal signs or altered mental status. Opening pressures should be measured and cerebrospinal fluid (CSF) should be sent for the standard analyses. Particularly important in these patients are the cryptococcal antigen assay (on serum as well as CSF), the India ink preparation, the VDRL, and culture for bacterial, fungal, and mycobacterial pathogens. Polymerase chain reaction of CSF for viruses and other pathogens is becoming increasingly available, but remains investigational (74).

1. Cryptococcal Meningitis

Cryptococcus neoformans, a yeast-like fungus, is the most common cause of meningitis in patients with HIV infection (75). Although the organism enters the body through the respiratory tract, pulmonary disease is present in fewer than 30% of patients with cryptococcal meningitis (37,76). Rarely, patients with cryptococcal meningitis will present with a mass lesion of the CNS, or "cryptococcoma."

In AIDS patients, abnormalities of the CSF, such as elevated protein, decreased glucose, and pleocytosis, are less reliable indicators of cryptococcal infection than in other patients, especially in patients with early, mild disease (35). Opening pressures are elevated to levels higher than 200 mmH$_2$O in about 70% of patients. Serum and CSF cryptococcal antigen titers are positive in more than 90% of cases. Fungal cultures of the CSF cultures are positive in essentially 100% of cases, and fungal blood cultures are positive in 60–80% (66).

Therapy should be initiated with amphotericin B, with or without flucytosine (5-FC). Flucytosine adds considerably to toxicity, especially bone marrow suppression (see Table 6; 77). However, it does lead to earlier sterilization of CSF and fewer relapses. Poor prognosis is associated with altered mental status, low CSF white cell count, high cryptococcal antigen titers, positive India ink preparation, and presence of cryptococcal disease outside of the CNS (78). Increased intracranial pressure has also been reported to be an important prognosticator of outcome (79). Serial lumbar punctures with removal of relatively large volumes of fluid (approximately 20 mL) will usually provide control of the increased pressure and will also alleviate headache and vomiting. Return of these symptoms indicates recurrence of increased pressure. If serial lumbar punctures do not control the pressure, shunt placement may be necessary. Glucocorticoids, osmotic agents, and acetazolamide are not generally recommended in the management of this condition.

2. Other Fungal Causes of Meningitis

Meningitis may also be part of disseminated infections with Histoplasma capsulatum and Coccidioides immitis. The CSF findings are nonspecific. As for pulmonary disease caused by these organisms (see Section V), diagnosis depends on preliminary serological tests, followed by confirmatory fungal cultures of blood and CSF (22,23). The mainstay of immediate therapy for disseminated histoplas-

Table 6 Therapy of Opportunistic Infections in Patients with HIV Infection

Disease	Drug	Dose	Route	Interval	Duration
Toxoplasmosis	Sulfadiazine plus pyrimethamine plus leucovorin	1–2 g 50–100 mg[a] 10–25 mg	PO PO PO or IV	q6h q.d. q.d.	Lifelong
	or				
	Clindamycin plus pyrimethamine	600 mg 50–100 mg[a]	PO PO	q6h q.d.	Lifelong
Cryptococcus	Amphotericin B with or without flucytosine	0.3–1.0 mg/kg 25 mg/kg	IV PO	q24h q6h	≥14 days ≥14 days
	or				
	Fluconazole[b] followed by fluconazole	400 mg	PO	q24h	≥14 days
Histoplasmosis	Amphotericin B followed by itraconazole	200 mg 0.5–1.0 mg/kg	PO IV	q24h q24h	Lifelong ≥28–56 days
Coccidiomycosis	Amphotericin B followed by Itraconazole	200 mg 0.5–1.0 mg/kg	PO IV	q12h q24h	Lifelong ≥56 days
	or				
		100–200 mg	PO	b.i.d.	Lifelong
HSV (mucocutaneous)	Amphotericin B	1 mg/kg	IV	q24h	Lifelong
HSV (encephalitis)	Acyclovir	200 mg	PO	5/day	≥7 days
VZV (dermatomal)	Acyclovir	10 mg/kg	IV	q8h	10 days
VZV (disseminated)	Acyclovir	800 mg	PO	5/day	7–10 days
CMV	Acyclovir	10–12 mg/kg	IV	q8h	7–14 days
	Ganciclovir followed by	5 mg	IV	q12h	14–21 days
	Ganciclovir	5 mg/kg	IV	q24h	Lifelong[d]
	or				
	foscarnet followed by	60 mg	IV	q8h	14–21 days
	foscarnet	90–120 mg	IV	q24h	Lifelong[d]

Infection	Regimen	Dose	Route	Frequency	Duration
PCP	Trimethoprim plus sulfamethoxazole	5 mg/kg with 25 mg/kg	PO, IV	q8h	21 days
	or Trimethoprim plus dapsone	300 mg 100 mg	PO PO	q8h q.d.	21 days
	or Pentamidine	3–4 mg/kg	IV (IM)	q.d.	21 days
	or atovaquone	750 mg	PO	q8h	21 days
	or Clindamycin plus primaquine	300–450 mg 15 mg	PO or IV PO	q6h q.d.	21 days
	or Trimetrexate plus leucovorin	45 mg/m^2 20 mg	IV PO or IV	q.d. q6h	21 days
	Severe PCP:[c] Prednisone	Tapering dose	PO	See footnote	See footnote
Candidiasis (oral)	Nystatin	5×10^5–$1 \times 10^6\mu$	PO	q6h	7–10 days
	or fluconazole	100–200 mg	PO or IV	q24h	7–10 days
Candidiasis (esophageal)	Fluconazole	100–400 mg	PO or IV	q24h	14–21 days
MAC	Clarithromycin plus	500 mg	PO	q12h	Lifelong
	ethambutol	15 mg/kg	PO	q24h	Lifelong[d]
	+/– Rifabutin	300–600 mg	PO	q24h	Lifelong[d]

[a] Therapy should begin with a single 200-mg–loading dose of pyrimethamine.
[b] Initial therapy with fluconazole is recommended only with very mild disease and favorable prognostic signs (see text).
[c] Prednisone is highly recommended as an adjunct in severe disease (see text). 40 mg q12h × 5 days, followed by 20 mg q.d. × 5 days, followed by 20 mg q.d. × 11 days.
[d] The 1999 revision of the USPHS/IDSA guidelines for the prevention of opportunistic infections acknowledges that discontinuation of primary prophylaxis (for PCP and MAI) and secondary prophylaxis (for CMV) may be appropriate under certain conditions (8).

mosis and coccidioidomycosis is amphotericin, which is then followed by lifelong therapy, usually with an azole antifungal agent (see Table 6).

3. Miscellaneous Causes of Meningitis

Meningitis caused by *M. tuberculosis* has been reported in the setting of HIV infection, as has syphilitic meningitis (80). Bacterial meningitis caused by *Listeria monocytogenes*, *S. pneumoniae*, *H. influenzae*, *Neisseria menigitidis*, and *Nocardia asteroides* occur and, in general, are managed similar to meningitis caused by those organisms in non–HIV-infected patients. Aseptic meningitis is not uncommon in the setting of HIV disease. It may occur either as part of the acute illness within several weeks of HIV infection ("acute retroviral syndrome"), or it may occur in late-stage HIV infection (81). Although the pathogenesis it is not entirely clear, the etiologic agent may be HIV itself. HIV has been isolated from the CSF of many of these individuals. Other CSF findings, typically mild mononuclear pleocytosis and mild elevation of protein, are nonspecific findings, as they also can be seen in HIV-infected patients in the absence of signs or symptoms of meningitis (82).

C. Viral Encephalitis

Personality and behavioral changes, somnolence, dementia, and headache are the most common symptoms associated with HIV-related viral encephalitis. The cause is usually viral.

1. Cytomegalovirus Encephalitis

Evidence of CNS infection with CMV is common in late-stage AIDS patients. Autopsy series indicate that approximately 25% of patients have evidence of diffuse CMV infection, but clinical illness attributable to such findings is less common (83,84). Antemortem diagnosis can be difficult, which has hampered clear definition of the clinical importance of CMV encephalitis in AIDS. Routine studies of the CSF are nonspecific, although a predominantly polymorphonuclear pleocytosis may occasionally be seen, a finding that is otherwise decidedly unusual in viral infection. Viral cultures of CSF for CMV are rarely positive. Occasionally, the infection is concentrated in the periventricular tissues ("ventriculitis"), which causes a characteristic pattern of periventricular signal enhancement on CT or MRI scans after administration of contrast (85). Improved diagnostic techniques such as PCR are helping to further define this entity (86). Although controlled clinical trials are lacking, treatment with both ganciclovir and foscarnet have been reported to be helpful in the treatment of CMV encephalitis (see Table 6; 87,88).

2. Herpes Simplex and Varicella–Zoster Virus Encephalitis

Encephalitis caused by HSV (both HSV-I and HSV-2) and varicella–zoster virus (VZV) have been reported, but are extremely unusual (89,90). VZV infection of the CNS is usually the result of dissemination of reactivated localized cutaneous infection. As with CMV, the clinical and CSF findings are nonspecific, and results of viral cultures are usually negative. The diagnosis is difficult, but PCR holds promise (74). In HSV encephalitis, diagnostic imaging may reveal lesions (often in the temporal lobe) that may provide guidance for biopsy. Treatment is with intravenous acyclovir (see Table 6).

D. Retinitis

1. Cytomegalovirus Retinitis

The retina is the most common site of clinically significant CMV disease. Symptoms depend on the site of the lesions: floaters may be the chief complaint in patients with peripheral lesions, whereas more central lesions are likely to cause scintillating scotomas and visual field defects. Rapid and pronounced decrease in visual acuity is associated with macular disease or disease of the optic nerve (91). On fundoscopic examination the lesions appear as perivascular whitish granular infiltrates with hemorrhage (''catsup and mustard'' lesions). Emergency ophthalmological referral is mandatory in any AIDS patient with new onset of visual symptoms.

Intravenous ganciclovir and foscarnet appear to be of equivalent efficacy in the treatment of CMV retinitis (92). However, foscarnet appears to offer a survival advantage that may be due to its inherent antiretroviral activity (93). This advantage may not be relevant in the era of highly active antiretroviral regimens. Oral ganciclovir, intravitrial ganciclovir implants, and cidofovir have markedly improved the long-term management of CMV retinitis (94,95). The goal of any of these therapies is to minimize disease progression (see Table 6).

2. Miscellaneous Causes of Retinitis

Although decidedly less common, retinitis other than that caused by CMV is seen in HIV disease (see Table 5). Differentiating one of these rarer causes of demands expert ophthalmological assistance (96,97).

IV. PULMONARY INFECTIONS

As in non–HIV-infected patients, the possibility of pulmonary disease in HIV-infected patients will usually be raised by symptoms such as fever, cough, dyspnea, and chest pain. These symptoms usually lead to a chest radiograph. Unlike other settings, in HIV a normal chest x-ray film does not effectively "rule out" pneumonitis: 10% of patients with confirmed pulmonary infections have no evidence of infiltrate at the time of presentation. Moreover, in patients with an abnormal chest x-ray film, the pattern of abnormality in HIV-infected patients is less likely to narrow the differential diagnosis than it does in their non–HIV-infected counterparts (98–100). Although common patterns predominate, HIV-associated pulmonary infections can present with uncommon radiographic patterns (Table 7; 101). PCP provides a prime example: besides bilateral diffuse infiltrates, focal infiltrates, lobar infiltrates, nodules, consolidation with air bronchograms, cavities, pneumatocoeles, bronchiectasis, pneumothorax, and pleural effusions, all have been described. In addition, biapical infiltrates have been described in patients receiving PCP prophylaxis with aerosolized pentamidine (102). Thus, in the setting of HIV, pulmonary symptoms in the presence of a normal chest x-ray film requires evaluation beyond that which is usual, and an abnormal chest x-ray film only provides documentation of an active pulmonary process requiring further evaluation (103).

A. Diffuse Interstitial Infiltrates

1. *Pneumocystis carinii* Pneumonia

Despite widespread use very effective prophylactic regimens, *P. carinii* remains the most common cause of pulmonary disease in late-stage HIV infection and the most common cause of bilateral diffuse infiltrates on chest radiographs (104). The most common presentation is an indolent onset of dry cough, malaise, fever, and night sweats that may be associated with weight loss (12). The diagnosis rests on the demonstration of organisms in sputum, bronchoalveolar lavage (BAL) fluid, or tissue, using special stains or immunofluorescence techniques (105,106). *Pneumocystis* is found in expectorated sputum in approximately 20% of AIDS patients with PCP, in induced sputum in approximately 80–90%, and in BAL fluid in more than 95%. The yield with transbronchial biopsy approaches 100%. However, yields vary from center-to-center depending on experience with the various diagnostic techniques. At many centers examination of expectorated and induced sputum is not routinely carried out, thereby making bronchoscopic BAL the diagnostic procedure of choice.

Treatment should begin as soon as the diagnosis, or presumptive diagnosis is made. In other than very mild disease, therapy should be instituted before definitive bronchoscopic diagnosis if that procedure is to be at all delayed (diagnostic yields are not affected by several days of treatment before bronchoscopy is performed). Mild to moderate disease may be treated as an outpatient with one of the recommended oral regimens and close monitoring (see Table 6).

Table 7 HIV-Associated Pulmonary Infections, by Radiographic Presentation

Diffuse infiltrate
  Common conditions
    Pneumocystis carinii pneumonia[a,b]
    Tuberculosis (common pattern in late-stage HIV disease)[b,c]
    Histoplasmosis (in hyperendemic areas)[b,c,d]
  Uncommon conditions
    Cryptococcosis[b]
    Coccidioidomycoses (in hyperendemic areas)[b,c,d]
    Cytomegalovirus pneumonia
    Mycobacterium avium-intracellulare pneumonia
    Legionella pneumonia
    Atypical bacterial pneumonia
    Herpes simplex pneumonia
Nodules and nodular infiltrate
  Common conditions
    Tuberculosis (common pattern in early-stage HIV disease)[b,c,d]
    Pneumocystis carinii pneumonia[a,b] (most common after diffuse interstitial pattern)
  Uncommon conditions
    Mycobacterium kansasii pneumonia[b]
    Toxoplasmosis
Focal infiltrate with or without consolidation
  Common conditions
    Bacterial "community-acquired" pneumonia[d]
    Staphylococcus aureus pneumonia[b,d]
    Gram-negative pneumonias (common only in late-stage disease)
  Uncommon conditions
    Rhodococcus equi pneumonia[b]
    Nocardiosis[b,d]
    Aspergillosis[b]

[a] May be associated with pneumothorax.
[b] May be associated with cavitary lesions.
[c] May be associated with hilar adenopathy.
[d] May be associated with pleural effusion.

For severe disease, treatment with either intravenous TMP–SMZ or IV pentamidine is recommended. Indicators of severe disease include marked hypoxia ($Pao_2 < 70$ mmHg on room air), a very wide alveolar–arterial gradient [$P(A-a)o_2 > 35$ mmHg on room air], severe abnormalities on initial chest radiographs, numerous organisms or the presence of greater than 5% neutrophils in BAL fluid, and an elevated serum LDH value (>300 U/L; 108). Severe adverse reactions necessitating discontinuation of pentamidine occur in approximately 40% of patients. Side effects of TMP–SMZ occur with similar frequency, but are much less severe and less frequently require discontinuation, making it the treatment of choice (see Table 6; 109).

Corticosteroids decrease the incidence of respiratory failure as well as overall mortality in patients with moderate to severe PCP (Pao$_2$ < 70 mmHg). A 3-week course of tapering doses of prednisone is a highly recommended therapeutic adjunct in this setting (see Table 6; 110).

Oxygen desaturation may occur 3–7 days after initiation of therapy and does not necessarily indicate treatment failure, as therapy may cause a transient increase in the inflammatory response in the lung. This response is blunted by the addition of steroids to the treatment regimen.

2. Pulmonary Histoplasmosis and Coccidioidomycosis

Diffuse interstitial infiltrate is also the most common radiographic pattern in pulmonary histoplasmosis and coccidioidomycosis in HIV-infected patients; nodular and cavitary lesions are much less common. As mentioned in Section IV.B.2, these infections are largely confined to endemic areas where they are important causes of pulmonary and disseminated disease. In certain metropolitan areas of the midwestern United States, histoplasmosis is more common than PCP in AIDS patients (22,23). Diagnosis is made by examination and culture of sputum and BAL fluid for fungi. Fungal blood cultures are also useful, as are specific serodiagnostic tests (coccidioides antibody and histoplasma antigen). Therapy is usually begun with amphotericin (see Table 6).

3. Tuberculosis

Tuberculosis is a common cause of diffuse interstitial infiltrate in late-stage HIV disease (111,112). This presentation is distinct from the nodular and cavitary disease (usually of the upper lobes) that is common in earlier-stage HIV infections as well as in non–HIV-infected individuals. Delayed-type hypersensitivity skin testing for *M. tuberculosis* is of little value in patients with advanced HIV infection, owing to their underlying defect in cell-mediated immunity. As in other settings, diagnosis is made by culture of clinical specimens. Specific regimens using standard drugs have been developed for HIV-infected patients (113).

4. Other Causes of Diffuse Interstitial Infiltrate

The role of CMV as a cause of pulmonary pathology in HIV-infected individuals has yet to be fully defined (114). Although virus can commonly be isolated from pulmonary secretions and tissue of patients with pneumonitis, other pathogens are also usually present (115). Examination of sputum or BAL fluid or tissue may reveal the presence of typical CMV viral inclusions in respiratory epithelium, but these findings do not always necessarily indicate a disease requiring specific treatment. In the absence of convincing data, it is probably prudent to assume that CMV alone may occasionally cause interstitial lung disease very late in the course of HIV infection, and that these patients may benefit from specific anti-CMV therapy (see Table 6). Pneumonia caused by HSV and MAC is also poorly defined. Legionnaires' disease, however, is well described (116).

B. Nodules and Nodular Infiltrates

1. Cryptococcal Pneumonia

The most common pathogen presenting as a nodular infiltrate in the setting of AIDS is *Cryptococcus neoformans* (37,76,117). Cryptococcal pneumonia usually coexists with cryptococcal meningitis. The serum cryptococcal antigen test result is usually positive with coexisting meningitis, but is often negative in the setting of isolated pulmonary disease (118). The diagnosis is made by examination of sputum and BAL fluid for the characteristic yeast forms; fungal cultures confirm the diagnosis. Initial treatment is usually with amphotericin (see Table 6).

2. Other Causes of Nodular Infiltrates

The differential diagnosis of nodular infiltrates also includes tuberculosis (early in the course of HIV infection), Kaposi's sarcoma (see Chapter 4), and lymphoma (see Chapter 5). PCP only rarely causes this chest radiographic pattern (102).

C. Focal Infiltrates

1. Bacterial Pneumonia

Community-acquired pneumonia (CAP) caused by *S. pneumoniae, H. influenzae, Staphylococcus aureus*, and *Branhamella catarrhalis*, is common at all stages of HIV infection (119,120). Gram-negative pneumonia, particularly that caused by *Pseudomonas aeruginosa*, generally occurs only very late in HIV disease (121). Focal infiltrate, sometimes with consolidation, is the most common presentation. Diagnosis is usually made by examination and culture of expectorated sputum; blood culture results are frequently positive (122).

Treatment is generally the same as that for the same infection in non–HIV-infected patient. When microbiological diagnosis is delayed, a second- or third-generation cephalosporin, a quinolone with adequate activity against gram-positive cocci, or a macrolide is most commonly employed as initial therapy on an empiric basis.

2. Other Causes of Focal Infiltrates

Two less common opportunistic organisms, *Rhodococcus equi*, a gram-positive rod, and *Nocardia asteroides*, a gram-positive filamentous bacteria, are well-documented causes of focal infiltrates in HIV-infected individuals. Both of these organisms tend to cause cavitary lesions. Prolonged combination antibiotic therapy (e.g., erythromycin and rifampin) is required for *Rhodococcus*; sulfonamides are the drugs of choice for *Nocardia* (123,124).

VI. GASTROINTESTINAL INFECTIONS

A. Esophagitis

Symptomatic esophagitis, usually caused by one of three opportunistic pathogens, will occur in approximately 50% of AIDS patients (Table 8). Primary symptoms are odynophagia and dysphagia.

1. Candidal Esophagitis

Candida albicans is the most common cause of esophagitis in AIDS patients (125). Odynophagia or dysphagia in the presence of oral thrush is often treated empirically with oral fluconazole (see Table 6). Endoscopy is usually undertaken when empiric therapy fails or one of the other causes of esophagitis is suspected. When carried out, endoscopy reveals shallow erosions, with overlying plaques or pseudomembranes. Fungal smears and cultures, a KOH preparation, and histology confirm the diagnosis.

2. Other Causes of Esophagitis

Three other common causes of esophagitis—HSV, CMV, and aphthous ulceration—cause localized pain owing to discrete ulcerative lesions. Biopsy is re-

Table 8 HIV-Associated Gastrointestinal Infections

Esophagitis
    Candida, cytomegalovirus, herpes simplex, idiopathic aphthous ulceration
Acute enterocolitis
    Salmonella, Shigella, Campylobacter
    Clostridium difficile (toxin-associated enterocolitis)
Chronic enterocolitis
    Cryptosporidia, Isospora, Microsporida, *Cyclospora*
    Cytomegalovirus, *Mycobacterium avium–intracellulare*

quired to differentiate CMV ulcerations from those caused by HSV. Although culture may assist in the diagnosis of herpes, CMV cultures are unreliable in this setting. The treatment for the former is acyclovir, for the latter, ganciclovir (see Table 6; 126). Esophagitis caused by idiopathic aphthous ulcer is diagnosed when no evidence of one of the other common pathogens can be found. Treatment with thalidomide or corticosteroids may be useful (127).

B. Acute Enterocolitis

Most HIV-infected patients experience episodes of diarrhea. The differential diagnosis of acute diarrhea, with or without fever, is not unlike that for non–HIV-infected patients (see Table 8) and the workup (i.e., examination of stool for ova and parasites and stool culture) is generally the same as for non–HIV-infected patient; however, blood culture results are frequently positive and should be obtained (128,129). Treatment for these enteric pathogens is similar to that used in other settings. However, *Salmonella* infections are particularly problematic in AIDS patients: bacteremia may recur following initial treatment and may require long-term suppressive therapy (130). Acute diarrhea caused by *Clostridium difficile* toxin is not uncommon in AIDS patients (131). Standard regimens with either oral vancomycin or metronidazole are recommended, but response to therapy may be less prompt in these patients.

C. Chronic Enterocolitis

Up to 80% of patients with chronic diarrhea (diarrhea persisting for more than 30 days) will have identifiable enteric pathogens. Such diarrhea is often a major contributor to the wasting syndrome associated with late-stage HIV infection (128,129). Most cases of infectious chronic diarrhea are caused by a distinct spectrum of pathogens (see Table 8).

Protozoa are probably the most common cause. Although certain of these infections (e.g., *Entamoeba histolytica* and *Giardia lamblia*) have an increased incidence in gay men, these parasites do not cause disproportionate disease among AIDS patients (132). However, other waterborne protozoa are important: *Cryptosporidia parvum, Isospora belli*, Microsporida, and *Cyclospora cayetanensis* (133–135). All commonly cause prolonged, profuse, debilitating watery diarrhea without fever. Diagnosis of cryptosporidiosis and isosporiasis is made by modified acid-fast staining of stool specimens or by special histology stains of tissue from bowel biopsy. Microsporidiosis is a more difficult diagnosis to make owing to the very small size of the organism. Electron microscopic examination of tissue obtained by small bowel biopsy has been the standard method of diagnosis, although a special trichrome stain of stool has been described and promises to facilitate the diagnosis (136).

Treatment of both cryptosporidiosis and microsporidiosis in the setting of AIDS is often unsatisfactory, although there are anecdotal reports of partial success with several drugs (paromomycin and clarithromycin for cryptosporidiosis; albendazole [for *Septata intestinalis*, but not for *Enterocytozoon bieneusi*], and atovaquone for microsporidiosis; 137,138). Isosporiasis and cyclosporiasis, however, are readily treated with trimethoprim–sulfamethoxazole or pyrimethamine (see Table 6).

Chronic diarrhea caused by CMV colitis is generally a very late-stage manifestation of HIV disease. Diagnosis is made by identification of characteristic CMV inclusion bodies on histopathological examination of biopsy specimens. Treatment is generally the same as for cytomegalovirus infection at other sites (see Table 6).

Gastrointestinal involvement with *M. avium* complex (MAC) is not yet well defined. In late-stage HIV-disease it is probably associated with chronic diarrhea, fever, night sweats, and weight loss. The major site of involvement appears to be the small intestine. MAC may also be associated with mesenteric or retroperitoneal lymphodenopathy, or both. Diagnosis is made by demonstration of typical acid-fast organisms in stool or on the mucosal surface of bowel biopsies. Treatment is the same as for systemic MAC infection (see Table 6).

Many AIDS patients who do not respond well to specific therapy for chronic diarrhea will respond at least partially to symptomatic treatment with agents such as diphenoxolate, loperamide, tincture of opium, or codeine. Octreotide, a synthetic analogue of somatostatin, has been reported to be of benefit in some patients with crytosporidial diarrhea (139).

Gut infections with CMV and cryptosporidia may involve the biliary tree, which can lead to obstruction associated with pancreatitis (140).

VII. BACTEREMIA AND SEPSIS

Fever is probably the most common symptom reported by patients at all stages of HIV infection (50). In late-stage HIV infection, fever with night sweats are common. Although most patients will have localizing signs and symptoms, fever without a specific locus of infection is not uncommon in this population. Small studies indicate that occult infections account for more than 80% of these episodes. Lymphoma and drug reactions account for less than 10%. PCP, MAC infections, CMV infections, sinusitis, and endocarditis are among the most common causes (56,11–143). Fever caused by HIV infection alone is felt to be rare and is a diagnosis of exclusion.

Bacteremia is common in both HIV-infected adults and children (144,145). Frank sepsis, however, appears to be less commonly associated with bacteremia in AIDS patients than in other settings. A source of infection in bacteremic pa-

Table 9 Recommended Prophylactic Regimens for HIV-Associated Opportunistic Infections

Pathogen	Major indications	Recommended regimen(s)	Alternative regimen(s) and *comments*
Pneumocystis carinii	CD4+ count <200, or oropharyngeal thrush, or prior PCP	TMP–SMZ (1 DS or SS tablet daily)	TMP–SMZ (DS tablet 3× per week) Dapsone (50 mg daily) + pyrimethamine (50 mg weekly) + leukovorin (25 mg weekly) Aerosolized pentamidine (300 mg monthly)
Mycobacterium tuberculosis	+PPD or close contact	INH (300 mg) + pyridoxine (50 mg) daily for 9 mo or INH (900 mg) + pyridoxine (50 mg) twice weekly for 9 mo	Rifampin (600 mg) q.d. for 4 mo; or rifampin or rifabutin (300 mg q.d.) + pyrazinamide (20 mg q.d.) for 2 mo. Rifampin is the agent of choice if exposure was to INH-resistant TB. Exposure to multidrug-resistant TB requires consultation with public health officials.
Toxoplasma gondii	IgG antibody and CD4+ <100	TMP–SMZ (1 DS tablet daily)	TMP–SMZ (1 DS tablet daily) Dapsone (50 mg daily) + pyrimethamine (50 mg weekly) + leukovorin (25 mg weekly)
Mycobacterium avium complex	CD4+ <50	Clarithromycin (500 mg b.i.d.) or azithromycin (1200 mg weekly)	Rifabutin (300 mg daily) Azithromycin (1200 mg weekly) + rifabutin (300 mg daily)

tients is not obvious in approximately 20% of patients. Gram-positive organisms, including *Strep. pneumoniae, Staph. aureus,* and other *Streptococcus* spp., are the most common isolates in all series. The most common gram-negative isolates are *P. aeruginosa, Salmonella* spp., and *Escherichia coli. Bartonella henselae* (formerly *Rochalimaea henselae*), the causative organism of cat-scratch disease, cutaneous bacillary angiomatosis, and peliosis hepatis, may also present as a ''fever and bacteremia'' syndrome (146).

Neutropenia (fewer than 500 neutrophils per cubic millimeter) has been reported to be associated with bacteremia in more than 20% of cases of bacteremia in AIDS patients. Indwelling intravenous catheters are being increasingly used in AIDS patients; as in other populations these devices are an important risk factor in the development of bacteremia and sepsis (147). Once cultures have been obtained, empiric broad-spectrum antibiotic coverage is generally begun, especially in the settings of sepsis or neutropenia. As in other situations, the antibiotic regimen is then modified once culture results are known and the patient's clinical status is reassessed.

VIII. PREVENTION OF OPPORTUNISTIC INFECTIONS

AIDS was first recognized as a distinct clinical entity through its remarkable association with PCP, which accounted for much of the morbidity and mortality during the first years of the epidemic (30,48,49). The first studies on the use of prophylactic agents in HIV-infected patients naturally targeted this entity (150). These studies, which ultimately demonstrated that PCP prophylaxis prolongs life and decreases morbidity, provided the framework for evaluation of prophylactic strategies for other OIs (151). In addition to efficacy, long-term safety, tolerability, ease of administration, and cost, all must be considered (152,153). Given such analyses, the U. S. Public Health Service makes recommendations for the routine use of prophylactic agents (Table 9). Vaccination with pneumococcal vaccine is recommended for all patients. Hepatitis B vaccine is generally recommended for susceptible patients (hepatitis B core antibody-negative patients). Annual administration of influenza vaccine is recommended, despite concern for inducing an increase in HIV viral replication. Hepatitis A vaccine is recommended for susceptible patients who have chronic hepatitis C (8).

REFERENCES

1. Fauci AS, Pantaleo G, Stanley S, Weissman D. NIH Conference: mechanisms of HIV infection. Ann Intern Med 124:654–663, 1996.

2. Pantaleo GP, Graziosi C, Fauci AS. The immunopathogenesis of human immuno-deficiency virus infection. N Engl J Med 328:327–335, 1993.
3. Centers for Disease Control. 1993 revised classification system for HIV infection and expanded surveillance definition for AIDS among adolescents and adults. MMWR Morbid Mortal Wkly Rep 41(RR-17), 1992.
4. Stein DS, Korvick JA, Vermund SH. CD4+ lymphocyte cell enumeration for pre-diction of clinical course of human immunodeficiency virus disease: a review. J Infect Dis 165:352–363, 1992.
5. Holmberg SD, Buchbinder SP, Conley LJ, et al. The spectrum of medical conditions and symptoms before acquired immunodeficiency syndrome in homosexual and bisexual men infected with the human immunodeficiency virus. Am J Epidemiol 141:395–404, 1995.
6. Moore RD, Chaisson RE. Natural history of opportunistic diseases in an HIV-infected urban clinical cohort. Ann Intern Med 124:633–642, 1996.
7. Taylor JM, Fahey JL, Detels R, et al. CD4 percentage, CD4 number, and CD4: CD8 ratio in HIV infection: which to choose and how to use. J AIDS 1:114–124, 1989.
8. Centers for Disease Control. 1999 USPHS/IDSA guidelines for the prevention of opportunistic infections in persons infected with human immunodeficiency virus. MMWR Morbid Mortal Wkly Rep 48, 1999. In press.
9. Phair J, Munoz A, Detels R, et al. The risk of *Pneumocystis carinii* pneumonia among men infected with human immunodeficiency virus type 1. N Engl J Med 322:161–165, 1990.
10. USPHS/IDSA Prevention of Opportunistic Infections Working Group. Guidelines for the prevention of opportunistic infections in persons infected with human immu-nodeficiency virus: disease-specific recommendations. Clin Infect Dis 21(suppl 1): S32–43, 1995.
11. Simonds RJ, Hughes WT, Feinberg J, et al. Preventing *Pneumocystis carinii* pneu-monia in persons infected with human immunodeficiency virus. Clin Infect Dis 21(suppl 1):S44–48, 1995.
12. Kovacs JA, Masur H. Prophylaxis for *Pneumocystis carinii* pneumonia in patients infected with the human immunodeficiency virus. 14:1005–1009, 1992.
13. USPHS/IDSA Prevention of Opportunistic Infections Working Group. Guidelines for the prevention of opportunistic infections in persons infected with human immu-nodeficiency virus: introduction. Clin Infect Dis 21(suppl 1):S1–11, 1995.
14. Kaplan LD, Abrams DI, Feigal E, et al. AIDS-associated non-Hodgkin's lymphoma in San Francisco. JAMA 261:719–724, 1989.
15. Lowenthal DA, Straus DF, Campbell SW, Gold JWM, Clarkson BD, Koziner B. AIDS-related lymphoid neophasia: the Memorial Hospital experience. Cancer 61: 2325–2327, 1988.
16. Knowlers DM, Chalmulak GA, Subar M, et al. Lymphoid neoplasia associated with the acquired immunodeficiency syndrome (AIDS): the New York University Medical Center experience with 105 patients (1981–1986). Ann Intern Med 108: 744–753, 1988.
17. Kaplan LD, Straus DJ, Testa MA, Von Roenn J, Dezube BJ, Cooley TP, Herndier B, Northfelt DW, Huang J, Tulpule A, Levine AM. Low-dose compared with stan-

dard-dose m-BACOD chemotherapy for non–Hodgkin's lymphoma associated with human immunodeficiency virus infection. N Engl J Med 336:16411648, 1997.

18. Piscitelli SC, Flexner C, Minor JR, Polis MA, Masur H. Drug interactions in patients infected with human immunodeficiency virus. Clin Infect Dis 23:685–93, 1996.

19. Johnson MP, Chaisson RE. Tuberculosis and HIV disease. In: Volberding PA, Jacobson MA, eds. AIDS Clinical Review 1993/1994. New York: Marcel Dekker, 1994:73–94.

20. Abouya YL, Beumel A, Lucas S, et al. *Pneumocystis carinii* pneumonia: an uncommon cause of death in African patients with acquired immunodeficiency syndrome. Am Rev Respir Dis. 125:617–620, 1992.

21. Luft BJ, Hafner R, Korzun, AH, et al. Toxoplasmic encephalitis in patients with the acquired immunodeficiency syndrome. N Engl J Med 329:995–1000, 1993.

22. Sarosi GA, Johnson PC. Disseminated histoplasmosis in patients with human immunodeficiency virus. Clin Infect Dis 14:S60–S67, 1992.

23. Wheat J. Histoplasmosis and coccidioidomycosis in individuals with AIDS. Infect Dis Clin North Am 8:467–482, 1994.

24. Fish DG, Ampel NM, Galgiani HM, et al. Coccidioidomycosis during human immunodeficiency virus infection. A review of 77 patients. Medicine 69:623–625, 1990.

25. Dehovitz JA, Pape JW, Boney M, et al. Clinical manifestations and therapy of *Isospora belli* infection in patients with the acquired immunodeficiency syndrome. N Engl J Med 315:87–90, 1986.

26. Pape JW, Verdier RI, Boncy M, et al. *Cyclospora* infection in adults with HIV: clinical manifestations, treatment, and prophylaxis. Ann Intern Med 121:654–657, 1994.

27. Zurlo JJ, Wood L, Gaglione MM, Polis MA. Effect of splenectomy on T lymphocyte subsets in patients infected with the human immunodeficiency virus. Clin Infect Dis 20:768–771, 1995.

28. Tappero JW, Mohle-Boetani J, Koehler JE, et al. The epidemiology of bacillary angiomatosis and bacillary peliosis. JAMA 269:770–775, 1993.

29. Glaser CA, Angulo FJ, Rooner JA. Animal associated opportunistic infections among persons infected with the human immunodeficiency virus. Clin Infect Dis 18:14–24, 1994.

30. Osmond D, Charlebois E, Lang W, et al. Changes in AIDS survival time in two San Francisco cohorts of homosexual men, 1983–1992. JAMA 271:1083–1087, 1994.

31. Lane HC (moderator). Recent advances in the management of AIDS-related opportunistic infections. Ann Intern Med 120:945–955, 1994.

32. Jacobson MA, Mills J. Serious cytomegalovirus disease in the acquired immunodeficiency syndrome (AIDS). Ann Intern Med 108:585–594, 1988.

33. Zurlo JJ, O'Neill D, Polis MA, et al. Lack of clinical utility of cytomegalovirus blood and urine cultures in patients with HIV infection. Ann Intern Med 118:12–17, 1993.

34. Kovacs JA, Hiemenz JW, Macher AM, et al. *Pneumocystis carinii* pneumonia: a

comparison between patients with the acquired immunodeficiency syndrome and other immunodeficiencies. Ann Intern Med 100:663–671, 1984.

35. Kovacs JA, Kovacs AA, Polis MA, et al. Cryptococcosis in the acquired immunodeficiency syndrome. Ann Intern Med 103:533–538, 1985.

36. Porter SB, Sande MA. Toxoplasmosis of the central nervous system in the acquired immunodeficiency syndrome. N Engl J Med 327:1643–1648, 1992.

37. Chuck SL, Sande MA. Infections with *Cryptococcus neoformans* in the acquired immunodeficiency syndrome. N Engl J Med 321:794–799, 1989.

38. Masur H. Prevention and treatment of *Pneumocystis* pneumonia. N Engl J Med 327:1853–1860, 1992.

39. Baughman RP, Dohn MN, Frame PT. The continuing utility of bronchoalveolar lavage to diagnose opportunistic infection in AIDS patients. Am J Med 97:515–522, 1994.

40. Powderly WG. Resistant candidiasis. AIDS Res Hum Retroviruses 8:925–929, 1994.

41. Kuppermann BD. Therapeutic options for resistant cytomegalovirus retinitis. J Acquir Immune Defic Syndr Hum Retrovirol 14(suppl), 1997.

42. Balfour HH, Benson C, Braun J, Cassens B, Erice A, Friedman-Kien T, Polsky B, Safrin S. Management of acyclovir-resistant herpes simplex and varicella-zoster virus infections. J Acquir Immune Defic Syndr 7:524–560, 1994.

43. American Thoracic Society. Treatment of tuberculosis and tuberculosis infection in adults and children. Am J Respir Crit Care Med 149:1359–1374, 1994.

44. Drew WL. Cytomegalovirus infection in patients with AIDS. Clin Infect Dis 14:608–615, 1992.

45. Tu JV, Biem HJ, Detsky AS. Bronchoscopy versus empirical therapy in HIV-infected patients with presumptive *Pneumocystis carinii* pneumonia: a decision analysis. Am Rev Respir Dis 148:370–377, 1993.

46. Vander Els NJ. Approach to the patient with pulmonary disease. Semin Respir Crit Care Med 16:240–250, 1995.

47. Gordin FM, Simon GL, Wofsy CB, Mills J. Adverse reactions to trimethoprim-sulfamethoxazole in patients with AIDS. Ann Intern Med 100:495–499, 1984.

48. Calenda V, Chermann JC. The effects of HIV on hematopoiesis. Eur J Haematol 48:181–186, 1992.

49. Youle MS, Gazzard BG, Johnson MA, Cooper DA, Hoy JF, Busch H, Ruf B, Griffiths PD, Stephenson SL, Dancox M, Bell AR. Effects of high-dose oral acyclovir on herpesvirus disease and survival in patients with advanced HIV disease: a double-blind, placebo-controlled study. AIDS 8:641–649, 1994.

50. Sullivan M, Feinberg J, Bartlett JG. Fever in patients with HIV infection. Infect Dis Clin North Am 10:149–65, 1996.

51. Broaddus C, Dake MD, Stulbard MS, et al. Bronchoalveolar lavage and transbronchial biopsy for the diagnosis of pulmonary infections in the acquired immunodeficiency syndrome. Ann Intern Med 102:747–752, 1985.

52. Katz SJ, Wenger NS, Shapiro MF. Diagnostic value of bacterial and fungal blood cultures in patients with the acquired immunodeficiency syndrome. Am J Med 88:28N–31N, 1990.

53. Cappell MS, Schwartz MS, Biempica L. Clinical utility of liver biopsy in patients

with serum antibodies to the human immunodeficiency virus. Am J Med 88:123–130, 1990.

54. Lebovics E, Thung SN, Schaffner F, Radensky PW. The liver in the acquired immunodeficiency syndrome: a clinical and histologic study. Hepatology 5:293–298, 1985.

55. Vazquez M, Rotterdam H, Vamvakas E. Diagnostic yields of surgical specimens from patients with AIDS or at risk for AIDS. Prog AIDS Pathol 2:187–194, 1990.

56. Prego V, Glatt AE, Roy V, et al. Comparative yield of blood culture for fungi and mycobacteria, liver biopsy, and bone marrow biopsy in the diagnosis of fever of undetermined origin in human immunodeficiency virus-infected patients. Arch Intern Med 150:333–336, 1990.

57. Zurlo JJ, Jeurstein IM, Lebovics R, et al. Sinusitis in HIV-1 infection. Am J Med 93:167–172, 1992.

58. Wachter RM, Luce JM, Turner J, et al. Intensive care of patients with the acquired immunodeficiency syndrome: outcome and changing patterns of utilization. Am Rev Respir Dis 134:891–896, 1986.

59. Rogers PL, Lane HC, Henderson DK, et al. Admission of AIDS patients to a medical intensive care unit: causes and outcome. Crit Care Med 17:113–117, 1989.

60. Friedman Y, Franklin C, Freeis S, et al. Long-term survival of patients with AIDS, *Pneumocystis carinii* pneumonia, and respiratory failure. JAMA 266:89–92, 1991.

61. Wachter RM, Luce JM, Safrin S, et al. Cost and outcome of intensive care for patients with AIDS, *Pneumocystis carinii* pneumonia, and severe respiratory failure. JAMA 273:230–235, 1995.

62. McArthur JC. Neurologic manifestations of AIDS. Medicine 66:407–437, 1987.

63. Levy RM, Mills CM, Posin JP, et al. The efficacy and clinical impact of brain imaging in neurologically symptomatic AIDS patients: a prospective CT/MRI study. J Acquir Immune Defic Syndr 3:461–471, 1990.

64. Bacellar JA, Muûoz A, Miller EN et al. Temporal trends in the incidence of HIV-1-related neurologic diseases: Multicenter AIDS Cohort Study, 1985–1992. Neurology 44:1892–1900, 1994.

65. Cohn JA, McMeeking A, Cohen W, et al. Evaluation of the policy of empiric treatment of suspected *Toxoplasma* encephalitis in patients with the acquired immunodeficiency syndrome. Am J Med. 86:521–527, 1989.

66. Oksenhendler E, Cadranel J, Sarfati C, et al. *Toxoplasma gondii* pneumonia in patients with the acquired immunodeficiency syndrome. Am J Med 88:5–18, 1990.

67. Cochereau-Massin I, LeHoang P, Lautier-Frau M, et al. Ocular toxoplasmosis in human immunodeficiency virus-infected patients. Am J Ophthalmol 114–130–135, 1992.

68. Berger JR, Kaszovitz B, Post J, et al. Progressive multifocal leukoencephalopathy associated with human immunodeficiency virus infection: a review of the literature with a report of sixteen cases. Ann Intern Med 107:78–87, 1987.

69. Whiteman ML, Post MJ, Berger JR, Tate LG, Bell MD, Limonte LP. Progressive multifocal leukoencephalopathy in 47 HIV-seropositive patients: neuroimaging with clinical and pathologic correlation. Radiology 187:233–240, 1993.

70. Bedro K., Weinstein W, Degregoria P, et al. Progressive multifocal leukoencepha-

lopathy in acquired immunodeficiency syndrome. N Engl J Med 309:492–493, 1983.

71. Hall C, Timpone J, Dafni I, Antonijevic Z, Millar L, Booss J, Clifford D, Cohen B, McArthur J, Hollander H. ARA-C treatment of PML in AIDS patients [abstr]. 4th Conference on Retroviruses and Opportunistic Infections, Washington, DC, Jan 22–26, 1997.

72. Safrin RS, Marra CM, Colson N, Jaffe HS. Cidofovir (CDV) therapy for progressive multifocal leukoencephalopathy (PML) in two AIDS patients [abstr]. 37th Interscience Conference on Antimicrobial Agents and Chemotherapy, Toronto, Canada. Sept 28–Oct 1, 1997.

73. Sacktor N, McArthur J. Prospects for therapy of HIV-associated neurologic disease. J Neurovirol 3:89–101, 1997.

74. Pollack H, Zhan MX, Safrit JT, et al. Diagnosis of central nervous system complications in HIV-infected patients: cerebrospinal fluid analysis by the polymerase chain reaction. AIDS 11:1–17, 1997.

75. Dismukes WE. Cryptococcal meningitis in patients with AIDS. J Infect Dis 157: 624–628, 1988.

76. Zuger A, Louie E, Holzman RS, Simberkoff MS, Rahal JJ. Cryptococcal disease in patients with the acquired immunodeficiency syndrome. Ann Intern Med 104: 234–40, 1986.

77. Van der Horst CM, Saag MS, Cloud GA, et al. Treatment of cryptococcal meningitis associated with the acquired immunodeficiency syndrome. N Engl J Med 337: 15–21, 1997.

78. Larsen RA, Leal M, Chan L. Fluconazole compared with amphotericin B therapy plus flucytosine for cryptococcal meningitis in AIDS. Ann Intern Med 113:183–187, 1990.

79. Denning DW, Armstrong RW, Lewis BH, et al. Elevated cerebrospinal fluid pressures in patients with cryptococcal meningitis and acquired immunodeficiency syndrome. Am J Med 91:267–272, 1991.

80. Theuer CP, Hopewell PC, Elias D, et al. Human immunodeficiency virus infection in tuberculosis patients. J Infect Dis 162:8–12, 1990.

81. Hollander H, McGuire D, Burack JH. Diagnostic lumbar puncture in HIV-infected patients: analysis of 138 cases. Am J Med 96:223–228, 1994.

82. McArthur JC, Cohen BA, Farzadegan H, et al. Cerebrospinal fluid abnormalities in homosexual men with and without neuropsychiatric findings. Ann Neurol 23: 534–537, 1988.

83. Petito CK, Cho ES, Lemann W, et al. Neuropathology of acquired immunodeficiency syndrome (AIDS): an autopsy review. J Neuropathol Exp Neurol 45:635–646, 1986.

84. Arribas JR, Storch GA, Clifford DB, Tselis AC. Cytomegalovirus encephalitis. Ann Intern Med 25:577–587, 1996.

85. McCutchan JA. Clinical impact of cytomegalovirus infections of the nervous system in patients with AIDS. Clin Infect Dis 21(suppl 2):S196–S201, 1995.

86. Cinque P, Vago L, Brytting M. Cytomegalovirus infection of the central nervous system in patients with AIDS: diagnosis by DNA amplification from cerebrospinal fluid. J Infect Dis 1408–1411, 1992.

87. Cohen BA. Prognosis and response to therapy of cytomegalovirus encephalitis and meningomyelitis in AIDS. Neurology 46:444–450, 1996.
88. Price TA, DiGioia RA, Simon GL. Ganciclovir treatment of cytomegalovirus ventriculitis in a patient infected with human immunodeficiency virus. 15:606–608, 1992.
89. Tan S, Guiloff RF, Scaravilli F, Klapper P, Cleator GM, Gazzard BG. Herpes simplex type 1 encephalitis in acquired immunodeficiency syndrome. Ann Neurol 34: 619–622, 1993.
90. Gray F, Belec L, Lescs MC, et al. Varicella–zoster virus infection of the central nervous system in the acquired immune deficiency syndrome. Brain 117:987–999, 1994.
91. Bloom JN, Palestine AG. The diagnosis of cytomegalovirus retinitis. Ann Intern Med 109:963–969, 1988.
92. Palestine AG, Polis MA, de Smet MD, et al. A randomized, controlled trial of foscarnet in the treatment of cytomegalovirus retinitis in patients with AIDS. Ann Intern Med 115:665–673, 1991.
93. Jabs D, the Studies of Ocular Complications of AIDS Research Group, in collaboration with the AIDS Clinical Trials Group. Mortality in patients with the acquired immunodeficiency syndrome treated with either foscarnet or ganciclovir for cytomegalovirus retinitis. N Engl J Med 326:213–220, 1992.
94. Jacobson MA. Treatment of cytomegalovirus retinitis in patients with the acquired immunodeficiency syndrome. N Engl J Med 337:105–114, 1997.
95. Masur H, Whitcup SM, Cartwright C, Polis M, Nussenblatt R. Advances in the management of AIDS-related cytomegalovirus retinitis. Ann Intern Med 125:126–136, 1996.
96. Jabs DA, Green WR, Fox R, et al. Ocular manifestations of acquired immunodeficiency syndrome. Ophthalmology 96:1092–1099, 1989.
97. de Smet MD. Differential diagnosis of retinitis and choroiditis in patients with acquired immunodeficiency syndrome. Am J Med 92:17S–21S, 1992.
98. Murray JF, Mills J. State of the art: pulmonary infectious complications of human immunodeficiency virus infection, Part II. Am Rev Respir Dis 141:1582–1598, 1990.
99. Meduri GU, Stein DS. Pulmonary manifestations of acquired immunodeficiency syndrome. Clin Infect Dis 14:98–113, 1992.
100. Wallace JM, Rao AV, Glassroth J, et al. Respiratory illness in persons with human immunodeficiency virus infection. Am Rev Respir Dis 148:1523–1529, 1993.
101. Suster B, Akerman M, Orenstein M, et al. Pulmonary manifestations of AIDS: review of 106 episodes. Radiology 161:87–93, 1986.
102. Goodman PC. *Pneumocystis carinii* pneumonia. J Thorac Imaging 6:16–21, 1991.
103. Murray JF, Mills J. State of the art: pulmonary infectious complications of human immunodeficiency virus infection, Part I. Am Rev Respir Dis 141:1356–1372, 1990.
104. Katz MH, Hessol NA, Buchbinder SP, et al. Temporal trends of opportunistic infections and malignancies in homosexual men with AIDS. J Infect Dis 170:198–202, 1994.
105. Glatt AE, Chirgwuin KC. *Pneumocystis carinii* pneumonia in human immunodeficiency virus-infected patients. Arch Intern Med 150:271–279, 1990.

106. Kovacs JA, Ng VL, Masur H. Diagnosis of *Pneumocystis carinii* pneumonia: improved detection in sputum with use of monoclonal antibodies. N Engl J Med 318: 589–593, 1988.

107. Katz MH, Baron RB, Grady D. Risk stratification of ambulatory patients suspected of *Pneumocystis* pneumonia. Arch Intern Med 151:105–110, 1991.

108. Kales CP, Murren JR, Torres RA, et al. Early predictors of in-hospital mortality for *Pneumocystis carinii*, pneumonia in the acquired immunodeficiency syndrome. Arch Intern Med 147:1413–1417, 1987.

109. Masur H. Prevention and treatment of *Pneumocystis* pneumonia. N Engl J Med 327:1853–1860, 1992.

110. Masur H, Meier P, McCutchan A, et al. Consensus statement on the use of corticosteroids as adjunctive therapy for *Pneumocystis* pneumonia in the acquired immunodeficiency syndrome. N Engl J Med 323:1500–1504, 1990.

111. Barnes PF, Bloch AB, Davidson PT, et al. Tuberculosis in patients with human immunodeficiency virus infection. N Engl J Med 324:1644–1650, 1991.

112. Fischl MA, Daikos GL, Uttamchandani RB, et al. Clinical presentation and outcome of patients with HIV infection and tuberculosis caused by multiple drug-resistant bacilli. Ann Intern Med 11:184–190, 1992.

113. American Thoracic Society. Treatment of tuberculosis and tuberculosis infection in adults and children. Am J Respir Crit Care Med 149:1359–1374, 1994.

114. Millar AB, Patou G, Miller RF, et al. Cytomegalovirus in the lungs of patients with AIDS: respiratory pathogen or passenger? Am Rev Respir Dis 141:1474–1477, 1990.

115. Bozette SA, Arcia J, Bartok AE, et al. Impact of *Pneumocystis carinii* and cytomegalovirus on the course and outcome of atypical pneumonia in advanced human immunodeficiency virus disease. J Infect Dis 165:93–98, 1992.

116. Blatt SP, Dolan MJ, Hendrix CW, et al. Legionnaires' disease in human immunodeficiency virus-infected patients: eight cases and review. Clin Infect Dis 18:227–232, 1994.

117. Cameron ML, Bartlett JA, Gallis HA, Waskin HA. Manifestations of pulmonary cryptococcosis in patients with acquired immunodeficiency syndrome. Rev Infect Dis 13:64–67, 1991.

118. Miller KD, Mican JA, Davey RT. Asymptomatic solitary pulmonary nodules due to *Cryptococcus neoformans* in patients infected with human immunodeficiency virus. Clin Infect Dis 23:810–812, 1996.

119. Polsky B, Gold JWM, Whimbey E, et al. Bacterial pneumonia in patients with the acquired immunodeficiency syndrome. Ann Intern Med 104:38–41, 1986.

120. Janoff EN, Breiman RF, Daley CL, et al. Pneumococcal disease during HIV infection. Ann Intern Med 117:314–324, 1992.

121. Baron AD, Hollander H. *Pseudomonas aeruginosa* bronchopulmonary infection in late human immunodeficiency virus disease. Am Rev Respir Dis 148:992–996, 1993.

122. Magnenat JL, Nicod LP, Aukenthaler R, et al. Mode of presentation and diagnosis of bacterial pneumonia in human immunodeficiency virus-infected patients. Am Rev Respir Dis 144:917–922, 1991.

123. Emmons W, Reichwein B, Winslow DL. *Rhodococcus equi* infection in the patient

with AIDS: literature review and report of an unusual case. Rev Infect Dis 13:91–96, 1991.

124. Kim J, Minamoto GY, Grieco MH. Nocardial infection as a complication of AIDS: report of six cases and review. Rev Infect Dis 13:624–629, 1991.

125. Bonacini M, Young T, Laine L. The causes of esophageal symptoms in human immunodeficiency virus infection: a prospective study of 110 patients. Arch Intern Med 151:1567–1572, 1991.

126. Wilcox CM, Straub RF, Schwartz DA. Cytomegalovirus esophagitis in AIDS: a prospective evaluation of clinical response to ganciclovir therapy, relapse rate, and long-term outcome. Am J Med 98:169–176, 1995.

127. Jacobson JM, Greenspan JS, Spritzler J, Ketter N, Fahey JL, Jackson JB, Fox L, Chernoff M, Wu AW, MacPhail LA, Vasquez G. Thalidomide for the treatment of oral aphthous ulcers in patients with human immunodeficiency virus infection. N Engl J Med 336:1487–1493, 1997.

128. Smith PD, Quinn TC, Strober W, et al. Gastrointestinal infections in AIDS. Ann Intern Med 116:63–77, 1992.

129. Bartlett JG, Belitsos PC, Sears CL. AIDS enteropathy. Clin Infect Dis 15:726–735, 1992.

130. Sánchez C, García-Restoy E, Garau J, et al. Ciprofloxacin and trimethoprim–sulfamethoxazole versus placebo in acute uncomplicated Salmonella enteritis: a double-blind trial. J Infect Dis 168:1304–1307, 1993.

131. Bartlett JG. Antibiotic-associated diarrhea. Clin Infect Dis 269:71–75, 1993.

132. Laughon BE, Druckman DA, Vernon A, et al. Prevalence of enteric pathogens in homosexual men with and without acquired immunodeficiency syndrome. Gastroenterology 94:984–993, 1988.

133. Pape JW, Verdier RI, Boncy M, et al. Cyclospora infection in adults with HIV: clinical manifestations, treatment, and prophylaxis. Ann Intern Med 121:654–657, 1994.

134. Wittner M, Tanowitz, HB, Weiss LM. Parasitic infections in AIDS patients: cryptosporidiosis, isosporiasis, microsporidiosis, cyclosporiasis. Infect Dis Clin North Am 7:569–586, 1993.

135. Weber R, Bryan RT. Microsporidial infections in immunodeficient and immunocompetent patients. Clin Infect Dis 19:517–521, 1994.

136. Weber R, Bryan RT, Owen RL, et al. Improved light microscopic detection of microsporidia spores in stool and duodenal aspirates. N Engl J Med 326:161–166, 1992.

137. Dietrich DT, Lew EA, Kotler DP, et al. Treatment with albendazole for intestinal disease due to Enterocytozoon bieneusi in patients with AIDS. J Infect Dis 169:178–183, 1994.

138. Anwar-Bruni DM, Hogan SE, Schwartz DA, Wilcox CM, Bryan RT, Lennox JL. Atovaquone is effective treatment for the symptoms of gastrointestinal microsporidiosis in HIV-1-infected patients. AIDS 10:619–623, 1996.

139. Cello JP, Grendell JH, Basuk P, et al. Effect of octreotide on refractory AIDS-associated diarrhea. Ann Intern Med 115:705–710, 1991.

140. Bonacini M. Pancreatic involvement in human immunodeficiency virus infection. J Clin Gastroenterol 13:58–64, 1991.

141. Bissuel F, Leport C, Perronne C, et al. Fever of unknown origin in HIV-infected patients: a critical analysis of a retrospective series of 57 cases. J Intern Med 236: 529–535, 1994.

142. Sepkowitz KA, Telzak EE, Carrow M, et al. Fever among outpatients with advanced human immunodeficiency virus infection. Arch Intern Med 153:1909–1912, 1993.

143. Miralles P, Moreno S, Perez-Tascon M, et al. Fever of uncertain origin in patients infected with the human immunodeficiency virus. Clin Infect Dis 20:872–875, 1995.

144. Krumholz HM, Sande MA, Lo B. Community-acquired bacteremia in patients with acquired immunodeficiency syndrome: clinical presentation, bacteriology, and outcome. Am J Med 86:776–779, 1989.

145. Krasinski K, Borkowsky W, Bonk S, et al. Bacterial infections in human immunodeficiency virus-infected children. Pediatr Infect Dis J 7:323–328, 1988.

146. Adal KA, Cockerell CF, Petri WA. Cat scratch disease, bacillary angiomatosis, and other infections due to *Rochalimaea*. N Engl J Med 330:1509–1515, 1994.

147. Raviglione MC, Battan R, Pablos-Mendez A. Infections associated with Hickman catheters in patients with acquired immunodeficiency syndrome. Am J Med 86: 780–786, 1989.

148. Gottlieb MS, Schroff R, Schanker HM, et al. *Pneumocystis carinii* pneumonia and mucosal candidiasis in previously healthy homosexual men: evidence of a new acquired cellular immunodeficiency. N Engl J Med 305:1425–1431, 1981.

149. Masur H, Michelis MA, Greene JB, et al. An outbreak of community acquired *Pneumocystis carinii* pneumonia: initial manifestation of cellular immune dysfunction. N Engl J Med 305:1431–1438, 1981.

150. Fischl MA, Dickinson GM, La Voie L. Safety and efficacy of sulfamethoxzaole and trimethoprim chemoprophylaxis for *Pneumocystis carinii* pneumonia in AIDS. JAMA 259:1185–1189, 1988.

151. Kovacs JA, Masur H. Prophylaxis for *Pneumocystis carinii* pneumonia in patients infected with the human immunodeficiency virus. N Engl J Med 14:1005–1009, 1992.

152. Gallant JE, Moore RD, Chaisson RE. Prophylaxis for opportunistic infections in patients with HIV infection. Ann Intern Med 120:932–944, 1994.

153. Powderly WG. Multiple opportunistic pathogen prophylaxis. AIDS 10(suppl): S165–171, 1996.

16

AIDS and Social Context

Mindy Thompson Fullilove
New York State Psychiatric Institute and Columbia University,
New York, New York

I. INTRODUCTION

Epidemics of diseases transmitted by needle-sharing and sexual intercourse spread through physically intimate networks. In a society divided by class, education, race, and other markers of social status, such a disease will flow largely— but not exclusively—within groups outlined by these markers. Acquired Immunodeficiency Syndrome (AIDS) is an important disease for many reasons, but not the least of these is that AIDS is a disease that reveals the ways in which important social markers order U. S. society and structure life chances. At every moment associated with illness, social context is highly influential. An understanding of these contextual issues can and should influence prevention, diagnosis, and treatment, in fact, every aspect of AIDS care within our society.

Obviously, the complete understanding of the sociology and anthropology of AIDS is beyond the scope of a single book chapter. Therefore, this chapter will examine a series of critical issues that are each important in and of themselves, but also serve as prototypes for understanding the range of social and contextual problems that surround the AIDS epidemic in the United States, with special reference to the cancers associated with AIDS. The first issue is that of community disintegration, which has placed whole neighborhoods at risk. The second issue is that of sex–drug settings that are linked to transmission of the virus. The third issue is that of social distance, which is a major obstacle to the provision of adequate care.

II. COMMUNITY DISINTEGRATION: THE CONTEXT FOR AIDS

The AIDS epicenters around the world appear to be markedly different kinds of places: wealthy enclaves of white homosexual men; destitute inner-city minority communities; rural villages of farm workers; countries torn by war; cities booming with sex tourism. But despite the seeming differences, an underlying similarity can be identified: in each of the AIDS epicenters, the integrity of community life has been shattered by powerful social upheaval. Gay men, for example, moved to urban centers because they could not be open about their sexuality while at home in "middle" America. As a source of disruption, the operation of homophobia on the lives of gay white men is quite different from the economic and physical damage done to inner-city communities, but the social and emotional outcomes are remarkably similar. The individual psychological process that follows displacement—from whatever cause—appears to include a set of universal elements that includes the loss of orientation, attachment, and identity associated with location. This set of psychological processes may predispose to secondary conditions, including an increased need for mind-altering experiences and the liberalization of community mores surrounding use of drugs and participation in sex.

We are postulating here a close link between *community life* and *individual health*, with specific emphasis on the negative effects of social upheaval. The fundamental feature of group life that promotes health is community integration; that is, interpersonal order and organization among those living in a given locale. Well-integrated communities order the social lives of their members in such a way that illness is prevented. When illness arises, orderly communities act to contain disease and restore individual and group well-being. Poorly integrated communities, by contrast, are unable to carry out these functions. Because there is no replacement the individual can make for the social capital created by group interaction, the loss of community order is a serious loss for the individual. To understand this better, let us examine the concept of community integration in more detail.

In 1990, McCord and Freeman published a paper in *The New England Journal of Medicine* that, among other shocking statistics, observed that African-American men in the Central Harlem community were less likely to reach age 65 than were men in Bangladesh, arguably one of the poorest nations on earth (1). AIDS is an important part of this picture of untimely death.

To understand the excess risk for mortality in Harlem, the U. S. Centers for Disease Control and Prevention (CDC) sponsored a study of the health of adult residents of the community. Preliminary results from the Harlem Household Study (HHS), which was conducted by the Harlem Center for Health Promotion and Disease Prevention, document widespread distress and difficult social conditions (2). For example, 51% of the respondents reported that they had not worked in the past year, 18% reported that they had no health insurance of any kind, and 61% reported that they had been a victim of violent assault. Human immunodeficiency virus (HIV) risk behaviors were common in the sample. Significantly, 46% of these surveyed reported having been tested for HIV, with 4% of those tested reporting that they were HIV-positive (4100.9:100,000).

These stark descriptors of a community that is now an AIDS epicenter stand in stark contrast to memories of "better days" reported by long-term residents of the area. Harlem, in its heyday from the 1920s to 1950s, was a world famous center for creative activities in art, music, literature, and theater. One resident, contrasting past and present, said:

> I was born and raised in Harlem so I have this romantic thing about Harlem. I find Harlem to be very people friendly. Sometimes I have to catch myself because of the romance of what it used to be. I liked Harlem when everybody was like "Good morning, how are you doing?" with a little Southern twang. The romance in Harlem was those of us who were born and raised, we remember the man with the cart who used to sell *TV Guide*, *Jet* magazine, *Amsterdam News*. The peanut man. He used to have the hot peppermints, the peppermints that melted in your mouth. That's what I mean about the romance of Harlem. The romance is that you didn't fear your neighbors, your kids didn't fear your neighbors, your neighbors were your safety . . . The romance in Harlem is gone. The love. The togetherness (3).

The question that arises is: what happened to alter the community? What was the process by which a supportive, exciting community became an unhealthy, hostile one? Understanding this process may assist community leaders in revitalization efforts. In searching for enlightenment on this issue, Leighton, one of the pioneers of social psychiatry, began by proposing that communities might be ranged on a continuum with a "model" community at one end, and a "collection" of unaffiliated individuals at the other (4). The model community might be thought of as a system of interdependent parts able to maintain itself despite changes in the surrounding environment. This self-integrating system, in his view, would be able to:

> Raise healthy children who were prepared to be productive adult members of the community
> Regulate the behaviors of its members
> Provide for a range of personalities
> Care for the ill and the infirm

Several forces can trigger disintegration of a model community. These include—but are not limited to—migration, epidemic disease, wars, economic decline, and housing destruction. Leighton and his colleagues identified the following as symptoms of communities that were falling apart:

Family fragmentation
Few and weak associations
Few and weak leaders
Few patterns of recreation
High frequency of hostility
High frequency of crime and delinquency
Weak and fragmented networks of communication

Harlem has experienced several of the triggers leading to disintegration. Economic decline, specifically the loss of unskilled jobs in manufacturing, has been severe. The area has also lost approximately a third of its housing stock in the years between 1960 and 1990. Marked outmigration of area residents has followed the loss of housing. The resulting pattern of social interaction fits closely with that predicted by Leighton's group. For example, only 16% of the adults reported that they were married at the time of Harlem Household Study survey; 27% reported they had been separated from their mothers for more than a year before age 18. Although African-Americans in the United States report very high rates of church membership, in the HHS only 42% of the respondents said they belonged to a church.

Reviewing the Harlem experience, we can hypothesize that the process of community collapse followed a downward spiral with identifiable stages, what we have called the "Stage-State Model of Community Disintegration" (Fig. 1). The initial stage, which we have termed "confusion," followed in the immediate aftermath of the first destabilizing events; in the case of Harlem, the destabilizing events were many microdisasters spread out over a period of many years. In general, people who have experienced some kind of disaster feel disoriented and unsure. At that point, rapid intervention may restabilize the community, ending the period of insecurity. However, if the community is not stabilized, these distressing feelings may become chronic, and people seek remedies. In the case of Harlem, some turned to drugs to alleviate their discomfort. Growing substance abuse acted as an additional destabilizing force, accelerating the downward spiral of the community.

Housing loss also aggravated the downward process in Harlem (5). The loss of housing worsens the distress experienced by community residents, initiating the second stage in community disintegration, which we have called "disorder." This occurs because the potential for order created by the built environment is undermined. Not only do people miss their neighbors, but also new, typically noxious, forces move into the abandoned areas. These include unwanted animals and plants, such as rodents, insects, and molds, as well as unwanted people, such as active drug users and homeless people.

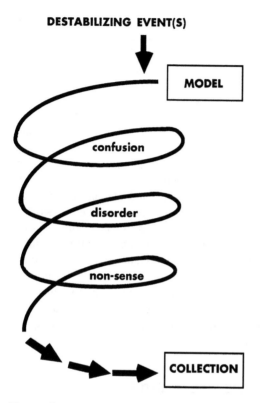

DESTABILIZING EVENT(S)

MODEL

confusion

disorder

non-sense

COLLECTION

Figure 1 Stage–state model of community disintegration.

The disorder in the environment increases the risk for trauma and violence which, in turn, add new momentum to the downward spiral. Trauma, for example, causes serious psychological injury. Traumatized people are less likely to trust others. They are also less likely to carry out the social behaviors that are needed for community integration. Widespread trauma and violence, in the context of a disorderly environment, create a condition of "non-sense," the third stage in community disintegration. An interesting aspect of non-sense is its close resemblance to surrealism.

These are tentative hypotheses about the process of community disintegration based on observations in the New York City area, and they cannot be generalized to other places in the United States or around the world without further research. Yet it is clear that understanding the integration–disintegration continuum is a useful way to characterize community context. It is intuitively obvious that AIDS treatment and prevention programs will need one set of parameters in a model community, but a different set in a non-sense community. Similarly, key institutions will have different strengths in different communities. Although churches are important to all communities, the density of their connections will not be the same at each point on the integration–disintegration continuum.

This model suggests a framework for determining where on the continuum between integration and disintegration a given community might lie. This can be thought of as a "Community Apgar Score" (borrowing from the pediatric assessment given to neonates), which consists of measures of five key components of community health: (1) degree of family fragmentation among residents; (2) number and strength of interpersonal associations among and between community residents; (3) number and quality of opportunities for recreation; (4) degree of intensity in expressions of crime, delinquency, and interpersonal hostility; and (5) strength or weakness of networks of communications among residents.

Any health care setting ought to be able to assess its catchment area from this perspective. The resultant understanding of social context will be useful in informing many kinds of treatment- and prevention-planning activities. Principally, institutions serving disintegrated communities should be aware that those communities are unable to supply many of the social support functions that exist in well-integrated communities. Therefore, the health care system in a disintegrated community will have to play a much more active role in supporting patients as they negotiate their illness.

III. SEX–DRUG SETTINGS: THE SITE OF INTIMATE CONTACT

The AIDS epidemic has been centered in disintegrated communities, but not all severely damaged communities have been equally affected. Detroit, which has suffered a major loss of housing infrastructure and has serious problems with drug addiction, reports rates of HIV infection below the national average. An additional factor, therefore, is necessary to explain the rapid and efficient spread of infection. That factor is settings in which large numbers of people engage with each other in intimate sex and drug-taking acts. These sex–drug settings take various forms in the United States. A heightened understanding of these settings is essential for understanding the spread of AIDS and many other sexually transmitted diseases (STDs).

This principle was well illustrated in the control of an outbreak of syphilis in Chester, Pennsylvania, a small town south of Philadelphia (6). The public health department noted a fivefold increase in cases of early syphilis in 1988 as compared with 1987. Epidemiological information identified cocaine use and prostitution as risk factors. The health department rejected the use of standard case-finding techniques, as likely to be ineffective in curbing an epidemic among drug users and their anonymous partners; instead they targeted intervention efforts to locations where sex and drugs were sold. The health department also decided to give empiric treatment to all persons at the time of screening.

The syphilis screening program was conducted for 6 days in April 1989. During the intervention, 136 people were screened and all of those who were sexually active were treated for syphilis. Twenty-five people were found to have syphilis. Among the intervention cases, there was a higher proportion of early latent syphilis cases than among routinely reported case-patients.

The health department noted a decline in cases after the intervention, suggesting that it may have played a role in halting the spread of infection. The authors of the study suggested that such targeted interventions had potential as a new tactic STD control efforts. What is important about the effort described here is that it employed the knowledge of the local sex–drug scene to plan an effective intervention. *Sex–drug scene* refers to the culture of a group of drug users within a defined geographic area. The users are situated in a sociogeographic space that can be mapped and studied. Furthermore, within that space, certain settings appear to be particularly important for encounters at which sex is negotiated. Finally, the culture of drug use will specify ways in which sex and drugs are mixed, including which drugs and which sex acts are acceptable under a given set of conditions. In the following sections, we will examine some of the key concepts guiding the study of STD epidemics that are related to drug use.

A. Sex-Drug Settings

A variety of linkages between drugs and sex have been observed. Drugs may be used by one or more of the parties as part of the sexual encounter. The use of alcohol as "social lubricant" may be the most common example of this phenomenon. Similarly, the use of amyl nitrate among gay men served to define sexual behaviors that were subsequently associated with diagnosis of Kaposi's sarcoma (KS). Second, people who are addicted to drugs may be involved in commercial sex work (prostitution) to obtain money for drugs. Drugs and sex may each be part of a cultural "scene," typically a place where people go to enjoy themselves. Bars, clubs, and bathhouses all fall into this category. All of these connections between sex and drugs can contribute to the spread of sexually transmitted disease, including the transmission of human herpes virus type 8 (HHV-8), associated with KS.

The sex–drug settings are perhaps particularly important because they can serve as points for large numbers of people to congregate. As the spread of disease is related to the density of the network of sexual partners, the settings that lead to the most effective mixing are those most likely to support new infections.

Work in Colorado Springs outlined some of the key features of the sex–drug setting as a supporting context for the spread of disease (7).

That study examined the network connections among people with gonorrhea in Colorado Springs and used two measures of connection. First, the researchers asked infected individuals to list up to six preferred sites for nighttime social activity. Second, they asked them to name all of their sexual contacts. By using these measures, they found that those with gonorrhea were closely linked on both counts. The cases were tightly clustered in four census tracts, including the major military base. Nighttime social activity was concentrated in drinking establishments. Among those with a preference a total of 1009 places were cited, but six establishments accounted for 516 (51%) of all citations. Cases were grouped in "sexual lots" (Potterat units, defined as sexually connected groups; that is, each person in the group had had sex with at least one other person in the group). Six lots contained 20% of the study population. The cases also tended to know their partners before sexual contact.

This study establishes several important features of drug–sex settings. First, within the heterosexual drinking culture in Colorado Springs, there were many establishments that catered to local tastes. Second, the clustering of cases in six locations suggests specific features of those locations that may be worth further investigation. Third, the social and sexual aggregation of the population shows a high level of organization, but relatively constant turnover of members.

B. Documentation of Settings

Describing sex–drug settings requires careful ethnographic research. It is critical that experienced observers document that manner in which sexual behaviors are intertwined with drug use in particular locales, as well as the connections among different locales in a particular drug subculture. In the mid-1990s, James Inciardi, an ethnographer who has studied the drug culture, conducted observations of the reemerging bathhouse scene among gay men in Los Angeles (8). He found that the bathhouses were a site where men took drugs (largely marijuana) and engaged in various kinds of sexual acts. Although the bathhouses offered condoms to clients, and displayed AIDS prevention posters, Inciardi observed a variety of unsafe sex acts of the kind linked to the spread of HHV-8 and development of KS.

The variety of settings is great and the dynamics of one milieu may not necessarily predict the patterns of behaviors that will be observed in another setting. As an example, an outbreak of STD among farm workers in Southern California was tied to visits by commercial sex workers to the areas where the men lived. Detailed description helps us to understand the context that supports unsafe sexual activity; this can be an essential element in planning epidemic control activities.

C. Trading Sex-for-Crack

Early in the 1980s a new drug, crack cocaine, was introduced into the drug scenes in a number of U. S. cities. As crack spread from one city to another, observers noted an accompanying spread of syphilis and gonorrhea. It took no great leap of the imagination to wonder: would users of this drug, so tightly linked to STDs, become a new AIDS risk group? To answer that question, it was critical to begin to understand the drug and the ways in which it was altering sexual relationships.

This cocaine-derivative was cheap and produced an intense state of euphoria that was rated by many users to be vastly superior to most other illicit drugs. The drug was short-acting: the effects of a "hit" lasted less than an hour. Its after effect was a dysphoria, nearly as pronounced as the high that had preceded it. The combination of intense high coupled with the need to avoid the painful crash drove the user to take another hit, followed by another, and so on. In early reports, users described that there was no "dose" of crack, the way there was a dose of heroin. "People take as much crack as they have money," a user explained. "If you have $200, you take that much crack. If you have a $1000, you take that much crack. If you have a house, you sell your house and then you smoke up the profit."

Crack defined a new era in drug-taking, one in which the "dose-you-could-afford" was the driving factor. The craving for crack was nearly insatiable. Many users who had disposed of their worldly possessions turned to other sources of money, most particularly they began to sell their bodies. But where an older generation of people addicted to heroin had developed a mannerly form of participation in commercial sex work, the bartering that developed in the context of the crack era was a no-holds-barred revision of what it meant to be engaged in sex work. Under the compulsion of addiction to crack, users had little ability to negotiate the niceties of place or price. Quickly, dealers discovered that those addicted to crack would do nearly anything for the promise of a hit. The perhaps apocryphal stories that began to circulate described dealers making outrageous sexual demands—oral sex with five men or intercourse with a dog—in exchange for a small dose of the drug. Not only were the sexual acts outrageous by community standards, but the sexual encounters were often carried out in public or semi-public places, such as alleys or hallways, violating existing conventions of public decorum.

Although some forms of these stories are undoubtedly exaggerated, a seven-city study of sex-for-crack found ample evidence of altered sexual relations in the context of crack use (9). Some consistent patterns emerged from city to city. First, in the context of crack, and unlike earlier drug epidemics, sexual favors were likely to be exchanged directly for drugs or for money to buy drugs. Often the actual amounts of money or drug were miniscule, undercutting the prices charged by other sex workers. Second, many kinds of acts could be included under the rubric of sex–drugs-exchanges. These ranged from casual sharing of drugs and sex by friends to the formal practices of crack houses where women and drugs were available for sale. Because individuals might engage in some or all of these practices, the sexual lots created in this context were large. Third, conditions of crack use contributed to risk of exposure to infection with sexually transmitted diseases. For example, crack smoking caused burns on the lips and gums that might facilitate infection. Similarly, crack, although marketed as an aphrodisiac, actually inhibited orgasm in men, contributing to prolonged erection and intercourse, which might irritate or tear the genital tissues of men or women.

The seven-city study offered a glimpse into the structure of institutions that formed the crack culture. Just as a network of drinking establishments formed the alcohol culture of Colorado Springs, so does a network of crack spots create the settings for drug use and sexual barter. Several kinds of crack spots were described, each of which contributes to the network. First, and probably most important from the perspective of disease spread, is the crack house. The crack house is a location dedicated to the consumption of crack. Crack houses often ''supply'' women as well as drugs. They are a place for people to meet each other and to socialize while becoming intoxicated. Crack houses may be deserted buildings, apartments, houses, or any other location taken over by dealers for the purpose of selling drugs. In addition to the houses, which are the most formal locations, are a second tier of homes where people gather to smoke crack. Such crack spots are more informal places. Users provide the host with a share of drug, in exchange for the use of the location.

The complex and diffuse organization of crack use, similar to the organization of drinking establishments, creates a social geography of the crack culture. Unlike legal establishments, cracks houses and crack spots are unstable. They may be closed by the police or destroyed in other ways. For example, in New York City, a deserted building that served as a crack house burned down as a result of a dispute between two users.

D. New Epidemics, New Places, New Problems

An important lesson learned from the crack epidemic is that the patterns of drug use are constantly changing. The infusion of a new drug alters the existing drug scene, but the patterns that will emerge cannot necessarily be predicted from previous experience. As an example, there was nothing about the heroin epidemics of the 1960s and 1970s that prepared inner city communities for women's engagement with crack cocaine.

Second, new drugs exert an attraction that is partly related to being ''new.'' New drugs tend to have a more positive aura than older drugs, largely because of the lack of reports of side effects. As experience accumulates and people become more and more aware of the downside of using a particular pharmacological agent, they will weigh decisions about its use with more caution. New drugs become connected to sexual behaviors through the development of a culture of users. As emphasized earlier, when new drugs are associated with STDs, the documentation of the supporting culture is an essential element in epidemic control.

Third, drugs arrive at a particular location as a result of market forces. This involves both marketers importing the drug and buyers purchasing it. The patterns of drug sales change constantly, a factor that will influence the growth and maintenance of sex–drug settings. The *New York Times* described the opening of drug shipment routes through Eastern Europe, beginning in the immediate aftermath of the collapse of Communist regimes there (10). Poland, for example, became an attractive site for drug shipments because law enforcement practices made it unlikely the drugs would be found or seized. Poland offered a convenient point for shipping to new markets in Eastern Europe, as well as to established markets in Western Europe and the United States. Such observations underscore the reality that market forces, with all the implied dynamics of the market, drive the drug trade and its attendant epidemics of sexually transmitted disease. Given the instability of markets, rapid and incessant shifts in drug cultures, and their sex–drug settings, may be anticipated.

IV. SOCIAL DISTANCE: THE FINAL BARRIER TO CARE

It can be inferred from the preceding sections that AIDS hit not the American mainstream, but rather those citizens living in some degree of disadvantage at the margins of U. S. society. It is common in university and public health settings for professionals to use the expression ''hard-to-reach'' when describing homosexuals, drug users, prostitutes, illegal immigrants, the homeless, and others who are at some social distance from themselves. In fact, the vast majority of people infected with HIV—living as they were at the social margins—fell into this group of the hard-to-reach.

But it must be noted that drug dealers find drug users all the time. Homeless people are often tightly networked ''on the street,'' able to share information about food, shelter, and other life necessities. Similarly, illegal immigrants form close networks within which they are able to help each other. None of these groups would view themselves as hard-to-reach.

This poses an important problem for the organization of treatment and prevention: the problem of social distance. The fervent wish of those in the mainstream to be isolated from those at the margins must not be underestimated as a factor undermining the provision of AIDS treatment and prevention services.

Social distance has very real geographic implications in U. S. society. Rich people place themselves at substantial physical distance from poor people. Many even feel the need to erect fences, to create "gated communities" to keep out the undesirables. The creation of housing that structures distance between the "haves" and the "have nots" is followed by the creation of care institutions that reinforce the ethos of exclusion. Hospitals and other health care settings are part of well-established systems of segregation that isolate people by various markers of social status. From their experiences with this care system, what the poor and the outsiders have come to expect is that the upper social groups do not care about them. They anticipate that they will be treated with disrespect and disregard. They avoid encounters with officialdom because such contacts are so often painful.

By way of illustration, let me describe a conversation that occurred during a group session at a drug treatment clinic where I conduct my research. A group of women were presented with a story and asked to discuss it. The story involved a problem in getting a bus transfer. The conflict with the bus driver escalated rapidly to an emotional confrontation between the passenger and the driver. The story made all the listeners tense. Immediately one woman after another recounted tales of similar contacts with bus drivers. All had been painful and humiliating. The women were clear that often the feasibility of a trip depended on getting a transfer. If the transfer did not come through, one could find oneself at some distance from home, without enough money to ride back.

This happened often enough, with serious enough consequences, that the women were quite agitated in thinking through the management of such episodes. An important aspect of such events was that the bus drivers treated poor women with contempt, never giving them a "second chance" or giving them the "benefit of the doubt." In fact, it seemed to be the opposite: a poor woman of color who needed a bus transfer was guilty until proven otherwise. Guilty of what? Scamming, cheating, needing: some desperate act of skimming from the public welfare for which they should be punished. None of the women in the group had a blemish-free past. But the judgment of their behavior was not made on the basis of their actions in the moment, but rather, on the basis of who they were as members of a low-status social group.

Obviously, it is impossible to provide decent health care based within systems of apartheid. But overcoming distance is not always easy: it requires the creation of a new kind of interaction between insiders and outsiders. *The Heart of the Matter* is a film that tackled this tough assignment. It is film about women and AIDS that features the story of Janice Jirau, an African-American woman who died of AIDS. Janice and her family worked with the producers to document many moments in her life, as well as her reflections on the past.

Janice spent most of her life feeling disenfranchised. She was sexually abused as a child, then rejected by family, friends, and church people because of the resulting pregnancy. This series of events taught her to bow to the needs of others, putting herself aside. When she learned that her husband was HIV-positive, she felt unable to insist on condom use. Later, when she learned of her own infection, she still put his needs before her own.

> When I found out I was HIV positive, I couldn't talk to my husband about it too much because he was dealing with his own anger and how I was going to accept being, you know, that he gave me this. I was so busy trying to make sure that he knew that I didn't blame him, that I really couldn't express all of what I was feeling to him. So I went in the bathroom—when I came home, I remember I went in the bathroom, and I got on my knees, and I just cried, and I asked God, I said, I can't ask you to take this away because you allowed this to happen to me, but if you will, if you will, please, let this—you know, I felt like Jesus Christ at the cross—let this cup pass if it's your will.

The film, however, became a vehicle for Janice to speak to others, demanding that they acknowledge her reality and her needs. Thus, the filmmakers were present when she spoke at an African-American church in New Orleans. Janice described to the congregation the rejection that marred her childhood:

> I came to the church, but because I was 13 and I had a baby, I was labeled a bad girl. They did not know that I gotten that baby as a result of dysfunction within my family, that I had been abused, that I came to them to embrace me, and they scolded me and threw me away.

The minister, a handsome and articulate black woman, had tears in her eyes and embraced Janice when she had finished speaking. "I'm so sorry that we were not there for you when you needed us," she told Janice. The congregation, too, through its attention and warm reception of her remarks, reached out to embrace Janice. It is a remarkable moment of overcoming social distance as a result of the efforts of insiders and outsiders to bridge years of exclusion and misunderstanding.

Such conversations are essential to health. They are also essential to the control of epidemics. Though the discourse on the marginalized—the concept "hard-to-reach," for example—would suggest that these distances are fixed and, therefore, impermeable, in fact, germs are no great respecters of such social niceties. Rather, they follow the often arcane, but always present, connections that link us all within our common ecosystem.

It is often pointed out by those who study social networks that the degrees of separation between any two people are rather small. The "middle" American, for example, is at most six people away from the President. Such calculations move in the opposite direction as well: most Americans are at most six people away from someone who is homeless, someone who is addicted, someone who is an illegal immigrant. Though separated by degree, Americans are not absolutely isolated from each other.

The first section of this chapter described the contribution of community disintegration to the spread of disease. It can be inferred that a society that accepts apartheid in daily affairs will forego some degree of health as a consequence. Social distance and its attendant geographic segregation, because they permanently disconnect parts of U. S. society from each other, therefore pose a substantial, long-term danger to the health of the nation. AIDS is a dramatic example of the problem, but neither the first nor the last that is likely to make the point.

V. CONCLUSION

Issues of social context influence every aspect of AIDS prevention and treatment. It may be useful, in these concluding remarks, to make some recommendations based on the observations presented here. First, despite the importance of context to the understanding of disease, this area has received relatively little support from major funding institutions. This hampers our ability to describe and manipulate the social realities of greatest concern. The creation of an appropriate body of knowledge is a matter of concern and some urgency. Second, what we do know makes clear that population-level issues having to do with the stabilization of communities are quite influential in the course of the epidemic in the United States and are likely to continue to exert major influence in years to come. The creation of appropriate treatments for illness may not stem the tide of infection if these larger social forces are not addressed. Third, the problem of social distance is an immediate and important barrier to care. Although other issues may appear to be outside of the scope of the medical enterprise, there can be no gainsaying the propriety of creating welcoming and hospitable centers of care. Apartheid, however it is evidenced, can be largely eliminated from care settings by the actions of providers and there is no need to hesitate in the implementation of such policies.

As an epidemic of intimate behaviors, AIDS has forced U. S. society to look at itself more honestly and more openly than it had heretofore. This is to the good, but we have paid a high price, in terms of unnecessary mortality, for these lessons. If we could learn from AIDS about the social roots of diseases, these sorrowful lessons might be worth the price we have paid.

REFERENCES

1. C McCord, H Freeman. Excess mortality in Harlem. N Engl J Med 322:173–177, 1990.

2. MT Fullilove, RE Fullilove. The effects of housing displacement and resettlement in Harlem. Paper presented at the U. S. Centers for Disease Control, Atlanta, Georgia, April, 15, 1996.

3. MT Fullilove. Psychiatric implications of displacement: contributions from the psychology of place. Am J Psychiatry 153:1516–1523, 1996.

4. AH Leighton. My name is legion: foundations for a theory of man in relation to culture. The Stirling County Study of Psychiatric Disorder and Sociocultural Environment. Vol 1. New York: Basic Books, 1959.

5. R Wallace, D Wallace, H Andrews, R Fullilove, MT Fullilove. Spatiotemporal dynamics of AIDS and TB in the New York City metropolitan region from a sociogeographic perspective: understanding the linkages of central city and suburbs. Environ Plann A 27:1085–1108, 1995.

6. JR Hibbs, RA Gunn. Public health intervention in a cocaine-related syphilis outbreak. Am J Public Health 81:1259–1262, 1991.

7. JJ Potterat, RB Rotherberg, DE Woodhouse, JB Muth, CI Pratts, JS Fogle II. Gonorrhea as a social disease. Sex Transm Dis 12:25–32, 1985.

8. CB McCoy, JA Inciardi. Sex, Drugs and the Continuing Spread of AIDS. Los Angeles: Roxbury Publishing, 1995.

9. MS Ratner, ed. Crack Pipe as Pimp: An Ethnographic Investigation of Sex-for-Crack Exchanges. New York: Lexington Books, 1993.

10. Bonner, R. Poland Becomes a Major Conduit for Drug Traffic. NY Times, 12/30/93, p. A3.

17

An Activist Perspective on the Gay Community Living with HIV, Primary Care, and Clinical Trials

Michael Marco
Treatment Action Group, New York, New York

I. INTRODUCTION

As a communicable disease the human immunodeficiency virus (HIV) does not discriminate. Any individual, regardless of race, gender, demographics, or sexuality is at risk. Nonetheless, at the beginning of the acquired immunodeficiency syndrome (AIDS) epidemic in 1981, gay men in urban centers—namely, San Francisco and New York—were the first "community" to die of AIDS. HIV had yet to be discovered; it was called GRID (gay-related immunodeficiency disease).

This chapter will discuss the response of the gay male community to AIDS over the past two decades, from the psychological toll of a mysterious disease, to their involvement in the medical establishment, and their attitude toward HIV treatment and clinical trials. It is important to note that the gay male community in the United States is heterogeneous; this perspective pertains mostly to white gay men with HIV living in a major urban center.

II. DEATH RAVAGES THE GAY COMMUNITY DURING THE EARLY YEARS OF AIDS

Pneumocystis carinii pneumonia (PCP) was the first and deadliest recognizable opportunistic infection to develop in homosexual men. In the 1980s, retrospective studies documented that between 45 and 64% of patients with severe PCP died of it (1,2). Nobody knew who was at risk. Gay men were entering hospitals complaining of fevers and shortness of breath, and within 2 weeks had died of PCP. Such rapid deaths in normal, seemingly healthy young men were terrifying the gay community.

Along with PCP, gay men in New York and San Francisco started developing epidemic, AIDS-related Kaposi's sarcoma (KS) at alarming rates. No one in the gay community—not even most doctors treating these men—had a true understanding of what it was. Maurice Kaposi was not a household name, and the disease he discovered was rarely discussed in American medical textbooks. It did not take long for the gay community to realize that KS was something very bad and a real threat to their survival. A startling article, "Gay Cancer," appeared in a 1981 issue of *MANDATE*, a gay male pornography magazine. Signaling that something deadly and ominous was overtaking the gay male community, Douglas Mayfair wrote:

> The numbers continue to climb, but final statistics are unimportant, especially to those who are unfortunate enough to have developed the disease. The important fact is that this cancer poses a very real and potentially lethal threat to segments of the gay culture. It is a menace that must be dealt with logically and quickly if we are to overcome it, and knowledge of the disease, its causes and effects, is our best weapon (4).

Mayfair was obviously speaking about KS, but he had little idea that KS would soon be recognized as one of predominant manifestation of HIV disease, and its incidence would soon be increased 100,000-fold compared with classic and African KS (5).

In fact, gay men in the United States own KS. No other AIDS-related opportunistic disease attacks and singles out one segment of the population as does KS in HIV-positive gay men. Numerous epidemiological studies in AIDS-related KS conducted over the past 15 years have documented this truism: men outnumber women approximately 95 to 5% (6); homosexual men who acquired HIV through gay sex outnumber heterosexual men who acquired HIV through heterosexual sex or intravenous drug use (IVDU) almost as significantly; and KS is extremely rare in hemophiliacs with HIV (7). In one major natural history study of hemophiliacs with HIV–AIDS, only 1 of 93 patients developed KS, and he happened to be a homosexual man (8).

In the 1980s when AIDS KS was much more prevalent and occurred as an original manifestation of AIDS, KS was the unique visual identifier that someone had "it." With its often rapidly progressive nature, appearing on one's arms, hands, neck, and face, many with KS felt like lepers because they were outcasts and people were afraid to be around them for fear of contacting the disease. Photographs that appeared in *Life Magazine*, *Time*, or *Newsweek* seemed to always depict a gay man with chronic and acute wasting, and of course, KS. If you are going to show the American public someone sick with a plague, they better look sick and very different than you. KS was the ultimate signifyer. Tom Hanks, in the movie "*Philadelphia*," won his Academy Award not so much for his acting, but for wearing fake, painted KS lesions so well. The general public walked away and said, "What a horrible disease, he looked so believable with those spots."

KS is different from most other cancers because KS lesions are easily identifiable. I can walk down a street and see someone with lesions and I know it is KS, but I am unable to recognize people with lung, colon, or prostate cancer. The trauma and disfigurement of the KS lesion, a social stigma and constant visual reminder of one's dual diagnosis of cancer and AIDS, can take a serious psychological toll on patients. Indeed, one clinician contends, "a patient's psychological distress may bear no relationship to the actual extent of cutaneous involvement by KS" (9). According to Steve Miles, a prominent AIDS oncologist from UCLA, "treating a patient with asymptomatic indolent lesions might be appropriate for some simply for its psychological benefit" (S. Miles, personal communication).

In 1982, gay men with HIV disease were also developing non–Hodgkin's lymphoma (NHL) at an alarming rate. This was first documented by the sensationally titled *Lancet* article, "Outbreak of Burkitt's-like Lymphoma in Homosexual Men" (10). It was not until 1985 that the U. S. Centers for Disease Control and Prevention (CDC) caught on and added NHL to the list of AIDS-defining illnesses. And similar to KS, it was not until those in the know realized that HIV caused severe immunosuppression, that it was widely speculated that patients with AIDS would be likely candidates for developing NHL. In fact, data reveal that in HIV–AIDS individuals, NHL is increased 230-fold (3).

III. THE PSYCHOLOGICAL TOLL ON THE GAY COMMUNITY

The constant deaths from PCP and KS took a psychologically devastating toll on the gay male community in major metropolitan cities. Mayfair's belief that KS (actually AIDS), was a "very real and potentially lethal threat to segments of the gay culture" was accurate. However, this threat to gay culture was plainly a loss of lives. A sense of panic spread through San Francisco and New York. Nobody knew who was infected with HIV or who would be next to die. Numerous gay men stopped having sex for fear that even a kiss would lead to sudden illness and death.

By the mid- to late-1980s, many gay men (usually older than the age of 30) had lost at least half of their closest friends to AIDS. In talking to older gay men about the early years of AIDS, one always hears the same tale about a person who has had to redo their address book every year because it was too difficult to see so many names of dead friends crossed or "whited" out. There are also those older, HIV-negative gay men who have "survivors guilt" (a psychological term given to many who survived Nazi concentration camps) for being alive. Some of these HIV-negative men still wonder why they are not HIV-positive and how they could have been "passed over" even though they were having repeated unprotected anal intercourse. Many believed the myth that HIV could possibly live in the body for as long as 15–20 years before antibodies developed. To them, a negative test meant nothing—it was a watchful-waiting numbers game. Today, however, we know full well that HIV enzyme-linked immunosorbent assay (ELISA) antibody tests are highly sensitive, and most people infected with HIV will develop antibodies within 3 months. If rapid results are needed, there is always a qualitative polymerase chain reaction (PCR) test.

IV. COUNTERING FEAR WITH ACTION

The intense fear that seemed to cripple the gay community in the early- to mid-1980s was countered by a small yet growing activist movement. One of the first leaders of this movement was Michael Callen. He and other activists—including Joseph Sonnabend, a stellar immunologist who treated some of the first HIV patients in New York City—started passing out condoms outside New York City bathhouses. This was due to the growing knowledge that HIV transmission was spread by semen and that the condoms would help prevent transmission. Most importantly, this fledgling, activist-driven, safe sex prevention campaign—the first of its kind in the United States—was done by these individuals because the Federal government—with its knowledge of HIV transmission—did nothing on the prevention front.

In 1983 Callen and colleagues established a self-empowerment movement at a meeting in Denver and established the Denver Principles which held that "people with AIDS had the right to representation and power within all organizations concerned with their well being" (11). Importantly, the universally acceptable term "people/person with AIDS" and its widely used acronym, PWA/s, was born.

Changing the vocabulary and creating a language for AIDS was just the first step in a growing activist movement. In 1987, a group of mostly gay men and a handful of lesbians founded the AIDS Coalition to Unleash Power (ACT UP) In New York City. Here again, power was in a voice, an angry voice used to call attention to the rapidly metastasizing AIDS pandemic. Thousands of ACT UP members took to the streets of New York chanting "ACT UP, fight back, fight AIDS."

According to one of its original members, Mark Harrington:

ACT UP, the AIDS Coalition to Unleash Power, was perhaps the most effective, and certainly the most noticeable, social change movement to occur in the USA during the Reagan–Bush years. Its tactics represented a unique fusion of strategies taken from the civil rights, women's and gay rights movements of the 1960s and 1970s with a new infusion of skills such as manipulating the media and generating the scientific understanding to play a role in scientific policy decisions within structures established by the FDA, the NIH and the drug companies (11).

Although many sought change: an end to government inaction on prevention and treatment research, and preventing AIDS discrimination in housing and in the work place, many took to the streets screaming "ACT up, fight back, fight AIDS" out of sheer fear and unbridled anger much the same way Peter Finch screamed "I'm as mad a hell and I'm not going to take it anymore" in Sidney Lumet's movie, *Network*. Even though many ACT UP members died of AIDS-related complications during its 6-year heyday, many believed their survival was greatly increased just by attending ACT UP general meetings and demonstrations. ACT UP gave numerous gay men with AIDS an outlet for anger, a sense of camaraderie, and a place of total acceptance.

As ACT UP grew over the years, many members began to collectively tackle and specialize in the various issues facing the "AIDS community": housing, insurance, clean needle exchange for intravenous drug users (its only real stab at prevention), and treatment. Possibly the most dynamic and successful group within ACT UP was its Treatment and Data Committee (T & D). T & D met weekly (and often times ad hoc in members' apartments) to learn the science of AIDS, understand the basics of biomedical drug development and U. S. Food and Drug Administration (FDA) regulatory issues, and advocate for the testing and rapid access to promising AIDS drugs.

AIDS treatment activism created the revolutionary patient advocacy movement. Patients were no longer subjects in clinical research without a voice, they were now consumers who were educated and wanted their voices heard and real-world concerns addressed. Gay men with HIV became educated about all facets of their disease and were able to dialogue with and challenge their physicians, rather than follow advice blindly.

Many of the nation's leading breast cancer advocates admit that ACT UP and its birth to treatment activism galvanized them to mobilize and demand their "place at the table." In fact, breast cancer advocates would never have been able to get Genentech to provide preapproval access to Herceptin (HER-2-neu) in 1998 if AIDS treatment activists had not first fought the FDA in 1989 to get preapproved "compassionate use" access to Bristol Myer's antiretroviral didanosine (ddI).

V. ALTRUISM VERSUS ACCESS

It is only recently that standard-of-care strategy studies have cropped-up in AIDS clinical research. Until the advent of protease inhibitors and highly active antiretroviral therapy (HAART), a majority of experimental, anti-HIV therapy studies (mostly nucleoside analogues, reverse transcriptase inhibitors) were conducted for the developer of the given agent. The HIV-positive gay male community seemed most interested in these unapproved, experimental drugs. Many needed to enroll in clinical trials because the older, approved antiretrovirals they had taken were no longer working and CD4 cell counts were dropping. Some just believed that new, unapproved therapies (the drug de jour) were better.

Most importantly, the gay male community (along with PWAs from minority communities) is attracted to AIDS clinical trials because, for the most part, they are free. Rarely are patients charged for any study medication and the cost of immunological monitoring and complete blood cell counts (CBCs) are often absorbed by the trial site. Open-label, single-arm studies with new therapies, or studies that have appropriate standard of care control arms are easily accruable. Many PWAs do not have insurance to cover the medications and laboratory costs, others cannot afford the copay, and some do not want their insurance companies knowing their HIV status.

This is not true, with most garden-variety phase III cancer studies. Cancer patients enrolled in clinical trials, most always older than the average AIDS patient, often have insurance and there is less of a problem with billing for cyclophosphamide, doxorubicin, vincristine, etoposide, paclitaxol, and routine CBCs. Many cancer patients in these phase III studies *do* realize they could be getting the same treatment (i.e., CMF, ABVD, and others) from their community oncologist, but seem to feel that they are either receiving better overall treatment (especially if they are at a prestigious university teaching hospital) or are helping advance cancer clinical research when they enter clinical trials.

This does not seem to be true for the gay male community when it comes to antiretroviral studies. One would hope that there are some who are altruistic, but for the most part, the gay male AIDS community views clinical trials as "access" and not "research." Those who are sophisticated often can tell what arm of the study they are on and sometimes tweak or augment the regimen (without informing the investigator) knowing full well that it's against study rules. Others have their CD4 lymphocytes and HIV RNA measured in their primary care physician's office and decide whether to stay on the study if they themselves are pleased with their laboratory numbers.

There are many barriers to clinical trials that investigators may not take into account when designing studies. The issue of blinding has recently been called into question because patients want to know what study medications they are receiving in case they are terminated from the study for reaching an endpoint.

This knowledge of what drugs one was taking is needed in this era of highly active antiretroviral therapy (HAART) so that an individual and his physician can select a new regimen based on treatment history and cross-resistance within certain classes of drugs.

Moreover, certain studies, with their cumbersome office visits and laboratory components, may not take into account a patient's lifestyle. One such study looking at interleukin-2 (IL-2) had to be redesigned because it asked that relatively healthy HIV-positive patients with 300–500 CD4 cells be admitted to a GCRC for a week every 8 weeks to receive intravenous infusion. Investigators may not have considered: How can a gainfully employed, seemingly healthy gay man with HIV (who has probably not disclosed his HIV status to his employer) ask for a week off every 8 weeks?

Another study in development plans to administer four to five antiretrovirals to newly HIV-infected individuals and has at least six laboratory intensive substudies. Granted, a person recently infected might want to begin antiretroviral therapy immediately, but does he or she want to be continuously giving lymph node and tonsil biopsies, semen or vaginal secretion specimens, when they are attempting to come to grips with their HIV diagnosis?

VI. THE DUAL DIAGNOSIS OF AIDS AND CANCER

The PWAs with AIDS-related malignant complications, such as KS or NHL, have an even more onerous task. For gay men, a dual diagnosis of AIDS and cancer is often the most unsettling. AIDS is still relatively new to many, but we all grew up knowing that cancer was bad and that many people, including our relatives, have died of cancer. A friend once said to me, "AIDS is bad enough, why do I also have to have cancer." Most HIV-positive individuals do not know the difference between renal cell carcinoma, colon cancer, or lymphoma. To them, cancer is cancer. The fact that a patient will have to leave the confines of the primary care doctor's office where they know the staff and are comfortable with the routine, and go see an oncologist ("a cancer doctor") at some ominous hospital is frightening. If they are lucky, they will see an experienced AIDS oncologist who is aware of the various treatment options and who knows the ins and outs of AIDS clinical management, but that is often not the case.

For gay men with KS and NHL, most do not have a clue about their treatment options. Whereas patients with HIV are now able to tailor their HIV antiviral regimen by choosing which well-advertised protease inhibitor fits their lifestyle best or which has the least objectionable toxicity profile, they have no idea what the acronyms ABV, CHOP, or m-BACOD mean. Unlike companies that market antiretroviral drugs, there are no slick advertisements from companies for chemotherapy or other agents in the treatment of AIDS malignancies.

Unfortunately, past AIDS malignancy studies were relatively void of "hot" or promising agents. Many patients with relapsed KS or NHL were referred to and enrolled in salvage therapy studies only because the arsenal of effective treatments was so limited. AIDS Clinical Trials Group 142, a study of approximately 200 patients comparing standard versus modified-dose m-BACOD in HIV-positive patients with NHL took almost 4 years to accrue (12). Although the question asked was extremely important and has helped develop our standard of care for treating AIDS-related NHL, most community oncologists decided not to refer their patients to this study and treated them with similar regimens in their offices.

For PWAs, the thought of cytotoxic chemotherapy in and of itself is a taboo subject. The general sentiment is, "the chemotherapy that this doctor is going to pump into me is going to make my hair fall out and make me vomit." Often, patients with progressive KS are content with a dermatologist freezing or injecting many individual lesions, when a few rounds of chemotherapy might really work. KS patients sometimes show up at an oncologist's office only when the KS has become visceral or edema prevents mobilization. Gay men with KS do not realize, possibly owing to the lack of adequate counseling, that there is a window of opportunity after the development of KS, and that clinical trials of experimental therapies are available. Also, if no treatment effect is seen, standard therapy can still be administered.

VII. THE MYTH THAT AIDS IS OVER

Since the advent of protease inhibitors in mid-1996, deaths of AIDS in the United States have decreased by approximately 50% (14). In fact, Donald Kotler (uber AIDS GI doc) now refers to the preprotease inhibitor era as "the dark ages." For many, AIDS has seemingly become a chronic and manageable disease. PWAs who were once concerned about how they would spend their dying years are now concerned with going back to work and even want to start investing for their retirement.

It is important for everyone, not just gay men with AIDS, to realize that HAART is not a cure. When some gay men hear the word "undetectable," they believe that they are cured or free of the virus. That is not true; several studies have recently documented that HIV proviral DNA persists at low levels in chronically infected cells (15). Likewise, various HAART regimens appear to render only 60–80% of HIV-positive patient undetectable for approximately 2 years. Once virus has become detectable, there is the growing anxiety over what will be one's second-line and third-line regimen. It is hoped that genotypic and phenotypic resistance testing will soon help us streamline choosing and switching antiretrovirals, but for now, it is often a guessing game.

It appears that the gay male community is able to benefit less from HAART than other communities affected with HIV because over the years so many HIV-positive gay men took every new antiretroviral approved by the FDA. Many are now multidrug-resistant and have difficulties assembling viable HAART regimens. In contrast, many PWAs from minority communities, who never before sought treatment, and are antiretroviral-naive, are able to choose from a myriad of drug combinations and have safe, effective second-line regimens as backups. This dilemma has caused some of the original AIDS treatment activists to wonder if flooding the market with new antiretrovirals and urging for unlimited preapproved expanded access actually harmed some PWAs. Advocating for PWAs who have exhausted all their treatment options, AIDS treatment activists are demanding that pharmaceutical companies test their new antiretrovirals in multiple protease inhibitor-resistant patients.

Probably the most surreal issue confronting the gay male HIV-positive community is a resurgence of unprotected anal intercourse, which is now referred to as barebacking. *POZ Magazine*, the nation's only magazine for HIV-positive individuals, is presently running a double cover story on barebacking (16,17). There are many gay men, both HIV-positive and negative, who no longer want to use condoms when having anal sex and who fetishize the sharing of semen.

Much of this barebacking craze has been fostered by those who now feel healthy and happy because of protease inhibitors. One man is quoted as saying, "Protease is helping me live longer, but gay men have finally had it up to here. After 18 years of living in doubt and crisis, men don't want to face a lifetime of wrapping themselves in latex" (17). The fact that we have no real clinical data telling us that reinfection occurs gives HIV-positive men who decide to have unprotected anal sex with each other an easy excuse. Many do not seem to realize that unprotected anal sex can lead to the transmission of HSV-1 and HSV-2, KSHV, and hepatitis B and C virus. These issues are rarely discussed and often ignored.

There are also some HIV-negative men who, stupid as it seems, are "barebacking" with known HIV-positive men. Some do not think they will get HIV because their sex partner is "undetectable." They do not seem to be aware that recent data have demonstrated that even if HIV RNA is undetectable in the blood and semen, some individuals, approximately 25%, are harboring replication-competent viruses in seminal cells capable of initiating primary infection (18). What angers so many older gay men who saw the early devastation of AIDS is that these HIV-negative gay men who are having unprotected anal intercourse with known positive men are, in fact, putting themselves at risk of receiving a protease-resistant virus (19). To the older generation of gay men, it is sad that protease inhibitors were not around to save the lives of their friend who died of AIDS. But, to now knowingly put oneself at risk of HIV and be unable to benefit from the best HIV antiretroviral therapy in 18 years, adds insult to injury. Many in the gay community need to give a wake-up call to these HIV-negative men who believe the myth that AIDS is a chronic and manageable disease like diabetes. Mortality is still a real and frightening fact.

RESOURCES

Organizations and Web sites

AIDS Action Council
Advocacy; information on public policy and treatment access. 1875 Connecticut Ave. NW, Ste. 700, Washington, DC 20009; 202-986-1300.

AIDS Clinical Trials Information Service (ACTIS)
Information in Spanish and English on federal and other clinical drug trials. 800-TRIALS-A; TTY/TDD 800-243-7012; www.actis.org

AIDS Education Global Information System (AEGIS)
Daily news updates, newsletters, trials, search engines; run by Sister Mary Elizabeth. www.aegis.com

aidsinfonyc.org
Cooperative site run by ATDN, PWA Health Group, Treatment Action Group (TAG), and other organizations. www.aidsinfonyc.org

AIDS Project Los Angeles (APLA)
1313 North Vine St., L.A., CA 90028; 213-993-1600; 204.179.124.76/apla/; Nutrition and Protease Inhibitors

AIDS Treatment Data Network (ATDN)
Clinical trials listing, many glossaries, ADAP, alternative treatments; also in Spanish. 611 Broadway, Ste. 613, NYC, NY 10012; 800-734-7104; aidsinfonyc.org/network

Critical Path AIDS Project
Treatment information, clinical trials, newsletter library. www.cripath.org

Gay Men's Health Crisis (GMHC)
Legal issues, prevention, treatment, counseling and support groups. 129 W. 20th St., NYC, NY 10011; 212-367-1000; Hotline 212-807-6655; www.gmhc.org

Gay and Lesbian Medical Association
459 Fulton St., Ste. 107, San Francisco, CA 94102; 415-255-4547

Heath Care Communications
A commercial web site with updates on conferences and physicians' and activist reports; www.healthcg.com

HIV/AIDS Treatment Information Service (ATIS)
Information in English and Spanish on FDA-approved treatments. www. hivatis.org

HIV Law Project
Legal advocacy; 212-674-7590

HIV Insite
A top-notch web site run by UCSF; hivinsite.ucsf.edu

HIV Net-Information Server. www.hivnet.org

Housing Works
Information, advocacy for HIV-positive homeless. 594 Broadway, NYC, NY 10012; 212-966-0466

Lambda Legal Defense and Education Fund
120 Wall St., 15th Fl., NYC, NY 10005; 212-809-8585

National Association of People With AIDS
Information, advocacy, referrals. 1413 K St. NW, 7th Fl., Washington, DC 20005; 202-898-0414

Project Inform
1965 Market St., Ste. 220, San Francisco, CA 94103; Treatment hot line 800-822-7422; 415-558-8669; www.projinf.org

PWA Health Group
Buyers' club that provides treatment information. 150 W. 26th St., Ste. 201, NYC, NY 10001; 212-255-0520; aidsinfonyc.org/pwahg

San Francisco AIDS Foundation
HIV information treatment, newsletter, referrals. P.O. Box 426182, San Francisco, CA 94142; 415-487-3000; www.sfaf.org

Publications

AIDS Clinical Care
Latest information on clinical HIV treatment. Published monthly by the Mass. Medical Society. P.O. Box 9085, Waltham, MA 02254; 800-843-6356

AIDS/HIV Treatment Directory
Comprehensive information on approved and experimental treatments, clinical trials, by AmFAR. 733 Third Ave., 12th Fl., NYC, NY 10017; 800-38-AmFAR

AIDS Treatment News
The ultimate resource, by John James. P.O. Box 411256, San Francisco, CA 94141; 800-TREAT12; aidsnews@aidsnews.org

BETA: Bulletin of Experimental Treatment for AIDS
e-mail beta@thecity.sfsu.edu; www.sfaf.org/beta.html

LAP Notes
By the Lesbian AIDS Project at GMHC. 129 W. 20th St., 2nd Fl., NYC, NY10011; 212-337-3532

Notes from the Underground
Alternative news, by the PWA Health Group

PI Perspective
Published four times a year by Project Inform

Positively Aware
Published six times a year by the Test Positive Aware Network. 1258 W. Belmont Ave., Chicago, IL 60657; 773-404-8726; www.tpan.com

POZ
Glossy bimonthly for HIV-infected and HIV-affected people; PWA profiles, news, opinion, and treatment information. 349 W. 12th St., NYC, NY 10014-1721; 212-242-2163; www.poz.com

SIDA Ahora
En español, by the People With AIDS Coalition. 50 W. 17th St., 8th Fl., NYC, NY 10011; 212-647-1415

TAG Line
Treatment newsletter by the Treatment Activist Group. 200 E. 10th St., Ste. 601, NYC, NY 10003; 212-924-3935; www.aidsinfonyc.org/network/tag

Treatment Issues
Published by GMHC

Treatment Review
Published six times a year by ATDN

Special Groups (see also Publications listings)

Children

Pediatric AIDS Foundation
1311 Colorado Ave., Santa Monica, CA 90404; 310-395-9051, 800-362-0071; www.pedaids.org

Newborn Testing Hotlinke
Run by the HIV Law Project; 800-662-9885

People with Hemophilia

Committee of Ten Thousand. (COTT) 800-488-COTT

Hemophilia and AIDS/HIV Network for the Dissemination of Information (HANDI)
c/o the Nat'l Hemophilia Foundation. 800-424-2634; en español, ext. 3754

Injection drug users

Harm Reduction Coalition
2 W. 27th St., 9th Fl., NYC, NY 10001; 212-213-6376

We the People
425 South Broad St., Philadelphia, PA 19147; 215-545-6868; www.critpath.org/wtp

Transgender

International Foundation for Gender Education
Transgender hotline, referrals. 781-899-2212; e-mail ifge@ifge.org

People of color

National Asian/Pacific Islander Consortium on AIDS and STDs
c/o Asian/Pacific Islander American Health Forum. 116 New Montgomery St., Ste. 531, San Francisco, CA 94105; 415-512-3408; e-mail etta @apiahf.org

National Black Leadership Commission AIDS
105 E. 22nd St., Ste. 711, NYC, NY 10010; 212-614-0023; e-mail kimblca@aol.com

Latino Commission on AIDS
80 Fifth Ave., Ste. 1501, NYC, NY 10011; 212-675-3288

National Minority AIDS Council
1931 13th St. NW, Washington, D.C., 20009; 202-483-6622

National Native American AIDS Prevention Center
134 Linden St., Oakland, CA 94607; 510-444-2051; www.nnaapc.org

Lesbians

Lesbian AIDS Project
A division of GMHC 212-367-1355 or 212-367-1363

Prisoners

American Civil Liberties Union National Prison Project
1875 Connecticut Ave. NW, Ste. 410, Washington, DC 20009; 202-234-4830

AIDS in Prison Project. www.aidsinfonyc.org/aip/index.html

Prisoners' Rights Project of the Legal AID Society
15 Park Row, 23rd Fl., NYC, NY 10038; 212-577-3530

Teenagers

Adolescent AIDS Program
Montefiore Medical Center, 111 E. 210th St., Bronx, NY 10467; 718-882-0023

AIDS Community Alliance
Works with HIV-positive and HIV-affected individuals. 44 North Queens St., Lancaster, PA 17603; 717-394-3380

Bay Area Young Positive
Youth-run, offers counseling, resources, newsletter. 518 Waller St., San Francisco, CA 94117; 415-487-1616; e-mail BAYPOZ@aol.com

Women

Sister Connect
Hot line for women with HIV. 800-747-1108

Women Alive
Treatment newsletter on the Web. 800-554-4876; www.thebody.com/wa/wapage.html

Project WISE
Newsletter available through Project Inform

World
Newsletter by and for HIV-positive women. P.O. Box 11535, Oakland, CA 94611; 510-658-6930

REFERENCES

1. Friedman Y, Franklin C, Rackow EC, et al. Improved survival in patients with AIDS, *Pneumocystis carinii* pneumonia, and severe respiratory failure. Chest 96:862–66, 1989.
2. Efferen LS, Nadarajah D, Palat DS. Survival following mechanical ventilation for *Pneumocystis carinii* pneumonia in patients with the acquired immunodeficiency syndrome: a different perspective. Am J Med 87:401–04, 1989.
3. Phair J, Munoz A, Detels R, et al. The risk of developing *Pneumocystis carinii* pneumonia among men infected with human immunodeficiency virus type 1. Multicenter AIDS Cohort Study Group. N Engl J Med 322:161–65, 1990.
4. Mayfair D. Gay cancer. Mandate, Dec 1981.
5. Biggar RJ. Epidemiologic clues to the etiology of cancer in AIDS [abstr S2]. 2nd National AIDS Malignancy Conference, Bethesda, MD, 1998.
6. Beral V, Peterman TA, Berkelman RL, et al. Kaposi's sarcoma among persons with AIDS: a sexually transmitted infection? Lancet 335:123–128, 1990.
7. Rabkin CS, Goedert JJ, Biggar RJ, et al. Kaposi's sarcoma in three HIV-infected cohorts. J Acquir Immune Defic Syndr 3(suppl 1):S38–S43, 1990.
8. Rabkin CS, Hilgartner MW, Hedberg KW, et al. Incidence of lymphomas and other cancers in HIV-infected and HIV-uninfected patient with hemophilia. JAMA 267: 1090–1094, 1992.
9. Schwartz JJ, Myskowski PL. New treatments for Kaposi's sarcoma. AIDS Reader July/Aug:129–132, 1992.
10. Ziegler JL, Drew WL, Miner RC, et al. Outbreak of Burkitt's-like lymphoma in homosexual men. Lancet 2:631–633, 1982.
11. Harrington M. Looking forward, looking back: AIDS treatment activism ten years on [Plenary]. 4th International Congress on Drug Therapy in HIV Infection Glasgow, Scotland, 8 Nov 1998.
12. Kaplan LD, Straus DJ, Testa MA, et al. Low-dose compared with standard-dose m-BACOD chemotherapy for non-Hodgkin's lymphoma associated with human immunodeficiency virus infection. N Engl J Med 336:1641–1648, 1997.
13. Nakamura S, Sakurada S, Salahuddin SZ, et al. Inhibition of development of Kaposi's sarcoma-related lesions by a bacterial cell wall complex. Science 255: 1437–1440, 1992.
14. Palella FJ Jr, Delaney KM, Moorman AC, et al. Declining morbidity and mortality among patients with advanced human immunodeficiency virus infection. N Engl J Med 338:853–860, 1989.
15. Cavert W, Notermans DW, Staskus K, et al. Kinetics of response in lymphoid tissue to antiretroviral therapy of HIV-1 infection. Science 276:1321, 1997.
16. Genden S. They shoot barebackers, don't they? POZ Feb: 48–51, 69, 1999.
17. Scarce M. A ride on the wild side. POZ Feb:52–55, 70–71, 1999.
18. Zhang H, Dornadula G, Beumont M, et al. Human immunodeficiency virus type 1 in the semen of men receiving highly active antiretroviral therapy. N Engl J Med 339:1803–1809, 1998.
19. Hecht FM, Grant RM, Petropoulos CJ, et al. Sexual transmission of an HIV-1 variant resistant to multiple reverse-transcriptase and protease inhibitors. N Engl J Med 339: 307–311, 1998.

18

National Cancer Institute Resources for AIDS Oncology Research

Ellen G. Feigal
National Cancer Institute, National Institutes of Health, Bethesda, Maryland

I. INTRODUCTION

The purpose of this chapter is to describe the programs and resources of the National Cancer Institute (NCI) as they relate to acquired immunodeficiency syndrome (AIDS) malignancies. These resources focus on the translation of basic research, the development of clinical research, and the creation of an infrastructure specific to the challenges of AIDS malignancies.

II. THE NATIONAL CANCER INSTITUTE

The National Cancer Institute, established under the National Cancer Act of 1937, is a component of the National Institutes of Health (NIH), a Public Health Service (PHS) agency in the Department of Health and Human Services (DHHS). The NCI's National Cancer Program is the federal government's principal agency for cancer research and training with responsibilities to disseminate new information and to assess the incorporation of state-of-the-art cancer treatments into clinical practice.

The NCI is described at the Directors home page, http://www.nci.nih.gov/klaus.htm. With a budget in 1999 of 2.8 billion dollars, the Institute

- Supports and coordinates research projects conducted by universities, hospitals, research foundations, and businesses throughout this country and abroad through research grants and cooperative agreements
- Conducts research in its own laboratories and clinics
- Supports education and training in fundamental sciences and clinical disciplines for participation in basic and clinical research programs and treatment programs relating to cancer through career awards, training grants, and fellowships
- Supports research projects in cancer control
- Supports a national network of cancer centers
- Collaborates with voluntary organizations and other national and foreign institutions engaged in cancer research and training activities
- Encourages and coordinates cancer research by industrial concerns where such concerns evidence a particular capability for programmatic research
- Collects and disseminates information on cancer
- Supports construction of laboratories, clinics, and related facilities necessary for cancer research through the award of construction grants.

The 1999 NCI budget can be found at: http://wwwosp.nci.nih.gov/osp/spp/bypass/bypass2000/04_request/4index.htm

III. CHALLENGES AND NEEDS IN HIV-ASSOCIATED MALIGNANCIES

The AIDS malignancy program, as with other programs within the Institute, represents the NCI's commitment to progress through science that would not exist without the resources to support it. The progress is driven by the creativity, dedication, and vigorous work of scientists and clinicians whose discoveries and ideas are tested to find ways to understand, prevent, detect, diagnose and treat AIDS malignancies. NCI has constructed a framework of support mechanisms, organizations, and networks that join scientists, facilities, and information.

The breadth of research efforts in AIDS malignancies begins with the basic sciences. They provide the new insights in cancer biology that can become hypotheses to test in epidemiological studies, leads in the development of treatment targets, and treatments to prevent and control AIDS malignancies. The basic science, even with associated drug development programs, would not make progress without clinical programs to test potential discoveries. Work in this area is necessarily collaborative and a major role of the NCI is to foster these collaborations, create research groups, and provide infrastructure from clinical trial support, to central specimen banking, to national scientific meetings, and new investigator training.

IV. COLLABORATION BETWEEN BASIC AND TRANSLATIONAL SCIENCE

A. Virology

Seroepidemiology is providing new insights in the modes of transmission of human oncogenic agents, particularly human herpes virus 8 (HHV-8; Kaposi's sarcoma [KS]-associated herpes virus), Epstein–Barr virus (EBV), and human papilloma virus (HPV). The understanding of the relation between new or reactivated latent infections and the development of precancerous conditions or cancers would have far-reaching significance, both in the presence and in the absence of human immunodeficiency virus (HIV)/AIDS. Investigators are being funded to study the role of coinfection of viruses, including human papilloma virus, human herpes viruses, hepatitis viruses, and HTLV-1/II in the etiology and molecular epidemiology of cancers and precancerous changes associated with HIV/AIDS, and the progression of HIV disease.

B. Epidemiology

The NCI's epidemiology programs support a range of studies that delve into the etiologic mysteries of AIDS malignancies. NIH-funded cohorts enroll HIV-infected persons and those uninfected but at high risk of acquiring HIV. They participate in prospective surveillance of the prevalence, incidence, molecular epidemiology, and temporal trends of all cancers, precancerous changes, and associated biological events. Linkage studies are being conducted with these cohorts and with population-based HIV registries and with tumor registries. Studies evaluating the cancers and precancerous changes occurring within the context of HIV/AIDS may address the temporality of observed events, including timing of first infection or reactivation of existing infections. Ongoing research is also trying to address mathematical-modeling and statistical methods useful for the development of the field of the epidemiology of HIV/AIDS-associated cancers and precancers.

Other challenges include discerning the effects of host genetics, immune functioning, hormonal changes, environmental conditions, and human behaviors on the epidemiology of HIV/AIDS-associated precancerous conditions and cancers.

C. Immunology

The scope of research topics includes the hematological malignancies, with special emphasis on those that occur as a result of congenital, iatrogenic, or acquired immunodeficiencies. The broad categories include cellular, genetic, and molecular aspects of immunology. The research covers areas such as the role of cytokines, B- and T-cell ontogeny, antigen receptors on B and T cells, lymphocyte activation and deactivation, and the effect of somatic mutations on lymphomagenesis.

D. Treatment and Prevention

1. Drug Discovery

The NCI has a strong tradition of leadership in retroviral research, dating back at least four decades. The program retains a very strong core of retroviral research, distributed among laboratories at Bethesda and Frederick among intramural and contract laboratories, as well as in the extramural grant program. Current anti-HIV research is directed at characterization and exploitation of molecular targets unique to this virus. New strategies to prevent and treat AIDS-associated malignancies and opportunistic infections are being developed from the rapidly expanding evidence for viral involvement. A major emphasis is on the development of novel molecular targets for drug discovery.

Many structural classes of anti-HIV compounds, previously unrecognized as antiviral agents, have been discovered. Detailed preclinical studies addressing formulation, pharmacokinetics, and toxicology have been pursued for promising compounds approved by a decision-making group within the NCI. Compounds with potential activity against drug-resistant virus or those that act through novel mechanisms are given high priority.

The NCI plays an active role in facilitating the work of grantees and other investigators. The structures and corresponding screening data on thousands of compounds not covered by confidentiality agreements and previously tested in the NCI screens have been released (http://www.dtp.nci.nih.gov). Information on how to obtain compounds or natural products from government-maintained repositories, either as single agents or plated on 96-well plates, is also being provided. The future emphasis will be to focus more on molecular targets and less on cell-based empirical-screening approaches.

Studies employing cDNA array technologies and combinatorial synthesis programs are examples of ways NCI is attempting to develop faster, cheaper, and smarter methods for the discovery of new agents. NCI is working with the National Institute of Allergy and Infectious Diseases (NIAID) to leverage and expand existing resources in drug discovery and development.

2. HIV Drug Resistance

Recent experience has revealed that newly developed antiviral therapies are highly effective at suppressing HIV replication in infected patients, but are time-limited in their effectiveness owing to the appearance of drug-resistant virus. To date, no single antiviral drug has been discovered to which the virus has not developed resistant mutants. The NCI has approached this problem by developing a program that will be able to use new and exciting opportunities for retroviral research not only to address basic problems related to viral diversity and drug resistance, but also to build on the existing strengths in retrovirus research in general to establish a major world center for retroviral research. The goals of this new program are the following:

1. To bring focus to the exciting NCI retroviral research programs and promote collaboration and communication among them.
2. To fill areas of need by recruiting the very best young and senior scientists in retroviral research, and providing an environment in which they can be at their most productive.
3. To create a strong programmatic focus on basic and translational research related to genetic diversity and drug resistance. Although drug resistance will be the major focus, the scientific problems addressed will touch on other relevant issues, such as vaccine development.
4. To provide a central resource for investigators worldwide interested in related problems.

Eventually, the program will comprise integrated and collaborative projects in a wide range of areas, which will include structural studies on target (or potential target) proteins, biochemical–mechanistic studies, basic virology, resistance studies in vitro, animal model studies, clinical virology, mathematical modeling of population dynamics, virus–host interactions, pathogenic mechanisms, and population genetics, epidemiological studies, translational–developmental studies, and informatics.

V. CLINICAL RESEARCH RESOURCES

Currently used AIDS and cancer treatments were at one time tested on patients with these diseases or at risk for their development. Even though trials often test the latest therapies, there is no promise that these will be better. A patient may choose to be part of a randomized clinical trial, and be randomly assigned to a control group of standard therapy. Another patient might opt to participate in an early-phase clinical trial in which the drug's effectiveness may still be unknown. Clinical trials provide patients access to cutting edge interventions and provide researchers with information that will ultimately lead to the use of more effective interventions for prevention and treatment of the AIDS and the cancer.

A strong clinical reseach infrastructure, including a comprehensive program of clinical trials in treatment, early detection, and prevention, is a vital component of NCI's research program. NCI's Cancer Centers, NIAID's Centers for AIDS Research (CFARs), NCI's and NIAID's Clinical Trial Cooperative

Groups and Community Clinical Programs in Cancer and in AIDS, respectively, and the AIDS Malignancy Consortium (AMC) are where findings from the laboratory are translated into new treatments, diagnostic tools, and preventive interventions, and where these measures can be first tested for safety and effectiveness. Clinical trials are supported through these and other research mechanisms, such as individual research project grants, program project grants, cooperative agreements, and contracts. To learn more about the Cooperative Group program visit the website at http://ctep.info.nih.gov/CoopGroup_Group_Prog.html.

Although the emphasis in each group varies from the 100% focus on AIDS malignancies of the AMC to the proportionately smaller efforts of the other groups, a rich network of opportunity exists at institutions participating in these groups to sponsor new clinical research studies and trials in AIDS malignancies.

A. AIDS Malignancy Consortium

The primary AIDS malignancy cooperative clinical trial group today is the AIDS Malignancy Consortium (AMC). The AMC replaced and expanded on earlier efforts, including the AIDS Lymphoma Network and the Small Clinical Trials programs funded in 1992. The NCI has funded AMC investigators since 1995 to develop hypothesis-driven early-phase clinical trials that utilize the expertise of NCI- and NIAID-sponsored scientists, and the role of the AMC has recently been expanded to conduct large, randomized phase III clinical trials. The AMC consists of clinical trial centers and one center for data management, operations, and statistical support. The diseases under study include non-Hodgkin's lymphoma, primary central nervous system lymphoma, Kaposi's sarcoma, anogenital dysplasia, and anogenital cancer.

The therapeutic approaches include biological therapy: interleukin (IL)-2, IL-12, interferon (IFN) alfa, monoclonal antibodies directed against B-cell targets, cytotoxic T lymphocytes directed against viral-mediated targets; as well as compounds that inhibit angiogenesis, and restore or improve immune function. In addition to assessing potential antitumor activity, and drug–drug interactions, the clinical trials are evaluating the effect of therapy on viral load and underlying immune function. The AMC also contributes toward the effort in AIDS-associated malignancies by collecting and donating specimens to the AIDS Malignancy Bank (AMB).

B. Centers for AIDS Research

Beginning in 1998, the Centers for AIDS Research (CFAR) program, previously supported by one NIH Institute, the NIAID, will now be cooperatively funded by six NIH Institutes. This is intended to encourage expansion of the scientific breadth of the CFAR, to stimulate multidisciplinary interaction and collaboration, and to strengthen the scientific synergy relative to AIDS. NCI participated in cofunding nine of these applications, including one on which it serves as primary sponsor. This is a mechanism that is complementary to the one in which supplements were provided directly to cancer centers to link them with CFAR investigators.

C. Cancer Centers

The centralized resources of the Cancer Centers benefit scientists who are supported by research grants dealing with cancer. Cancer Centers proactively stimulate scientific interactions, and all research members of a Center have access to Cancer Center resources (e.g., DNA-sequencing cores, flow cytometry cores, animal facilites). The Cancer Centers Program has periodically awarded one-time supplements to existing grants to stimulate research in AIDS-related malignancies. A supplement initiative was supported in 1996 to assist Cancer Centers in developing integrated research programs in AIDS-related malignancies. These programs, once established, can be sustained as part of a Cancer Center's formal research program structure.

VI. INFRASTRUCTURE TO FACILITATE RESEARCH

A. Clinical Collaborations

The U. S. Office for Protection from Research Risks and the European Organization for Research and Treatment of Cancer (EORTC) reached an agreement that should improve the ability of NCI-sponsored clinical trial groups to collaborate with the EORTC and other international cancer research groups. The agreement was created to strengthen the protection of patients in international clinical trials. The impact is anticipated to decrease duplicative research efforts in the United States and abroad, improve the ability to conduct international large-scale trials, and increase the recruitment of patients into trials for rare cancers. A desired effect is to speed the transfer of laboratory findings to clinical trials and ultimately take those promising findings into clinical practice.

NCI is working closely with NIAID's drug discovery, development, and clinical trials expertise and resources to have a more fully integrated NIH plan in these areas. Information on NIAID's adult and pediatric clinical trials networks, the Centers for AIDS Research, and the Terry Beirn Community Programs for Clinical Research in AIDS (CPCRA) can be found on Web site http://www.niaid.nih.gov.

B.   AIDS Malignancy Bank

The AIDS Malignancy Bank (AMB) consists of 5 main member institutions and approximately 30 affiliated institutions. Started in 1994, it was established to provide access for the research community at large to well-characterized tumor tissue, biological fluids, and demographic and clinical data from HIV-infected patients with malignancies. Information on the AMB, an updated database, and application forms are available on the Internet (http://cancernet.nih.gov/amb/amb.html). Proposals to utilize the AMB are reviewed three times a year by the Research Evaluation and Decision Panel (REDP) of the AMB. Specimens from the AMB have been distributed to a wide variety of researchers with proposals approved by the REDP. These specimens are from patients with AIDS-related lymphoma, KS, anogenital disease, and lung cancer, to name just a few. The types of specimens available include tumor-involved and matched-control frozen tissues, multisite autopsy, blood cells and serum, and frozen and fixed biopsy specimens.

C.   Conferences and Workshops

The National AIDS Malignancy Conference is an annual international meeting that began in 1997 to serve as a forum for the dissemination of scientific information focused on the biology, virology, epidemiology, prevention, and therapeutic intervention aspects of AIDS malignancies and related fields. It is a multidisciplinary gathering of scientists, clinicians, other health care workers, and community advocates from around the world. Summaries and abstracts are located on the Internet, World Wide Web site http://hiv.medscape.com/conference/malignancy3, and plenary talks have been published in monographs.

NCI also has held conferences on the immunobiology of AIDS NHL, a workshop on the sensitivity and specificity of assays for the detection of KSHV/HHV-8, and a joint conference cochaired by NCI and NIAID: New Approaches to Identifying Infectious Etiologies of Chronic Disease.

D.   AIDS Oncology Resource Handbook

The *AIDS Oncology Resource Handbook* (Web site address http://ctep.info.nih.gov/AIDSOncoResources) is a compendium of NCI-sponsored research in AIDS and AIDS malignancies, updated annually since 1997 and available in hardcopy and on the Internet. It provides an accessible and comprehensive listing of the intramural and extramural clinical and laboratory research resources that receive NCI AIDS funds. Principal investigators from the NCI intramural program provide a brief synopsis of their research studies and recent accomplishments. NCI program directors or the program scientific liaisons describe the broad research questions and major highlights of the extramural research programs. The contact persons for each of these areas are listed to facilitate access for questions, as well as to foster collaborations.

E. AIDS Malignancy Working Group

The AIDS Malignancies Working Group (AMWG) consists of 25–35 extramural and internal NIH scientists, clinicians, and community advocates representing a spectrum of disciplines currently working in or with an interest in AIDS malignancies, and those conducting research that may have relevance for these cancers. The purpose of the group is to identify and prioritize important research opportunities and approaches, and to provide advice to and participate in decision making at the NCI. The AMWG held its first meeting in 1996, and continues to meet on an annual basis, addressing questions in epidemiology and databases; virology, immunology, and cancer biology; and cancer prevention and treatment. Summaries can be found on http://deainfo.nci.nih.gov/advisory/pog/other_wg/aids/index.htm.

VII. EXTRAMURAL RESEARCH FUNDING AND SUPPORT

A. Research Project Grants

The main pool of funds for grants to extramural scientists and clinicians is known as the Research Project Grant (RPG) pool. These funds foster the creativity of talented scientists by providing them with the freedom to pursue the best ideas that will yield progress against cancer.

The NCI funds two main types of research project grants: Single Research Project Grants, awarded to institutions on behalf of individual principal investigators; and Program Project Grants, funded to foster collaborations among groups of scientists involved in related research projects. These grant awards constitute the single largest category of annual NCI investment. Collectively, the Single Research Project and Program Project Grants span the full range of basic, clinical, and population-based studies on etiology, biology, prevention, detection, diagnosis, and treatment.

A complete listing and description of NCI's grant mechanisms and the review process is described in Table 1. Additional information can be found at http://deainfo.nci.nih.gov/flash/awards.htm.

B. Role of NCI Extramural Research Staff

The NCI's extramural research programs include the Divisions of Cancer Biology, Cancer Treatment and Diagnosis, Cancer Prevention, and Cancer Control

Table 1 National Cancer Institute Funding Mechanisms

Program	Purpose
Fellowship programs: F series	Provides supervised research training in health and health-related areas leading to a research degree (predoctoral fellows), and provides postdoctoral research training to broaden the scientific background and extend the potential for health-related research.
Career development programs: K series	Fosters scientists' career development at different career stages: The young scientist with outstanding potential for a career of independent research in a health-related field The midcareer clinician needing protected time to devote to patient-oriented research and to act as a mentor for beginning clinical investigators; Established investigators with a proven track record of high competence that will enable institutions to finance such investigators in a manner favorable to their intellectual growth and research productivity
Research program projects and centers: P series	Supports multidisciplinary or multifaceted research programs that have a focused theme including planning grants, specialized shared resources, and center grants. Specialized center grants may support any part of the full range of research from the very basic to clinical. The spectrum of activities comprises a multidisciplinary attack on a specific disease entity or biomedical problem area.
Research projects: R series	Grants awarded to institutions on behalf of a principal investigator to facilitate pursuit of a scientific focus or objective in the area of the investigator's interest and competence. Institutional sponsorship assures the NIH that the institution will provide facilities necessary to accomplish the research and will be accountable for the grant funds. Awards include small, limited grants for pilot projects, funding for conferences, and exploratory–developmental grants.
Cooperative agreements: U series	Similar to grants in that they are awarded to assist and support research and related activities; however, they differ from grants in that the NIH has substantial involvement in carrying out the project's activities.

and Population Sciences. A key component of the extramural research program is the NCI's program staff. Their scientific expertise and national focus in a given research area enables them to work effectively with NCI-funded scientists in academia and industry to facilitate research progress. They synthesize the state of the science in important areas, identify priorities for new research directions, foster collaborations among scientists, keep abreast of the research program through active communication with investigators, organize scientific meetings to promote the interchange of information among investigators, and secure supplemental funds for meritorious projects. Program staff members are a resource for researchers, educating them on NCI policies and procedures; advising scientists, clinicians, and other investigators new to the NCI system on the preparation of research grant applications; and reviewing and identifying gaps in the research portfolio that may lead to new areas of research emphasis. They monitor the progress of extramural grants through contact with individual investigators and annual research progress reports.

C. Intramural Research

The Intramural Research Program consists of more than 400 principal investigators in the Divisions of Basic Sciences, Cancer Epidemiology and Genetics, and Clinical Sciences.

The Epidemiology and Genetics Division serves as a national program for population-based studies to identify environmental and genetic determinants of cancer. It supports epidemiology and interdisciplinary research, building on ongoing discoveries in molecular genetics and cancer biology, and broadening them through population-based studies into the etiology of cancer and its prevention.

The Clinical Sciences Division conducts its research principally in NIH's Clinical Center. It provides the opportunity for patients around the country to be treated in cutting edge research protocols. The HIV and AIDS Malignancy Branch focuses on the development of therapies for patients with AIDS or AIDS malignancies. For more information on the NIH clinical center, visit http://www.cc.nih.gov.

VIII. TRAINING PROGRAMS

Training the next generation of clinician scientists is one of the most critical challenges in cancer research, including AIDS malignancies research. Clinician scientists of the future will need to incorporate new modalities and ways of thinking to keep abreast with the rapid pace of scientific discovery and advances in technology. Novel methods of educating, training, and advancing clinician scientists are essential to integrate technological advances rapidly into the research pro_cess, and ensure that investigators are equipped to work together to solve the myriad factors contributing to AIDS malignancies.

Rapid advances in understanding the pathogenesis of cancer and AIDS and improvement in therapeutic interventions have occurred over the past decade. The ability to bring these new discoveries to the communities and clinics where they benefit patients and those at risk for developing disease depends on well-trained scientists and clinicians. NCI is committed to building a cadre of trained cancer researchers by continuing to provide critical training to the scientific and medical workforce.

The goals of NCI's 1999 strategic plan in training programs and career development are to build and sustain a critical mass of basic, clinical, population, and behavioral scientists capable of taking full advantage of the vast spectrum of future cancer research opportunities; to create new models for educating and training scientists who can interact effectively in translating basic knowledge into productive cancer prevention, detection, diagnosis, and treatment strategies; to attract into cancer research scientists whose unique disciplinary orientations or special technical skills can be integrated with those of more traditionally trained scientists in biology and medicine to generate novel, more powerful approaches to cancer research; and to increase the participation of underrepresented racial and ethnic minority scientists and scientists from medically underserved areas and populations in cancer research.

The NCI supports career development awards focused on the area of AIDS-related malignancies. In 1998, the NCI awarded grants to five institutions to train AIDS Oncology Research Scientists. The Clinical Scientist Development Program Award supports institutional, multidisciplinary, training programs focused on the HIV/AIDS oncology field. The goal of this program is to train a cadre of clinicians with the highly specialized skills necessary to address the clinical and research problems associated with AIDS-related malignancies. There is an important need for trained AIDS–oncology specialists to exploit research opportunities, conduct patient-oriented research, and provide the clinical management skills necessary for advancement in this field. As part of the same initiative, supplements were awarded to five cancer centers to train young investigators in clinical research in AIDS and oncology.

NCI has created career tracks offering a continuum of opportunities that stabilize the training and career development of basic scientists, physicians (MDs) pursuing basic science careers, MDs pursuing clinical science careers, individuals pursuing population science careers, individuals working in or from underserved areas, and individuals from underrepresented racial and ethnic minority groups pursuing careers in any field of cancer research.

Individual "mentored" awards, bridging awards, transition awards, established investigator awards, and institutional program awards strategically link career tracks. Establishing these career tracks and implementing the other strategies described in the foregoing are NCI's most recent efforts directed at achieving its training, education, and career development objectives.

IX. NCI'S INFORMATION SERVICES

Many persons, from health professionals to cancer patients and their families, and to the general public, benefit from NCI's menu of information and public education services. A physician searches a database and identifies several clinical trials that have an excellent chance of helping a patient. Worried patients visit a Web site for information that will help them weigh their treatment options.

By using methods ranging from basic printed materials to sophisticated Internet technology, NCI provides millions of persons each year with the comprehensive and reliable information they need to make decisions about prevention, detection, treatment, and follow-up care.

A. Cancer Information Service (CIS)

This newly improved cancer information and education network receives more than 2000 calls per day. By calling one, toll-free number, 1-800-4-CANCER (1-800-422-6237), cancer patients, their families and friends, persons at risk, and health professionals can receive information to help them find information on treatment options, including clinical trials; learn about strategies for dealing with varied aspects of cancer treatment; or learn how to start health-promoting behaviors, such as quitting smoking or getting a screening test. Callers with TTY (teletype for the hearing impaired) equipment can dial 1-800-332-8615. Every call is kept confidential, and trained CIS staff answer questions in English or Spanish.

B. PDQ Database

The Physician Data Query (PDQ) database contains current, peer-reviewed cancer information summaries on treatment, screening, prevention, and supportive care. It has a comprehensive, computerized cancer database that provides descriptions of active clinical trials and directories of physicians, health professionals who provide cancer genetics services, and organizations involved in cancer care. Information is available in technical and nontechnical versions and in English and Spanish. It is updated monthly and is reviewed by cancer experts. Most PDQ information is available on the CancerNet Web site; selected information is available by facsimale (fax) from NCI's Cancer Fax service (301-402-5874).

C. NCI's Internet Services

The public and research community with access to the Internet may search for information about cancer on the following World Wide Web sites.

> NCI's Web site (http://www.nci.nih.gov) or the International Cancer Information Center's CancerNet Web site (http://cancernet.nci.nih.gov).
> Cancer Trials (http://cancertrials.nci.nih.gov) is a new clinical trials resource that provides information about ongoing prevention, detection, diagnosis, and treatment clinical trials. This site includes links to databases of ongoing studies and general information about clinical trials.
> CANCERLIT is a bibliographic database with over 1.4 million records on cancer literature from 1963 to the present. It is updated monthly and can be accessed from the CancerNet Web site.
> PDQ/CANCERLIT Service Center provides customized searches from the PDQ an CANCERLIT databases to health professionals. Requests are through a toll-free telephone service (1-800-343-3300), e-mail or fax.
> CancerMail is a service that allows one to order PDQ information summaries, CANCERLIT searches on selected topics, and other cancer information through e-mail. Write to cancermail@icicc.nci.nih.gov with the word "help" in the body of the message. Users receive a content list and ordering instructions by return electronic mail.

D. Print Publications

NCI produces about 600 publications and audiovisual materials in Spanish and English. Designed for people of diverse cultures and literacy levels, these materials address a wide range of cancer-related topics, from coping with the emotional burden of cancer, to suggestions for health-promoting changes in the diet, to understanding clinical trials. They are available from the toll-free number 1-800-4-CANCER or from the NCI Web site.

X. AIDS MALIGNANCY FUNDING

One metric to assess NCI's commitment to AIDS-associated malignancies is the level of financial support. NCI funding for AIDS in 1998 was nearly 226 million dollars, of which 97 million was for AIDS malignancies. The breakdown by funding mechanism is shown in Figure 1.

XI. CONCLUSIONS

The National Cancer Institute offers a wide array of resources that can be utilized for the basic, translational, and clinical study of AIDS malignancies. Several of

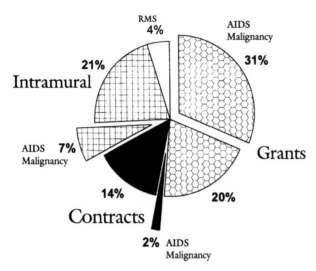

Figure 1 1998 National Cancer Institute AIDS/AIDS malignancy dollar funding: $225,991,000 total ($97,011,000 AIDS malignancy).

the resources are specific for AIDS malignancies, but many are general mechanisms that can be readily adapted to the study of these entities. Many collaborative group opportunities have been created; however, a specific idea, translated into a research question and hypothesis usually still require the efforts of a single investigator or small research team to design and conduct the research needed, and multiple resources are available for the pursuit of these ideas. AIDS-associated malignancies offer a chance to understand etiology from the unique interplay of viral and immunological pathogenesis.

Index

Page numbers in boldface indicate an extensive discussion of the topic.

419

About the Editors

ELLEN G. FEIGAL is Deputy Director of the Division of Cancer Treatment and Diagnosis at the National Cancer Institute, Bethesda, Maryland. The author or coauthor of over 70 professional papers and abstracts, Dr. Feigal leads the National Cancer Institute's extramural efforts in AIDS-associated malignancies including the formation of clinical trials groups, specimen banks, and annual international meetings on HIV and malignancy. She received the B.S. (1976) and M.S. (1977) degrees from the University of California, Irvine, and the M.D. degree (1981) from the University of California, Davis.

ALEXANDRA M. LEVINE is Chief, Division of Hematology, University of Southern California (USC) School of Medicine and Medical Director, USC/Norris Cancer Center, Los Angeles. The author or coauthor of over 160 peer-reviewed publications, more than 160 abstracts, and over 50 book chapters, Dr. Levine is a member of the American College of Physicians, the American Society of Hematology, and the American Society of Clinical Oncology. She received the B.A. degree (1966) from the University of California, Berkeley, and the M.D. degree (1971) from the University of Southern California, Los Angeles.

ROBERT J. BIGGAR is International AIDS Coordinator in the Viral Epidemiology Branch of the National Cancer Institute, Bethesda, Maryland. Dr. Biggar is the author or coauthor of over 200 publications in peer-reviewed journals, and is a Fellow of the American College of Pediatrics, the American College of Epidemiology, and the American Public Health Association. He received the B.A. degree (1964) from Pomona College, Claremont, California, and the M.D. degree (1968) from the Baylor College, Houston, Texas.